KEY TO PSYCHIATRY

A TEXTBOOK FOR STUDENTS

THIRD EDITION

Key to Psychiatry

A TEXTBOOK FOR STUDENTS

Third Edition

MAURICE J. SAINSBURY, M.B., B.S. (SYDNEY),
F.R.A.N.Z.C.P., F.R.C.PSYCH., D.P.M.

Director, The New South Wales Institute of Psychiatry

*Former Chief Examiner in Psychiatric Medicine,
New South Wales Nurses Registration Board*

JOHN WILEY & SONS
Chichester • New York • Brisbane • Toronto • Singapore

First edition 1973
Second edition 1976

Third edition published in 1980 by
AUSTRALIA & NEW ZEALAND BOOK CO PTY LTD
23 Cross Street, Brookvale, N.S.W. 2100, Australia

Exclusively published and distributed throughout the World, except Australia, New Zealand and USA, by
JOHN WILEY & SONS LTD
Baffins Lane, Chichester, Sussex, England
ISBN 0 471 26009 6

Computer photocomposed by Computer Graphics Corporation Pty Ltd, Adelaide, and printed at Griffin Press Limited, Netley, South Australia

FOREWORD

Dr Sainsbury has had extensive experience in psychiatry, particularly in hospital settings, and in recent years has added to his clinical skills and experience by his involvement in teaching psychiatry at both undergraduate and postgraduate levels.

Psychiatry is essentially a practical discipline, being learned over a period of years spent in managing and coming to know at first hand, people with psychiatric problems. Though it is not possible to learn psychiatry from books alone, it is necessary to build one's practical experience on a sound basis of theory.

This is what this book is all about; theory and practice. The book is directed primarily to nurses, but students of psychiatry no matter what their discipline will find this book a valuable introduction to their subject.

Of particular interest to practitioners of psychiatry will be the explanation of the roles of the various members of the treatment team. Nothing is more destructive to out patients than to be on the receiving end of inter-disciplinary conflict between professionals, whether this be about means or ends. If this volume is used properly, it will make its own contribution to minimising conflict by directing our attention away from our over-valued ideas back to the patients and the facts they present to us for observation and understanding.

WILLIAM A. BARCLAY
M.B., B.S., B.Sc. (Med.) Sydney, M.S. (Admin. Med.) Columbia, F.R.A.N.Z.C.P., D.P.M.

Former Commissioner for Personal Health Services, Health Commission of New South Wales.

CONTENTS

ACKNOWLEDGEMENTS

The Author's first thanks are to Miss Lorrie Solomons of the Health Commission of New South Wales for the patient and painstaking correction of drafts and manuscripts at each stage. Miss Solomons, with her wide experience in nursing, her interest in teaching, and her understanding of the psychiatric nurse's needs, helped the Author clarify the presentation in areas that otherwise may have remained nebulous and confusing.

Dr G. M. Nicholls of the University of New South Wales and a lecturer at the New South Wales Institute of Psychiatry, kindly corrected some of the Author's misconceptions in the section dealing with heredity, and also produced the initial schema for Figure 7. Dr Brian Turner is thanked for his advice on chromosome abnormalities and screening tests for metabolic disorders.

The initial descriptions of clinical conditions have been drawn freely from Glossary of Mental Disorders reprinted from the Report of the 64th Session of the National Health and Medical Research Council, April, 1967, and the chapter on Child Psychiatry will be seen to quote freely from *Synopsis and Critique of the G.A.P. Classification* written by Dr M. Freeman and mentioned in the Bibliography.

Typing of drafts and final manuscript was performed by Miss Kelsie Williams and Mrs Pam Allen, and the efforts of both are greatly appreciated.

The encouragement of and the interest shown in the completion of this book by Mr D. J. Mooney, Chairman of the New South Wales Institute of Psychiatry, are gratefully acknowledged, as is the forebearance of the Author's wife, Erna.

The Author thanks the Publishers very sincerely, for their patience, cordiality and assistance.

PREFACE

FIRST EDITION

This book covers a syllabus suitable for a comprehensive course for students in psychiatry. It is directed towards workers of all disciplines in psychiatry.

It deals with psychiatric medicine, and is not intended to be an omnibus edition attempting to encompass psychology and psychiatric nursing as well, though many aspects of both are covered. Certain practical details are directed to medical students and doctors and not specifically to nurses. No apology is made for this as nurses were for too long regarded merely as handmaidens to the doctor, and even if they do not issue instructions relating to treatment, they should know what lies behind decisions made by doctors concerning the patient's management. The author trusts that as well as meeting the needs of students in their training and vocation, this book will serve as a practical guide to doctors working both inside and outside the hospital setting.

The roles of various members of the therapeutic team are dealt with in Chapter 2. With the concept of such a health team rightly gaining greater momentum, a greater understanding of the roles of colleagues in a variety of disciplines working with psychiatric patients becomes paramount. In this respect it is hoped that this work will fulfil the need for a straightforward text for the psychologist, social worker, occupational therapist, and other 'health team' members, thus facilitating stronger cohesion within the team. This concept of the team approach is apparent throughout the text.

In order to discuss nursing roles and nursing relationships in close proximity, Chapter 4 precedes a discussion of personality and human dynamics in Chapters 5 and 6. 'The Nurse as a person' will be more meaningful to readers without a basic knowledge of personality and human dynamics, if these latter chapters are read first.

The classification of psychiatric disorders used throughout the text is that of Section V of the World Health Organisation's Eighth Revision of the International Classification of Diseases.

A deliberate effort has been made to restrict the use of cross references within the text, and an adequate index has been provided to facilitate necessary cross references.

It is worth stating that students of psychiatry are dealing with people and there is no literary substitute for first hand experience with people. It will be found that the symptoms of many patients will not fit neatly into the conditions described. This merely shows how complex is the human mind, and it should not dismay us, but cause us wonder.

1973 MAURICE J. SAINSBURY

SECOND EDITION

Not a great deal of time has elapsed since the first edition of this book was published and hence one would not expect to find any great changes in content. However, in the light of helpful comments by reviewers and other readers alterations and additions have been made.

To give a balance in theories of personality development comment has been made on those of Erikson and Adler as well as that of Freud. The section on psychotherapy has been expanded to include a number of theoretical approaches to this treatment modality. With the growing interest in behaviour therapy a segment has been introduced on this topic, and the section on psychopharmacology has been updated. Anti-psychiatry, child health clinics and new approaches in the management of alcoholism and drug dependence are mentioned. Some small changes have been made in setting out material, and the chapter entitled 'Psychoses' under which the Organic Brain Syndromes were previously dealt with has had a name change with appropriate explanation.

The major new features in this second edition are the inclusion of two additional chapters, one entitled 'Admission Ward Psychiatry' which lends itself to a coverage of a number of problems in patient management, and the other entitled 'General Hospital Psychiatry' in which are mentioned the effects of hospitalisation on patients and stresses on staff. This chapter has also been used as a vehicle to look at some areas of thanatology, namely death and dying, and bereavement.

It is hoped that what has been produced will add further dimensions to students' understanding of a fascinating speciality with improved patient care as the ultimate goal.

1976 M.J.S.

THIRD EDITION

Few authors of technical subjects can be satisfied with their endeavours, both immediately after writing, and in the light of growing knowledge in their field. This author is no exception, and it is hoped that his dissatisfaction has produced something more balanced in the presentation of a fascinating subject. Perhaps his feelings of inadequacy as a purveyor of ideas could have been tolerated longer but for the introduction of a revision of the World Health Organisation's International Classification of Diseases. In a sense, while not rendering previous editions completely obsolete, the Ninth Revision of the I.C.D. weighed heavily on an author desirous of conforming to something that should improve communication and a more general understanding of psychiatry. The glossary of I.C.D. has been quoted freely, and it is hoped that this adds to, rather than detracts from, a text aimed at leading to better patient care.

1980 M.J.S.

1

AN HISTORICAL SURVEY OF ATTITUDES TO MENTAL ILLNESS, INSTITUTIONALISATION AND SOME NURSE PIONEERS

Introduction

It is most difficult to define specific periods when the majority of people held particular views about mental illness. Some writers divide public attitudes towards mental illness into stages, at the end painting a rosy picture that everybody is now thoroughly enlightened. However, one has but to converse with members of the general public to see that the various opinions expressed through the ages still linger in some form or other in sections of so-called civilised communities, and truly archaic attitudes exist among present day peoples who have little contact with western civilisation. I do not think that people living in Sydney in the last two decades would have much faith in the concept that mental illness was due to a man walking on a spot where someone had urinated or that mental illness can be helped by swinging the poor sufferer with ropes attached to the ankles from a Moreton Bay fig tree in the Botanical Gardens. Yet this type of thinking and treatment is reported by Professor G. M. Carstairs as being carried out in one particular Indian culture studied by him in recent years.

So we see there are individual attitudes in a particular culture and a wider divergence of attitudes in differing cultures. However, certain periods can, in fact, be described when the attitudes of those responsible for treating folk with mental illness underwent successive changes.

The following does not pretend to be a detailed historical account, but serves to illustrate some attitude changes throughout the ages.

Early period

Since the beginning of recorded history there appear to be references to mental illness in both Eastern and Western civilizations. In western cultures up to the middle ages and later, mental illness was ascribed to such factors as sin, possession by demons, witchcraft or evil spirits sent by the local deity or God.

The Greeks and Romans some 2,000 years ago appear to have

approached the problem of mental illness in a scientific manner but their treatments entailed more the art than the science of medicine.

Hippocrates (460-375 B.C.) and his followers taught that the brain was the seat of the mind, talked of bodily humours which produced particular temperaments, and rejected the then held belief that epilepsy was due to sacred or supernatural causes. Yet both he and the Greeks before him regarded conversion reactions (page 218) as being due to wandering of the uterus (hysteria).

The Middle Ages

The Middle Ages in Europe saw a reversion to belief in demon possession and witchcraft as causes of mental illness. The mentally ill were rarely seen as people who were sick. Some regarded them as people to be feared or venerated, others felt they should be punished. In hospitals established by the Church, the priest took a principal role in the management of sufferers from mental disorders. Exorcism by 'bell, book and candle' was administered to the mentally ill and to sufferers from epilepsy. Immersion in sacred wells was practised, and outside the church hospitals, in a less kindly vein, if a person was accused of witchcraft, a ducking in the local village pool was one of the milder measures meted out by the local population.

The Bethlem Hospital in London was used for the mentally ill from A.D. 1377 and Guys Hospital had a 'lunatic' ward in 1728. Conditions generally were deplorable. The populace paid a subscription to view the lunatics at the Bethlem Hospital. Emetics, purges, floggings and immersions in cold water were the order of the day. Camisoles or straight jackets were in common use. Dungeons and chains were considered appropriate for the sufferers. In America, the Pennsylvanian General Hospital had wards for the insane in 1756 and conditions there were not dissimilar.

Era of humane treatment

An era of humane treatment began as an aftermath of social changes emanating from the French Revolution. Philippe Pinel removed the chains from patients housed in the Bicêtre in Paris in 1798. In England, William Tuke (1732-1822) opened the York Retreat in 1796. He replaced punishment and solitary confinement with humane methods of treatment including various occupational measures. John Connolly (1794-1866) at Hanwell in 1839, stimulated further reforms with the abolition of restraint. It was Connolly who is credited with some of the earliest practical thoughts on the role and training of nurses who were then referred to as attendants, but the first known set of lectures to psychiatric nurses was delivered by Sir Alexander Morison at the Surrey Asylum (now Springfield Hospital) in 1843-44. In 1854 W. A. F. Browne, at the Crichton Royal Hospital, gave a course of thirty lectures primarily to the officers and attendants (nurses), but also to some of the patients who had belonged to the medical profession. 'In these lectures,' he says, 'mental disease was viewed in various aspects; the relation of the insane to the community, to their friends and to their custodians were described; treatment so far as it depends upon external impressions and the influence of sound mind was discussed; and it was attempted to impart attraction by illustration and narrative and by examples drawn from the actual inmates'.

This statement, made more than twelve decades ago, is certainly applicable to psychiatric training today.

Institutionalisation

The impetus of the earlier reforms appears to have waned and the latter part of the 19th Century and early 20th Century saw large mental hospitals built some distance from the centres of large cities, sufficiently far away to keep the mentally sick at a 'respectable' distance from the rest of the community. London is a typical example, being ringed by psychiatric hospitals, in general some 8 to 12 miles or more from the hub of the city, with observation wards or admission centres more centrally situated. These hospitals, many of them containing 2,000 beds and more, were an attempt to provide a reasonable standard of care for the mentally ill. Similar institutions, often very much larger, appeared in the United States of America. The type of care in these hospitals was essentially custodial and the outcome of such care is well portrayed in a book by Denis Martin entitled *Adventure in Psychiatry.* Martin describes the traditional system of patient management in hospitals in the first half of this century as being benignly authoritarian. The authoritarian regime came into being in order to care for the mentally sick and to control the socially unacceptable expressions of mental disorder.

The satisfactory running of these hospitals depended upon the submission of the patients to authority with a minimum of resistance; that is, a so-called authority-submission formula operated. Repressive controls were used, namely, locked doors, restraints, segregation of the sexes, heavy sedation, ECT, prolonged sleep, leucotomy. In their place most of these measures are legitimate treatment procedures but some were frequently used as punitive measures. Patients were threatened with these 'treatments' if they did anything to disturb the peace or the tidiness of a ward. So there came to exist in patients fear of such treatments, and on top of this, the fear of being moved to a disturbed ward with a resultant loss of privilege from the staff. The patients tended to blame the nursing staff entirely for such attitudes, and would not dare to convey their state of oppression to the doctor for fear that further 'punishments' might be inflicted by nursing staff.

The doctors were not blameless; they gave consent to such repressive measures, doing their ward rounds hurriedly in the morning and going off to their game of golf in the afternoon. Blame cannot legitimately be attached to nursing staff for operating within an accepted pattern. There was a clear-cut hierarchy from the Physician Superintendent, Matron, Chief Male Nurse, Secretary or Manager, in their respective departments with orders passed down the line. In other words, communication was downwards, and the further downward the orders were passed the less clear it became why they were given in the first place. Last in the line of people receiving orders was the patient, and he was expected to submit to authority with no way of expressing any sense of injustice felt, save through disturbed behaviour or social withdrawal.

This sounds like a terrible situation for patients to find themselves in; however, this same authority was a benevolent one as long as the patient submitted to it. Entertainments, cinema, outings, sports and other activities were provided, and the hospital afforded security. Patients had no need to think for themselves in anything but the least important trifles. They became more dependent and lost their initiative and sense of responsibility. The final result was what has been termed 'institutionalisation' (D. V. Martin 1955) or 'institutional neurosis' (Russell Barton 1959).

Both the authority-submission formula and the hospital acting as the providing parent, leading to greater dependency in patients, help to produce this state of institutionalisation. An extract from Martin's original article in the *Lancet* (1955) paints a clear picture of the end result achieved:

> Well-institutionalised implies that the patient has ceased to rebel against, or to question the fitness of, his position in a mental hospital; he has made a more or less total surrender to the institution life. When the nurses are asked about the progress of an institutionalised patient, the usual reply is, 'He gives no trouble, doctor, he is very cooperative.' Here 'cooperative' usually implies that the patient does as he is told with a minimum of questioning or opposition. This response on the part of the patient is very different from that true cooperation, essential to the success of any treatment in which the patient strives to understand, and work with the doctor and other staff members in efforts to cure.
>
> The 'well-institutionalised' patient, resigned and cooperative, who has ceased to question his position as a patient, and who has become too passive to present any problem of management, has in the process lost much of his individuality and initiative.

The nurse under the traditional authoritarian system

What about nurses under the old regime?

They, too, were placed in their own hierarchy. Orders were passed down the line. There were rules for most contingencies. It was comfortable to know exactly what to do in a given circumstance. The main emphasis was on nurses exercising control over their patients and guarding them against injury to themselves. The nurse's role was custodial and directive. There was a relationship of authority-submission between nurses and patients, and nurses were expected to direct and manage patients in all their activities. The criterion of the nurses' efficiency was the quietness and tidiness of the ward, rather than the therapeutic atmosphere and the quality of their relationship with their patients.

Orders were passed down to the junior nurses who usually did not know why decisions were made, and who dared not express an opinion. They could not express up the line of authority any sense of injustice they may have felt. Pockets of tension, frustration and anxiety developed which could not be reduced except through the undesirable channels of gossip and rumour.

It is hoped that too grim a picture has not been painted of doctors and nursing staff under the old traditional regime. They simply fitted into the prevailing system, but were not wicked ogres. Traditionally, hospital staff are expected to be kind, sympathetic and understanding, and there is no doubt they were, even in custodial days.

Occasionally a patient in a long-stay ward after years of hospitalisation would somehow become miraculously socialised and be able to re-enter the outside community. It was generally found that a nurse had taken a particular interest in him or her, establishing communication and some form of helpful relationship, which appears to have brought about the change. This leads us to the subject of our next chapter, 'The Therapeutic Community'.

Before embarking on this important topic, it is worthwhile looking at the part nursing staff have played in some of the major attitude changes to mental illness that have taken place. The following paragraphs contain extracts or paraphrases from Dr Alexander Walk's presidential address given at the Cane Hill Hospital to the Royal Medico-Psychological Association in July, 1960.

It is often assumed that Pinel's act of liberation of patients from chains at the Bicêtre in Paris was a dramatic one. It came only after years of patient work against opposition and with the collaboration of what we would call a chief male nurse, Jean-Baptiste Pussin. M. Pussin was not appointed by Pinel but was in office before Pinel became Physician to Bicêtre, and prior to Pinel's arrival, was already bringing into action principles with which Pinel thoroughly agreed. Pinel had a tremendous respect for M. Pussin as well as for his wife Mme. Pussin, who presided over the female staff with the title of 'Governess'. Her sphere of work was not confined to the female side and in fact all the anecdotes related by Pinel concern her work among the male patients. Pinel himself writes of these times: 'The harmful effects of the use of chains had given me much concern during the time I carried out the duties of Physician to Bicêtre, and it was not without extreme regret that I found myself unable to witness the termination of this barbaric custom (because of his transfer from Bicêtre to the Salpêtrière), but on the other hand I felt quite confident, trusting as I did in the skill of the Superintendent* (M. Pussin), whose heart was as set as my own on putting an end to this negation of the true principles of treatment. Success was happily achieved by him two years later, on the 4th of Prairial, year 6 (May 1798). Forty unfortunate patients, who had languished in irons for various lengths of time, were set at liberty and allowed to move freely about the airing courts, with their movements merely controlled by the use of the straight-waistcoat.' The same result was achieved three years later (1801) at the Salpêtrière, again with the assistance of Pussin, who had been transferred at Pinel's special request.

It is interesting to note that Pussin himself had been a patient at Bicêtre possibly suffering from a depression in early manhood, and it was not

* The words 'keeper', 'attendant', 'nurse', and sometimes 'Superintendent' were used interchangeably at this period, except that 'nurse' was generally confined to women.

unusual for him to select as his assistants, both at Bicêtre and the Salpêtrière, recovered or convalescent patients.

During the first part of the 19th century, it was customary to have married couples occupying the roles of Chief Male Nurse and Matron as we now understand these terms. Katherine Allan and her husband George Jepson, became the first 'matron' and 'chief male nurse' at the York Retreat. George Jepson is given the credit for the introduction of methods of moral treatment for which the Retreat became famous. In Samuel Tuke's *Description of the Retreat* of 1813, examples are given of Mr Jepson's inventiveness in the art of gaining the patient's confidence, the introduction of outdoor occupations, the use of a liberal supper in promoting sleep, and the social value of Mrs Jepson's tea parties.

A further indication of the tremendous importance placed on the nursing role can be seen in a passage from John Connolly's *Indications of Insanity,* published in 1828: 'Every patient should have a superintendent or keeper with him during a great part of each day, so long as there remains a hope of cure . . . every opportunity should be taken of effecting the restoration of the patient to mental health . . . to converse with, to amuse, to instruct the patient is the great business of each day'.

Many other examples could be given of the part played by nursing staff in initiating and carrying out changes in hospital systems. Denis Martin, with his conviction that patients were people, and with the quiet solid backing of the then Physician Superintendent, John S. Harris, catalysed a great social change in Claybury Hospital with its 2,000 beds. Martin first worked through the problems entailed in the concept of the mental hospital as a therapeutic community with members of the nursing staff, and would be the first to acknowledge the important part that many nurses played and are still playing in implementing the change from a traditional mental hospital.

The foregoing is but a brief historical survey of attitudes towards mental illness and the process of institutionalisation. Some attention has been given to the part nursing staff played and are playing in initiating and implementing changes in management programmes. Such changes in management programmes do have their impact upon community attitudes to mental illness.

Attitudes of individuals to mental illness (and particularly to hospitalisation) vary tremendously. The psychiatric nurse, in her work and her private and public life, can do much to help throw light into the superstitious and fearful corners of thought still present in more than a few members of our community.

Whilst this chapter deals with institutionalisation in the hospital setting, one should be alert to the fact that the process can occur in practically any organisation. It has even been shown that hospital out-patients may become institutionalised.

With the current thrust towards the development of community resources such as community health clinics, half-way houses, boarding houses, and other extramural facilities, it is well to remember that it is not the location nor the architecture of such facilities that prevents the development of the institutionalisation process in clients and patients, but the attitudes of staff of all disciplines working within and from them.

2

THE HOSPITAL AS A THERAPEUTIC COMMUNITY

Before 1950, hospitals were run on extremely custodial lines with a strict hierarchical authoritarian structure. As previously stated, even under this type of regime, some long-stay hospital patients made apparently miraculous recoveries to once again enter the outside community. It was frequently found that members of the nursing staff had taken a personal interest in and formed healthy relationships with these patients, giving them the opportunity to express themselves, and in short accepting them as individuals with the same inalienable rights as people outside the hospital walls. Where this type of interest becomes part of the hospital atmosphere or milieu we are on the way to developing a therapeutic community.

ORIGINS OF THE THERAPEUTIC COMMUNITY

One of the earlier attempts to serve the individual, the group and the community was made by army psychiatrists with neurotic military casualties at the Northfield Army Neurosis Centre in England. Here, for the first time a hospital was conceived as, and took the form of, a therapeutic community.

An Englishman, Dr T. Main (1946) was responsible for the concept and the term 'therapeutic community'. One of his former staff members, Dr Maxwell Jones applied therapeutic community principles to the conduct of an ex-POW Settlement Unit and later was instrumental in developing a therapeutic community in the section of the Belmont Hospital now known as the Henderson Hospital, in Surrey, England. His influence later spread to the United States of America.

The importance of social factors in treatment procedures was emphasised by Stanton and Schwartz (1954) who described the result of three years work at the Chestnut Lodge Sanitarium, Maryland. They looked at the hospital as a total culture, emphasising how events in one area affected others. They described in some detail what they termed the 'triangular conflict' wherein the players consisted of a demanding patient and usually two staff members of peer status with differing views on the management of the patient, one of whom becomes unduly involved with the patient. Stanton and Schwartz showed how communication froze and tensions built up, eventually leading to the final collapse of a staff member. They also showed that early confrontation of two such staff members, and the opening and facilitation of free verbal face-to-face communication between them served to resolve such difficulties.

Many more references to social factors operating in mental hospitals are described by David Clark (1964). From such observations, it became obvious that adverse social factors had deleterious effects on patients in terms of the process of institutionalisation, and on staff members in terms of tensions, frustrations and disillusionment. The therapeutic community approach does much to obviate this unhappy, if not crippling, state of affairs.

A simple definition of a therapeutic community, derived from the concepts of Denis Martin and Maxwell Jones is as follows: *'A therapeutic community is one in which a conscious effort is made to employ all staff and patient potential in an overall treatment programme, according to the capacities and training of each individual member'.* 'All staff' means staff at all levels in the hierarchical scale and staff of all disciplines. It covers, in fact, everybody who comes into contact with a patient in the course of a patient's day; and all such staff should be involved in the treatment programme. This is a radical departure from the authoritarian regime where communication is essentially downwards throughout the medical, nursing and managerial lines, and more radical still in that patients are afforded the opportunity to have some say in their own management. In a therapeutic community, communication, as well as being down the line, develops in an upwards direction, and in becoming a two-way affair, breaks down the authority-submission formula and counteracts the process of institutionalisation. The development of a degree of what is termed permissiveness, as opposed to an authoritarian approach, also takes place.

MISCONCEPTIONS

Before dealing with the aims of the therapeutic community and the means whereby these aims are achieved, three misconceptions about the therapeutic community will be pointed out:

1. There is the misconception that the nurse must dedicate all efforts towards making the patient's stay in hospital as pleasant as possible. To some, 'make the place as home-like as possible' and variations on this theme are synonymous with the concept of the therapeutic community. There is no doubt that the aesthetic qualities of the grounds and interior appointments, the way food is served and the social programmes are important, but if the emphasis is on pleasantness in contrast to activities which foster emotional growth, the patient may become more fixed in his infantile attitudes of retreat and dependency, and on leaving hospital may be even more vulnerable to the complications of life outside hospital.

2. It is wrong to assume that a hospital or a ward constitutes a therapeutic community just because group psychotherapy is conducted there. Group psychotherapy may be carried out in practically any inpatient or outpatient setting. It is a therapeutic tool employed in many therapeutic community settings, but it is not synonymous with a therapeutic community.

3. There are some who assert that their particular brand of therapeutic

community is the only effective one. Such people unwisely shut their eyes to workable variations on a theme. A little thought will show that the degree of patient involvement, for example in management committees, will depend on the nature of the patients and their ability to become involved. However, the principles entailed in Maxwell Jones' and Denis Martin's definition—that a therapeutic community is one where a conscious effort is made to employ all the staff and patient potential in an overall treatment programme—can be applied in a variety of situations. A crucial fact to remember is that the extent of one's permissiveness is dependent on the mental state of the patient, and *the worker in the therapeutic community is as permissive as the patient's mental state will allow*, for one has responsibilities to the patient, his family and the community.

Many different types of hospitals employ therapeutic community techniques. Units especially interested in family and community psychiatry, admission centres, 'long-stay' wards, special neurological investigation units and surgical and rehabilitation centres are numbered among these. In fact, therapeutic community principles may be applied to any situation in which patients are investigated and treated.

AIMS OF THE THERAPEUTIC COMMUNITY

1. The opening up of new opportunities for the most liberal communication between staff and patients and amongst staff of different grades and disciplines.

This is the most important single change that is fostered in developing a therapeutic community. If this aim can be realised, the upward communication developed from junior staff and patients exposes authority to constant correction by the whole community, so preventing it from acting in an autocratic and uninformed fashion. Also, the creative contributions of patients and junior staff are incorporated into the total life of the community and are not suppressed, therefore eliminating a degree of frustration. It follows that people in positions representing authority at all grades must be able to accept suggestions and criticism from all staff without making their juniors feel out on a limb.

2. The creation of an atmosphere of acceptance of disturbed behaviour with understanding, rather than attempting to control it by arbitrary authority and rule.

The question the staff should first ask themselves is 'What does this behaviour mean?' rather than 'How can we control it most easily?'.

3. The development of independence and the ability of patients to make decisions to the maximum degree their illness will permit.

To this end, *nothing is done for patients which they can reasonably be expected to do for themselves or for one another.*

THERAPEUTIC COMMUNITY ORGANISATION

Staff meetings

All members of the ward or unit staff must first learn to express themselves as freely as possible. They must themselves experience the permissiveness inherent in the system and deal with their own anxieties produced by change or evolution also inherent in the system, before they can extend the approach to patients. The staff meeting is the fundamental step in first developing a therapeutic community and is just as important to maintain in the established evolving therapeutic community, as neither staff nor patients' needs are static.

Meeting of the functional therapeutic unit

Such a unit may be the ward or a system of two or more small wards with similar therapeutic goals and situated in close geographical proximity. It may be that within this functional treatment unit there are a number of sub-sections dealing with groups such as geriatrics, young people, patients with similar problems, or family groups. Whatever staff and patients there are in the evolving treatment unit should meet regularly in an atmosphere of acceptance with encouragement to speak freely about anything or anybody. In such a meeting the patients' or junior staffs' suggestions for running the unit should be implemented if they are acceptable. A variety of patients' and staff subcommittees or committees of management can be set up where the need arises within such a system.

In a large well-established psychiatric hospital such as Claybury where there is already differentiation of ward functions, at least to the extent of allocating patients to wards in terms of length of illness, age and to some extent diagnostic categories, Martin found the ward to be the best functional therapeutic unit. Meetings of from twenty-five to fifty or sixty patients are found to be worthwhile, though there is little doubt that one should aim at treatment units of thirty to forty patients at the outside if one wishes to gain the maximum involvement of patients in meetings, keeping in mind the économic staffing of a ward.

With larger units or wards, and where the composition of the patient population is such that widely differing needs are presented, the unit meeting is still of utmost importance in terms of developing and maintaining a community atmosphere, even though maximum involvement is impossible in large groups. It is necessary however, for smaller subgroups to meet to deal with intrapersonal and interpersonal difficulties at a more intense level.

Mixed sexes

The mixing of the sexes in socially acceptable ways is a prerequisite for adequate functioning of the therapeutic community. As Martin puts it, 'Many of the emotional problems underlying mental disorders are bound up with the relationship between the sexes and express themselves in disordered sexual function, marital disharmony and compulsive avoidance of emotional involvement with the opposite sex. Strict segregation robs the patient of the opportunity of meeting these problems in the treatment situation, where help is available to understand them and work them out'.

Integration of the sexes means integration of staff as well as patients. It is traditional for a female to nurse patients of both sexes, and not until recent years has it become commonly acceptable for males to undertake both physical and psychiatric nursing care of female patients. A disquiet still exists however, inasmuch as male nurses may be wrongfully accused of improper conduct by some female psychiatric patients; and as such accusations are possible it is well to have a female nurse in the vicinity when nursing procedures are being carried out by males.

The therapeutic team

This is a natural outcome in hospitals where therapeutic community principles are applied. Membership of such a staff team will, of course, depend on the available staff. One would see at least the following as being desirable in any such team: doctors, nurses, clinical psychologists, social workers, welfare officers, occupational therapists, recreational officers, physiotherapists in units where they are required, the hospital chaplain, at times a nursing instructor or tutor, and a person perhaps not employed within the hospital but functioning essentially in the outside community. An example of such a person would be a social worker, welfare officer or domiciliary nurse, for though the therapeutic community is essentially an internal hospital organisation, the hospital must strengthen its links with outside community agencies and facilities if it is going to have any real impact on community health. Each member of the team has a specialised role to play, a role for which each individual is trained or is in training. Roles do overlap to some extent, a situation which may cause some degree of emotional friction. This friction can be minimised if every attempt is made to delineate roles clearly and if each team member is free to discuss difficulties as they arise.

In some psychiatric hospitals, voluntary mental health workers under guidance play a substantial role in areas of patient care and social rehabilitation, and appropriate measures should be taken to build this valuable group into the therapeutic team. The same may be said of the art therapist and music therapist where these positions are on the hospital establishment.

Special sections deal later with the roles of psychiatrist and nurse. At this point, with apologies to the team specialists who might hold different opinions, views on the roles and functions of a number of personnel frequently forming part of our therapeutic teams today will now be given.

The Psychologist

The psychologist has four main theatres of operation:

(a) He administers to patients batteries of psychological tests which throw light on intellectual functioning, attitudes of patients and the patient's inner mental mechanisms and fantasies, many of which are not at all apparent at clinical interview. As well as aiding in a diagnostic appraisal, he can often delineate areas of difficulty with which the patient can later be helped to deal.

(b) He may be called upon to undertake patient counselling or to utilise more formal psychotherapeutic or behaviour modification techniques.

(c) His special training in statistical and research methodology places him in a position where he can design and carry out research projects dealing with diagnostic, treatment and other clinical procedures. He may undertake studies relating to staff selection and ward programmes, administrative difficulties, and problems relating to community psychiatry.

(d) He has a teaching role wherein he can apply himself to both remedial teaching of patients with certain educational handicaps and the training of other staff members in psychological concepts which will help these fellow workers in their management of patients.

The Social Worker

Traditionally the social worker is the team member par excellence who functions both inside and outside the hospital.

In the hospital setting she is generally seen as the person who deals with the problems of the patient's environment and who, on the whole, works with the healthy parts of a patient's personality. Some hospitals require their social workers to take a full social history on every patient admitted, a truly herculean task where there are large numbers of admissions. This is a duplication of work in many instances, as a good history taken by the doctor should cover many points relevant to such social histories. It is perhaps more meaningful if the doctor, nursing staff and other members of the therapeutic team refer to the social worker, patients who show indications of having social problems. Much of the social worker's time is spent in helping individual patients and their relatives. She interprets the hospital procedures and gives guidance in such matters as social services, pensions, child welfare allowances and other available services. She must be able to assess the relatives, be able to gauge the type of relationships that exist between them and the patient and assess the potentiality of the whole family for making a proper social adjustment. She may have the training and special ability to act as counsellor or psychotherapeutic agent. The patient's rehabilitation begins upon admission. The social worker maintains contact with employers or with officers of relevant employment services, with hostels, nursing homes, rehabilitation centres, and other agencies who may be able to help in housing and resettlement. In some hospitals, the overtures concerned with, and the placement of patients in suitable employment constitutes a separate role, that of work advisor.

All these functions are traditional ones for the social worker. In the therapeutic community, per medium of staff meetings, she becomes more closely involved in decision making and in the management of the patient and the family unit. The social worker is able to observe the interaction of patients in group settings, and with suitable training, her own ability as a group leader enables her to function with family groups, groups of patients requiring encouragement to leave or who are about to leave hospital, and many other types of groups that arise in treatment situations.

Outside the hospital the social worker carries out case work with patients' families. She is able to see at first hand, the conditions under which families live and is in a position to tap the resources of welfare agencies to alleviate problems on the home front. The family may need help in adjusting to the patient's hospitalisation, and the presence and advice of the social worker may prevent the premature closing of the family's ranks which would militate against the reacceptance of the patient.

Many social workers now find themselves fully community-based, working in and from community health centres.

The Occupational Therapist

Like other team members the occupational therapist has undergone training in a specialised field. The application of the occupational therapist's skill in the earlier days of this speciality was aimed at diverting the patient's attention from his inner conflicts. Interesting, relaxing and soothing occupations were the order of the day. In most instances, particular occupational activities were actually prescribed by the doctor in the same way as he might order an X-ray. It was believed, on the basis of little or no evidence, that certain types of activities benefited patients with particular psychiatric conditions. The activity itself was regarded as therapeutic, and little cognizance was given to the dynamic aspects of personal and group relationships which developed in the occupational situation.

The present aim of occupational therapy is to consciously use the personal relationship between the therapist and patient, and between patients themselves, that develop within the framework of occupational activities, in a way that will help patients gain an understanding of, and modify if necessary, their particular patterns of behaviour.

The location of such activities will vary with the particular needs of patients, and occupational therapy can be effective either in the ward setting or in a special building set aside for the purpose. Craft work with certain individuals, still has its rightful place and can give the patient a sense of achievement and satisfaction. However, in order to understand and help the patient in his interpersonal relationships, the trend towards patients working in group situations has now become established.

The type of occupational activity varies according to patients' needs. Long-stay patients may require re-education in such pursuits as housework, cooking, shopping, and beauty care. It is a terrifying experience for some long-hospitalised, and usually institutionalised, patients to walk into a busy street. They are often surprised at current prices, and lacking in confidence, they require encouragement to face the salesmen or saleswomen.

Patients with specific physical handicaps may have specially designed jobs to re-educate affected muscle groups. Here the advice and cooperation of another team member, the physiotherapist, will be necessary.

Some patients have speech difficulties, and if the hospital does not have the services of a speech therapist, it may fall to the occupational therapist to devise activities to encourage speech. At a more advanced level she may involve patients in play readings and psychodrama.

In many patients recently admitted to hospital, failure in daily work and activities is due, not to disuse of skills and lack of practice in them, but to emotional conflict. The occupational therapist plays her part along with other team members in the treatment of emotional difficulties that hinder work efficiency.

A fairly recent development in psychiatric hospitals is that of industrial therapy. In this activity the occupational therapist becomes Works Manager, Personnel Officer and clerk rolled into one. Industrial therapy provides something that is not far away from a normal work situation. If the type of work is graded, patients can progress from one grade of work to another and can derive pleasure, improve the length of periods of concentration and receive some sort of remuneration which increases their sense of independence.

Mention might be made of the teaching role of the occupational therapist. This pertains particularly to the treaching of some of her skills to nursing staff in hospitals where there are insufficient occupational therapists for large numbers of patients. Before the advent of the occupational therapist, specialist psychiatric nursing staff carried out most of the traditional functions now performed by the occupational therapist, and some of our older psychiatric nurses will wonder at this swing of the pendulum. They will wonder, too, at the more active role the occupational therapist team member takes as a counsellor or psychotherapeutic agent.

The Physiotherapist

The physiotherapist is an indispenable body in admission centre psychiatry, and in more specialised areas in psychiatric hospitals dealing with medical and surgical problems. Her attendance at regular team meetings is necessary in order to gain a background knowledge of psychiatry and psychology which is essential if she is to function efficiently in a psychiatric setting. If she does not attend the team meetings, she loses the opportunity of hearing about and discussing methods of managing patients that she will meet in the hospital situation.

The role of the physiotherapist may be seen as follows:

(a) *Physiotherapy expert.* In her specialised physiotherapy role, she will deal with:

(i) problems coincident with the patient's psychiatric illness and this includes anything from flat feet to bronchiectasis.

(ii) conditions directly or indirectly caused by the patient's psychiatric condition such as nerve lesions from severed wrists in suicide attempts, bronchopneumonia occurring in the elderly and in patients suffering from temporary brain dysfunction such as occurs in an epileptic fit or acute alcoholic states.

(iii) conditions inextricably bound up with the patient's psychiatric state, for example some cases of asthma; brain dysfunction, congenital or traumatically acquired, which involves both mental and physical disabilities; arthritis, which may precipitate depression, which in turn produces a greater degree of immobility in a patient leading to further disuse and freezing of joints.

(b) *Psychotherapeutic role.* The physiotherapist must be aware of the patient's psychiatric condition to know how much cooperation she might expect and also so that any communication she makes with the patient is in line with the therapeutic plan developed at the therapeutic team meeting. A very depressed patient may require much support and encouragement whereas some antisocial personalities require little or no support and should be given little opportunity for manipulation. The opportunity will frequently present itself for the physiotherapist with understanding to make some interpretation of a patient's behaviour. Physiotherapy itself may be extremely therapeutic. The psychotically depressed patient and the withdrawn schizophrenic patient, for example, benefit from the physiotherapist's daily sessions, and her interest in them, along with her pleasant encouraging remarks, may be more beneficial than the few lungs full of air she may persuade them to take.

Team ball games and calisthenics in a group may do much to break down barriers in patients showing social withdrawal.

(c) *Advisory role.* The physiotherapist is in a position to advise on the most beneficial form of physiotherapy for a particular patient and such treatment can be dovetailed into the general management programme for that patient. She may be consulted about the value of conducting long physical rehabilitation programmes particularly on patients with brain damage, frequently caused through trauma or following strokes.

(d) *Liaison work.* This may involve contacting other doctors or previous treatment centres to ascertain the actual extent of original disabilities and the actual work already put into rehabilitation programmes so that a more accurate prognosis as to eventual outcome can be made.

If proper fitting orthopaedic shoes are required, the physiotherapist approaches the social worker about ways of paying for these, arranges for a fitter to come to the hospital and finally sees that the right shoes reach the right patient.

(e) *Teacher.* Physiotherapists, unlike nursing staff, are not present in treatment areas twenty-four hours a day. Procedures such as postural drainage, supportive coughing, fitting calipers and walking exercises should be taught to the nursing staff so that they can be carried out on a 'round the clock' basis.

These then are short descriptions of the functions of some of the team members. Space does not allow us to deal with the roles of all. The essential principle is that each member has a specialised training and function, each has contributions to make both in assessment and management of patients and can extend their influence into the family situation and community where this is necessary.

A therapeutic team should meet at regular intervals, preferably daily, but this will vary with the hospital admission rate and other commitments, though time spent in such meetings is generally found to save time in the long run, and it enables members to learn techniques from each other, to learn how each member can function to the greatest advantage of the patient. Responsibility for assessment and management becomes a shared one, though the final responsibility must be accepted by the team leader. He, however, can make more informed assessments and can initiate more rational treatment programmes with the cooperation of his team.

Our definition of a therapeutic community speaks of involvement of 'all staff and patients in an overall treatment programme'. No mention has been made of patients in this constitution of the therapeutic team, and I do not see how they can have any place in such a team where matters of a confidential nature are discussed among team members. Patients have every right to choose when and how they disclose their difficulties to fellow patients. The usual codes of professional secrecy are maintained in the therapeutic team, and having patients as members would be contrary to this principle.

Patients, however, are encouraged to be members of activities committees, parliamentary committees, social committees, disciplinary committees or whatever functional committee develops in the therapeutic community. Staff members should also form part of such committees, if only in an advisory or limit-setting capacity, and should not entirely relinquish their responsibilities to the patient population. They should however, encourage patients to accept responsibility and to use their own initiative to as great an extent as possible.

It is important to note that the therapeutic community concept should not imply that group techniques of treatment are used exclusively. There may be some units within a hospital where other forms of therapy are not required, but any rational form of therapy including drug therapy and physical treatments may also be employed within the therapeutic community setting.

TOTAL HOSPITAL AS A THERAPEUTIC COMMUNITY

So far, we have talked only of functional treatment units run as therapeutic communities. A hospital is a group of such units or wards, and anything happening in one ward of a hospital is likely to have repercussions on other wards and on the general management of the hospital, either directly or indirectly. Hence it is important to open up lines of communication laterally to other wards and special units and to the executives in the medical, nursing and managerial lines.

In a hospital which functions adequately as a total therapeutic community, apart from communication developed at functional unit level, the minimum requirements appear to be meetings of the following groups:

1. Executive staff, with representation from the medical, nursing and managerial staffs.
2. Executive nursing staff, senior charge nurses and charge nurses, nurse educators, medical and managerial senior executives.
3. The total medical staff of all functional units, from medical superintendent to the most junior doctor.
4. There must be every facility for the heads of paramedical staff to meet with the manager and medical executive, and in some instances this may be achieved at a regular meeting.

Other meetings of sections of the hospital community may rise and fall according to the need at the time. In some hospitals, patient representatives from all areas of the hospital have formed a patients' committee to discuss matters with the hospital executive staff.

The structure and function of the meetings suggested as minimal requirements are open to variation to suit local needs. The important principle is to open up lines of communication laterally and both up and down the hierarchical lines in order that an understanding of why things are done can be increased. This makes work more meaningful, with ideas from all levels and disciplines being brought to light and, if acceptable, being used in the total management programme. Meetings take time, but it is usually found to be time well spent and extremely valuable in terms of hospital policy making. They are a right step in producing a community where there is utilisation of all staff and patient potential in an overall treatment programme according to the capacities of each member of the community.

PERMISSIVENESS; 'HIERARCHICAL PROMOTION'; RESPONSIBILITY AND AUTHORITY

In this section it is intended to look at possible traps into which one may fall while working in a therapeutic community, and to stimulate thought on the questions of responsibility and authority.

The concept of permissiveness has been touched upon, and the point made that one is as permissive as a patient's mental state will allow. There is a tendency to overlook the implications of this and to develop a laissez faire attitude with respect to individual patient requirements and management. The general therapeutic community umbrella, with in-built group therapy sessions, is hidden under, ostrich-like, by some staff as if this milieu will completely protect potentially sucidal patients or those grossly disturbed by delusional thoughts. It helps, but it is not enough for these patients. Specific treatment programmes may not be suitable for all patients in the therapeutic community, and more flexibility may be required in providing programmes for different groups of patients within the therapeutic setting. This is an important point to bear in mind, particularly if working in an admission area.

One other pitfall, contrary to therapeutic community principles, is the tendency of some enthusiasts to superimpose a system that has been developed in another therapeutic community on to a new situation, without giving staff and patients the opportunity to work through its implications and to create their own optimal treatment and living conditions.This smacks of 'hierarchical promotion', a phrase used by Dr T. Main to describe a state that can occur in a developed therapeutic community. Briefly, it refers to the application to future situations, of decisions 'worked through' in a therapeutic community. In this way something discussed fully at a point in time, and suitable to conditions at that point in time, is given the status of a rule or law which is later imposed in an authoritarian fashion. If the therapeutic community is to retain its vitality and therapeutic potential, this tendency must not be allowed to develop.

A few thoughts now on responsibility and authority. It is a fair administrative tenet that responsibility and authority go hand in hand. Changing the direction of communication so that it travels upwards and laterally, as well as downwards, is, in the words of David Clark, achieved by 'flattening the authority pyramid'.

If, indeed, authority is used in the sense of being on top of an hierarchical structure, forsaking authority at top levels should mean lessening the responsibility of top executives or team leaders. To be realistic however, final responsibility does rest squarely on the shoulders of the medical team leader, no matter how much it has become a shared responsibility, involving shared leadership with other disciplines or decision-making by consensus. This being so, if the afore-mentioned administrative tenet be correct, the team leader's position must be associated with comparable authority, whether it be by virtue of his position, or, more healthily, by virtue of him being the person he is.

This might sound heretical in terms of therapeutic community thinking, and one might be accused of delegating authority to junior staff and patients with tongue in cheek, and asked, 'What of the concept of patient government that is bandied about?'.

Two points will be made. One is that a team leader can have authority without being authoritarian, and the other is that one does not run a therapeutic community to create anarchy, or to produce a democracy, or any other political system. One is merely giving patients and junior staff the opportunity to make their relevant contributions according to their capabilities and training, thus offsetting the unhealthy social situation brought about by the application of the 'authority-submission' formula. One gives them the opportunity to contribute and to develop their personalities, preventing the insidious onset of a state of institutionalisation in staff and patients alike.

It is hoped that these comments will show that a therapeutic community is not a static formulation, but a situation in which one must constantly question the appropriateness of the current status quo.

3

THE ROLES OF THE PSYCHIATRIST AND THE PSYCHIATRIC NURSE

We have looked together at the parts certain disciplines play in the therapeutic team. In this chapter we shall focus on the psychiatrist and the psychiatric nurse, endeavouring to see where each fits into the scheme of things.

THE PSYCHIATRIST

People working with psychiatrists are often perplexed by the multitude of different approaches utilised by different members of this profession. There appears to be no consistent role adopted by all psychiatrists, and the role assumed is often not consistent over a period of time in the one psychiatrist. We shall now try to throw some light into this area of confusion.

A psychiatrist is a qualified medical practitioner who has made a specialised study of psychiatry or psychological medicine.

It is important that he be, first and foremost, a doctor because many conditions of medical nature produce or are associated with mental symptoms, and on not infrequent occasions a knowledge of general medicine is found to be a prerequisite for a thorough clinical appraisal of a patient.

Psychiatrists may develop interest and expertise in particular areas of their specialty, for example psychotherapy and, more specifically, analysis of the psychoanalytical (Freudian) or Jungian school. These psychiatrists undergo a personal analysis and are supervised in the techniques of dealing with patients undergoing analysis. A training analysis of this type may entail a five day per week personal analysis, the analysis of a patient, and regular sessions with training analysts, the whole process lasting for some years. Such training is expensive and time-consuming and it is little wonder that only a small percentage of psychiatrists enjoy the benefits of psychoanalytical training. In passing, it might be mentioned that 'lay analyst' is the term applied to people outside the medical profession who have undergone a training analysis.

Other special interests developed by psychiatrists lie in the fields of group, family and social psychiatry, child psychiatry, psychogeriatrics, behaviour therapy, drug therapy and other physical methods of treatment, or the psychiatrist may have special research interests. This list could be expanded, and the nurse in her daily experience will possibly meet psychiatrists with one interest or another, or perhaps a mixture of a number. Some specific interests may be the outcome of personality factors in the psychiatrist, or he may find that he can handle particular age groups or particular conditions better than others, and the tendency will be to concentrate on these.

Whether a psychiatrist deals with children, adults or geriatric patients, or favours the management of certain specific problems, it will become evident to people working in psychiatric situations that two divergent though disappearing views still exist in psychiatry, namely, the physiological or biological and the psychological or dynamic. It behoves the nurse not to be wooed too early into either camp, but to appreciate that the enthusiasts in both camps have opened new doors in the management of the psychiatric patient, and that both approaches have their place.

With developments in knowledge of neurochemistry and neurophysiology it seems likely that significant correlations between psychological and physiological aspects of behaviour will eventually become apparent and the dichotomy of views may become a thing of the past. As things stand, the modern psychiatrist with a broad-based training is more able to integrate both viewpoints into his theoretical and practical framework. To utilise concepts from both psychological and physiological standpoints is referred to as adopting an *eclectic approach* to psychiatry, though the concept of eclecticism goes further than this, taking into consideration biological, psychological, sociological and cultural factors—the body, mind, group and culture as described by Cawte and Brown.

It has become obvious that the psychiatrist's role may be an extremely varied one; however, we shall attempt to indicate broadly the role of the psychiatrist in a modern psychiatric hospital run on therapeutic community lines. Such a psychiatrist may have any of the leanings mentioned above, depending on factors in his personality and on his particular training and experience, but in a therapeutic community it is his responsibility to assume leadership of the therapeutic team. Arising out of his training, firstly in general medicine and then in psychiatry, he should be the one most able to make a valid clinical diagnosis and to formulate a plan of management for a patient. However, in this he is frequently dependent upon the skills of the members of his team, which may include the psychologist, the nursing staff, social workers and welfare officers, occupational therapists, physiotherapists, the hospital chaplain and perhaps others. The psychiatrist must serve as a catalyst in his team, and he must know how the members' skills can be utilised in the assessment and management of patients. It may take some time, particularly for the young psychiatrist to learn how to lead and to use his team effectively. Some doctors, through their training in traditional surgical hospital type medicine and through an inability to delegate and share responsibility and authority, find such an approach a difficult one, and these doctors must adapt to the new circumstances before they can function effectively in the modern psychiatric hospital.

A most important aspect of the psychiatrist's role is the teaching one.

It is encumbent upon him to teach in the work situation at every available opportunity, as better-informed staff mean smoother-running wards and hence a better atmosphere in which patients may recover from their psychiatric disabilities.

In short, the psychiatrist's role in a modern psychiatric hospital is a tripartite one, that of specialist, team leader and teacher.

THE NURSE

A start will be made by drawing a picture of the traditional nurse. It is a dangerous practice to generalise, as many general nurses do not fit the pattern presented, and regrettably some psychiatric nurses do. However, at the risk of offending some, the traditional general nurse will be described.

The traditional general nurse

Most people have some sort of stereotype or imagined picture of the typical nurse. Usually this picture is associated with the general nurse and it frequently goes something like this: 'A busy little golden hearted person doing things for sick people—and usually in a hurry'. I am aware that most general nurses would throw up their hands in horror at this description. However, these aspects of 'doing things for' and 'in a hurry' are a true picture of nursing in many general hospitals.

The nurse is busy on technical details of her work, is often too busy to talk to a patient and is frequently discouraged from doing so. (One would hope that the senior nurses who look reproachfully at their juniors, asserting that they are wasting time when they talk to patients are a vanishing race.) However inadequate and grotesque the above picture of the traditional nurse is, the fact remains that there is a tendency in some unenlightened areas of general nursing to maintain the old surgical hospital formula; far too much is 'done for' a patient (the emphasis being on the particular condition) thus fostering dependency needs, and almost paradoxically, too little notice is taken of the person as a whole. In one general hospital, a male patient was in status asthmaticus for several days. All the then known physical therapeutic measures including cortisone had been tried, and as a last resort, as not infrequently happens, a psychiatrist was asked to see the patient. He merely allowed the patient to get certain matters of conflict off his chest and within a short time the patient was breathing freely with no distress. Such a simple 'procedure' could have been carried out by the resident doctors or nursing staff if they had formed a satisfactory relationship with the patient and had been aware that a whole man was with them, not just a chest containing constricted mucousy bronchioles. One appreciates that patients with severe medical conditions do, on frequent occasions, require complete nursing care and the nurse must needs do everything for the patient. But frequently this 'doing things for' is carried over into unnecessary situations. That this tradition still exists in many general hospitals is evidenced by the guilt and anxiety initially experienced by general trained nurses when they come to work in a psychiatric setting where the work pace and demands are different.

It must be remembered too, that patients with physical conditions have frequently made satisfactory social adjustments in the community, and perhaps some short-term mothering will not unduly foster dependency needs. On the other hand, psychiatric patients frequently have made poor social adjustments and it is much easier for them, often starting with dependency needs, to regress into more childish dependent attitudes if too much is done for them.

If the general nurse appears to have been wronged in an effort to make a point, I apologise, but the role of the psychiatric nurse is different from that of the still-surviving traditional general nurse. Wherein lie the differences? They will, it is hoped, become apparent in the next section.

The psychiatric nurse

The various sub-roles of the modern psychiatric nurse may be seen as follows:

1. Parent substitute.
2. Socialising agent.
3. Teacher.
4. Psychotherapeutic agent or counsellor.
5. Manager.
6. Technician.
7. Communicator.

There are times when these sub-roles may overlap to some extent, but the good nurse should always be aware of her sub-role at any particular time.

It is important for a nurse to know that she serves as a model to the patients, demonstrating an approach to the problem of living. This applies in all sub-roles which we shall now look at in more detail.

Parent substitute

This sub-role may be compared with the role of a parent and involves such acts as feeding, bathing, dressing, comforting and supporting patients and setting limits to their behaviour. Patients who are acutely physically ill do, in fact, require things to be done for them in the same way as an infant requires care from a parent. Many psychiatric patients also show immature (or regressive) behaviour patterns which necessitate mothering or fathering patterns in the nursing staff. The nurse must be conscious that she is functioning in this sub-role as a necessity arising out of the patient's state at the time, and should not be beguiled into assuming this sub-role when it is no longer necessary. If a parent maintains for an unnecessarily long time, a protective attitude to a child it is likely that the child will later have difficulty in being independent. In the same way, a nurse may foster dependency needs in patients, something that happens particularly when he or she has some inner need to be a good parent. Knowing when to relax one's support of a patient, a necessary step somewhere along the line to recovery, is an art that sometimes takes a deal of experience to acquire.

As a general rule in psychiatry nursing *one does nothing for a patient that he can reasonably be expected to do for himself.*

On the question of limit setting, though a permissive attitude is the rule in a therapeutic community, one must not assume that being permissive means the abrogation of responsibility for aiming at reasonable standards of behaviour in patients. A mother would surely not allow her child, innocent of danger, to enter a dangerous situation, nor would she countenance his wilful damage of property or person. At some stage of a patient's illness, arising out of an abnormal mental state he may be in similar situations. In such circumstances a nurse would be expected to exert some degree of control over a patient.

The rule here is: *The nurse is as permissive as a patient's mental state will allow.*

Socialising agent

Many writers lay too much stress on the 'professional role' of the nurse, important as it is, to the exclusion of this important sub-role which, among other things, implies sharing activities with patients, such as playing indoor and outdoor games, watching and discussing TV, etc. A number of psychiatric illnesses, and unfortunately still, the attitude of families, friends and the community to such illnesses, cause the patient to lose confidence, to feel inadequate or insecure in social situations. Nursing staff are with patients twenty-four hours of the day and it seems reasonable that part of this time is spent away from the rigours of more strict therapeutic regimes in the process of re-learning, or learning for the first time, the give and take of social intercourse. The patient, using the nurse as model, will learn the rules demanded by society. He will also learn to become freer in interpersonal relationships and thus gain greater confidence in day to day living. Before he can relate widely, it is frequently the case that he has to learn to relate socially as an equal to an individual—the nurse. She must step out of her other sub-roles for a time for this relationship to develop.

The development of a social relationship with a patient is not without its dangers, especially if the nurse is not aware of her own motives or is unable to deal with her feelings, both of which may lead to the development of unhealthy involvements. Good psychiatric nursing, however, requires the utilisation of this sub-role. It is not easy, but a nurse should make every effort to develop skills in dealing with the ramifications of this sub-role. Certain general rules may help:

1. Once a patient shows signs of better social functioning in the individual sense with a nurse he should be encouraged to relate to another patient or group of patients.
2. If this sub-role produces anxieties in a nurse she should discuss these with her colleagues or members of the ward team.
3. Similarly, the ward team or other colleagues, and not the patient, should be the recipient of the nurse's current personal problems. Two things may happen if a nurse discusses her private life with a patient:
   (a) It may distress a patient further.
   (b) Certain patients may use the material discussed to blackmail or manipulate the nurse into a compromising situation.

Only after a great deal of experience will a nurse become expert in knowing when to utilise this sub-role and how much of herself to give to it. A chronic regressed schizophrenic patient may not respond well to pressures to enter activity programmes, but may require a period in which the nurse has but to sit and talk with him and later engage in some activity herself in the presence of the patient. Such a patient may, after identifying with the nurse, commence a similar activity. Again, it would be unreasonable to expect a severely retarded psychotically depressed patient to play croquet or enter into games requiring concentration with the rest of the group. On the other hand, some patients require and can take a deal of stimulation to enter into social programmes.

Teacher

This sub-role involves namely: communicating ward routines to patients; helping to inculcate acceptable habits with respect to dressing, eating and toilet in regressed or deteriorated patients. The importance of speaking to patients, and especially children, while such activities are in progress cannot be overemphasised.

The nurse gains some degree of specialised knowledge in anatomy, physiology and numerous other topics during her training. It is sometimes helpful to correct wrong views held by patients with respect to many aspects of life and living. A nurse should be able to set aside a short period of time daily to discuss and answer questions put to her by patients.

There is another aspect to consider apart from the teaching of patients, namely the teaching of other staff members. This is not just the responsibility of institutes, training schools, charge nurses or senior nurses. Any nurse at any stage of training, by virtue of her particular experience, may colloquially have the edge on a colleague in terms of knowledge. Such knowledge should be imparted at every available opportunity.

The good psychiatric nurse is conscious of her place in teaching both patients and staff, the latter including nursing, paramedical and medical staff, many of whom are in training and none of whom, however experienced, know all the answers.

Psychotherapeutic agent or counsellor

This sub-role has proved a conflicting one for many working in psychiatry. Some stoutly maintain that a nurse should never be interpretative of patients' behaviour and there are those at the other end of the scale who give nurses unlimited responsibility in this sphere, often when they are not sufficiently trained or mature enough to accept this responsibility.

Just as among psychiatrists there are immense differences in psychotherapeutic ability (and even in acceptance of psychotherapy as a treatment measure), so nursing staff have greater or lesser aptitude for functioning in this sub-role. Every nurse, however, should be helped to develop her potential in this specialised field.

The prime requirements are to *be a good listener* and *to show genuine acceptance of the patient as a person.* The nurse may hear much that is unacceptable to her in terms of her own upbringing and particular sub-culture, but she should be wary about moralising. It is more important to look into the reason for untoward behaviour than simply to pass judgment on it. You may be offended for example if a patient masturbates. Such an act (which incidentally is infrequently observed) may result from strong feelings of insecurity and this latter point is one to take up with the patient, not the fact that you personally may consider the act right or wrong.

When talking with patients, avoid using terminology that is obscure to you. It will be even more obscure and confusing to a patient. Encourage the patient to delineate clearly the focal point or meaning of his communications. Be honest. Do not look as if you understand to whom or what the patient is referring when he talks about 'him' or 'they' or some other vague or erroneous concept, as this will foster sloppy habits of thinking in your patient. Also, he may regard you as a mind reader or pretty quickly assume you are neither interested nor genuine. If the patient is vague, ask him to whom he is referring or say something like this: 'I don't follow precisely what you are getting at. Let's look at it again'.

Being human, the nurse may have a tendency to accept a patient's statement in a way that pleases her most. For example, if a patient says: 'You are the only understanding nurse in the hospital', a nurse may be inclined to feel and accept the fact with pride that she is a cut above her colleagues in this respect. However, such a statement by a patient may have a number of meanings. It may be a plea by the patient for approval, perhaps following an altercation with other patients. It may be a 'blarney stone act' used with all nurses in order to manipulate them into doing some favour. The patient may feel lonely or isolated and may employ this overture to elicit sympathetic understanding. This is but one example of the way that one statement may indicate a number of different things, and it is the nurse's job to elicit the valid one. In the instance quoted, a nurse may do well to comment as follows, 'I'm sorry to hear that you feel misunderstood. Would you like to tell me about it?' or the nurse may make some comment about loneliness if she sees this as the possible problem. Such comment opens the way for further clarification, whereas the acceptance of the statement at its face value closes any further communication. *Moral—do not uncritically accept patients' statements at their face value.*

It may be that a particular nurse may not advance past this clarification role. But, if she can but do this properly, her contribution as a psychotherapeutic agent or counsellor will be great, for it will help patients to focus more clearly on their problems.

When you are out of your depth, admit this to yourself and usually also to the patient and encourage him to raise the problem with the psychiatrist individually or in a group situation. You are soon spotted as phoney if you pretend erudition when it is not there.

It may be a fact that you are indeed the only person with whom a patient feels he can communicate freely. You are entrusted with a person's inner hopes, fears and secrets. *Do not break this trust* by broadcasting such facts as you know, without first obtaining the patient's permission. If you do, the patient loses confidence in you, communicates no more and probably suffers more as a consequence. Of course, every effort should be made to get the patient to tell such facts to the psychiatrist or to the patient therapy group. If this is done, mountains often become molehills and fearful skeletons in cupboards become innocuous bags of bones when shared in the light of day.

One further comment will be made, and this on patients showing the mental symptoms of delusions and hallucinations. I cannot think of any circumstance where it is necessary to agree with a patient's delusions or delusional system. It is right and proper to accept the delusion, indicating to the patient that you know it to be a very real experience to him, but that it is not your experience. The delusion is an inner experience of the patient projected on to the external world. Unless everybody else is out of touch with reality, it must be conceded that the patient is not seeing the world outside himself realistically, and it is your job to paint the true picture for the patient in order that he may make some attempt to adjust to reality. In one of our hospitals a patient would not do anything unless she was wound up at the back, and the nursing staff went through the imaginary motions of winding her up when they wanted her to do anything. This may be a far-fetched example, but if this woman believed she was some sort of clockwork apparatus the action of the nurses merely underscored this false belief. Another long-stay patient in an English hospital insisted that she was Lady . . . and her rather grandiose manner fitted this appellation. The hospital staff played up to this known falsity and referred to her as 'Lady . . .'. On her death bed she stated she was not Lady . . . and chuckling said she had fooled the doctors and nursing staff for years.

In the same way, the nurse must accept the fact that hallucinatory experiences are real to a patient, but she must not for instance agree that she hears the same voices.

It is probably worthwhile to discuss with patients the nature of the hallucinatory experiences and to look for possible reasons for the content of such hallucinations.

In summary, points to be remembered in functioning in the role of psychotherapeutic agent or counsellor may be listed as follows:

1. Be a good listener.
2. Show genuine acceptance of the patient as a person.
3. Be wary about moralising.
4. Clarify communications and be precise yourself.
5. If out of your depth, admit it to yourself and encourage the patient to discuss material with the psychiatrist or to bring it up at a group therapy meeting.
6. Do not break a patient's trust in you.
7. Do not go along with patients' delusions or hallucinations.

Manager

This sub-role may not feature largely in the junior nurse's frame of reference but will develop as she progresses and assumes greater responsibility in a ward situation.

A good manager will have a sound knowledge of her patients, her staff and her stocks. With regard to patients, a knowledge of their mental state will be necessary in order to position them in wards and make decisions regarding limits of freedom. If a nurse in a position of authority and responsibility is to get the best from her junior staff, she must know their strengths and weaknesses, roster them in most advantageous situations in the ward, rotate them for purposes of training and encourage them in areas of work where they are weak. Stock includes dispensary and C.S.D. (Central Sterilising Department) requirements, oxygen, laundry, crockery, and all other ward equipment and furniture. Both requisitioning for new supplies and for repair of equipment are managerial functions.

Seeing that patients' clothing and property are properly stored and made available when required, distributing meals and special diets, co-ordinating the duties of the domestic staff, maintaining a satisfactory relationship with visitors to the ward (for example, the Magistrate, technicians, artisan staff, medical and paramedical staff, chaplains and patients' friends and relatives), the proper preparation of patients and the smooth organisation of facilities for the carrying out of special procedures and investigations are further managerial functions that add to the smooth running of a ward.

In a therapeutic community setting, the nurse's contribution to the planning of therapeutic programmes and her part in carrying them out are of utmost importance.

As indicated earlier in this section, the managerial sub-role may not feature much in the early days of psychiatric nursing, but situations do arise where it may be necessary to assume the cloak of authority and responsibility in a ward situation much earlier than one expects, so some knowledge of this sub-role should be gained early in training by taking good note of all routines in the ward situation.

In summary, the sub-role of manager involves all activities and routines aimed at producing a smooth-running ward and hence a total environment maximally conducive to the patients' recovery.

Technician

The psychiatric nurse finds herself involved not only in conditions emanating from disturbances originating above eye level, but sees the patient as a total person with a body as well as a mind. Psychiatric patients have their share of physical disabilities, both associated and unassociated with mental symptoms. Bodies need attention as well as minds and 'total care' should be the watchword. Dressings may be required, injections given, bladders emptied and special investigations carried out. Any of the technical procedures common in general hospitals, including a variety of emergency procedures, may fall to the lot of the nurse in a modern psychiatric hospital. As well as these, there are certain investigation and treatment procedures more commonly encountered in psychiatric hospitals. Included among these are abreactive techniques and electroplexy, and the nurse must be au fait with the equipment and the techniques used. She must know her nursing procedures, know how to set up trays for special purposes and have a thorough working knowledge of principles of asepsis. The list could be lengthened greatly but enough has been said to indicate that the sub-role of technician is as important in psychiatric nursing as in any other nursing discipline.

Communicator

The importance of passing on and recording information resulting from one's observations of patients cannot be overemphasised.

Keeping in mind the fact that it is unwise to break a patient's trust in you by passing on privileged communications arising from your special psychotherapeutic sub-role without the patient's permission, facts arise every day which need to be discussed with other members of the therapeutic team or entered in relevant report books or progress notes. For example, if a patient has indicated that he feels suicidal or intends to absent himself without leave, appears to be becoming involved in some unhealthy way with another patient or spends his time avoiding entering into the therapeutic programme, these observations should be shared with all who have any degree of responsibility in his management. Communication is important at all times and it goes without saying that failure to pass on information at change of working shifts to one's opposite numbers coming on duty could be to the detriment of one's patients.

CONCLUSION

To be effective, the nurse must develop skills in functioning in these various roles so necessary for the patients' welfare.

4

THE NURSE AS A PERSON

Chapter 3 dealt with the sub-roles of the psychiatric nurse in the work situation. Examples were given of some attitudes and behaviour on the part of nursing staff that could be unhelpful to patients, and mention was made of certain difficulties inherent in one's professional role. We should not shut our eyes to the fact that psychiatric nursing makes singular demands on those working in this field, particularly demands at an emotional level which are not met to the same degree in other branches of nursing.

It is important, therefore, to study the nurse as a person with her own drives, motives, reactions and attitudes, and to study more closely interpersonal relationships both between staff members and between staff and patients. Before we can do this meaningfully, it will be necessary to develop a concept of the phenomena of transference and countertransference, as both these unconscious mechanisms are at work in all interpersonal relationships. As these two terms emanate from psychoanalytic literature our initial description of them will be in the narrow confines of the individual psychoanalytical treatment situation. It will be shown later that the phenomena have much wider implications than this.

Transference

Transference consists of the projection of feelings, thoughts and wishes on to the analyst who comes to represent to the patient someone from his (the patient's) past. It is believed that all such feelings, thoughts and wishes transferred to the therapist were present in the patient's infantile and childhood relationships with his parents. For example, the child who saw his father as a threatening authoritarian figure may see the therapist as a similar threatening authoritarian figure.

There may perhaps be intermediate figures in time between the patient's parents and the therapist, and the transference of feelings, thoughts and wishes may appear to be occurring fundamentally from these intermediate figures to the therapist. It is stated, however, that the emotions and attitudes directed towards such intermediate figures, are, or were, themselves the outcome of transference to them of the emotions and attitudes previously held towards parents.

When we study the unconcious mental mechanism of repression wherein unacceptable ideas, memories, feelings, drives and unresolved conflicts are automatically removed from conciousness and thrust back into the unconscious realms of the mind (page 59), we shall see that such repression occurs during the stages of psychosexual development as well as operating throughout life as an ego defence mechanism. As oral, anal and phallic stages in psychoanalytical theory normally commence at the ages of six months, one year and four years respectively, it must follow that material repressed at such early ages will be at an infantile level of feeling and thought. In psychoanalysis, this repressed and unconscious material is revived and the analyst becomes the recipient of the same emotions and attitudes that were consciously or unconsciously directed towards the parents in the patient's infancy. In short, such attributes as the patient in his infancy imputed to his parents and the emotions involved in the relationships with parents are transferred on to the person of the therapist. Being at an infantile level of feeling and thought, such transference reactions are intense, ambivalent, changeable, infantile and frequently quite inappropriate. Transference feelings may be so intense that they give rise to a transference neurosis, in which the patient perceives the therapist almost entirely on the basis of early neurotic feelings and reactions.

The therapist may be seen as all-powerful and all-knowing, and the patient may react submissively or rebelliously towards him. The transference may involve all the anxiety and other emotions associated with libidinal drives or aggressive impulses formerly directed towards parents.

As well as the part parents or parent substitutes play in the transference phenomenon, one's siblings may also come into the picture, giving rise to what is known as *sibling transference.* In this situation, emotions and attitudes previously entertained towards brothers and sisters come to be transferred to the therapist.

Transference may be described as:

1. *Positive transference* wherein the patient overvalues or loves the therapist without adequate or realistic reasons.
2. *Negative transference* when the patient dislikes or even hates the therapist, again without a rational basis.

The reason for saying that transference is unrealistic is that the emotions and attitudes directed towards the therapist are not the result of reactions produced in the patient by the therapist (that is, if he is a competent therapist), but they result from feelings appropriate to other situations involving parents and siblings.

So far, we have looked at transference limited to the psychoanalytical treatment situation. It should be pointed out quite firmly that, as well as existing between patient and analyst, transference can exist between people completely divorced from treatment situations. In a hospital, the phenomena can exist between patient and patient, between staff and patients and between different members of staff of all disciplines. We should ignore for the moment the strong initial psychoanalytical assertion that ultimately all transference phenomena are related back to infantile emotions and attitudes held towards parents, because from a practical point of view, transference does also occur from extrafamilial intermediate figures such as teachers and doctors.

Broadly therefore, transference may be defined as *the unrealistic transferring of emotions and attitudes held towards some person(s) in the past on to a person or persons in the present.*

Let us come closer to home, to our working situation in the hospital or in the outside community, and remember that not all emotions and attitudes evidenced in people are unrealistic transference phenomena. As staff working with psychiatric patients, we are prone to be ostriches and to see all patient behaviour as resulting from transference, without looking at the possibility that our behaviour and attitudes may be the factors producing what are realistic reactions in patients, and not reactions resulting from transference. The mechanism of transference may indeed be determining patients' attitudes to staff, but all staff should be wary of laying the blame at the feet of parents and some unconscious mechanism before excluding the possibility that they themselves are engendering particular reactions in patients. On the other side of the coin, staff may accept patients' attitudes at their face value when such attitudes have transference as their basis. This point will be touched upon when we deal with countertransference and again when we focus on the nurse, the person.

Countertransference

Just as patients develop transference to their therapist so may the therapist develop transferences to patients. The name given to the transference reaction of the therapist to his patient is termed countertransference. (Counter in the term countertransference means 'complementary to' and not 'opposite to'.) In a strict sense this countertransference involves inappropriately intense feeling and unconscious displacement (page 60) of such feeling from a person in the therapist's past on to the patient.

There are two sources, however, from which the feelings of the therapist are derived. Firstly, there are feelings which are based on the reality of the patient's appearance, his personality and character, and the conflicts he presents—essentially a conscious process. Secondly there are feelings derived from the therapist unconsciously assigning to the patient attributes of people in his (the therapist's) past. This has the same basis as a transference reaction being derived from unconscious needs and conflicts, this time in the therapist and not in the patient.

It is most probable that countertransference emotions, arising out of short-lived identification (page 63) with the patient, are necessary to more fully understand the patient's communications. The competent therapist has through his training learned to understand the basis for the emotions produced in himself and is able to control and use them constructively in the treatment situation.

It is well to point out here that some authorities speak of countertransference only when repressed (therefore unconscious) infantile wishes are involved, and others include both the conscious and unconscious reactions of the therapist to the patient. Still again, others limit the term countertransference to the unconscious reaction of the therapist to the patient's transference. As there can be a degree of fluidity in what is unconscious and what is conscious, depending on developing insights, it seems reasonable to adopt a broader view in which countertransference involves both conscious and unconscious reactions of the therapist to: the patient's appearance, personality and character; the conflicts presented; the treatment situation itself; and the patient's transference to the therapist.

Obviously it is easier for the therapist to deal with the enemy he knows, the conscious aspects of the therapeutic relationship, than with conflicts within himself of which he is still unconscious. A thorough training is intended to minimise such blind spots, thus enabling the therapist to deal with a wider variety of problems in patients.

A number of undesirable countertransference reactions may occur in therapy:

1. If a patient produces material which is akin to the therapist's own unresolved conflicts the therapist may use his usual defences in the therapeutic situation and become unable to accept such material. Thus, he cannot help the patient in particular problem areas.
2. Certain deeply ingrained personality disturbances in the therapist may seriously impede effectual psychotherapy. For example, a passive masochistic therapist may accept a patient's abuse of him at its face value rather than seeing it as a transference phenomenon and interpreting or commenting on it. On the other hand, unconscious aggression in the therapist may produce anxiety in him which does not allow him to be definite and firm because to him such attitudes are aggressive and must be avoided at all costs. A paranoid attitude in the therapist may lead to his seeing or even trying to unearth in the patient, qualities he cannot accept in himself. This is an example of projection—the therapist projects his own unwanted qualities on to the patient.
3. If the treatment situation largely represents a source of narcissistic gratification to the therapist, he will be prone to see himself as the great omnipotent healer or fixer of people's lives. When he does not get the desired results, or in other words therapeutic returns, as quickly as his own needs demand, there may be a tendency for him to become hostile or even rejecting towards his patient.

These examples could be extended considerably, but enough has been said to indicate how unconscious conflicts and needs in a therapist can lead to unhelpful countertransference adversely affecting the treatment of a patient.

It has been pointed out that transference occurs outside the analytical treatment setting. The same may be said of countertransference, which can also exist in any situation where two people relate; and from our point of view, we must be aware that in hospitals it occurs between patients and patients, staff and patients and between different members of staff.

The nurse the person

So far in this chapter, both the patient and the analyst have been laid somewhat bare. If nursing staff and others working in a psychiatric setting are to be effective, then an honest look at themselves is also essential. To a large extent the general public, and to some degree people within the profession, build up a stereotype of the nurse, a pattern which the nurse often feels she must fill, as unrealistic as it may be. Let us remember that nurses too are human; they have the same basic needs, conflicts, motives, reactions and attitudes that are common to man. The individual nurse's personality is the outcome of factors mentioned in Chapter 5. She has had to make, and is making, adjustments in the business of living. She, too, demonstrates unconscious motivation, experiences anxiety and defends against it (Chapter 6). Let us at this point place the nurse in a similar situation to that in which we have already placed the analyst. For, although the nurse does not practise psychoanalysis, she meets with similar problems in her day-to-day contact with psychiatric patients, and the mechanisms of transference and countertransference are operating in varying degrees, depending to a large extent on the type of psychiatric nursing currently engaged in. Examples of such mechanisms are legion and we shall look at a number in order to get a slightly clearer picture of their operation, at least in the hospital work situation, and in terms of staff-patient and staff-staff relationships.

Staff-patient relationships

Mention has already been made that patients may react in a realistic fashion to behaviour of, or attitudes apparent in, nursing staff. The patient who says that Nurse Jones is either the most friendly or the least helpful nurse on the ward, may be making an appropriate assessment of Nurse Jones at a point in time. Such attitudes however, may arise out of transference feelings derived from a loving person (positive transference) or a hateful person (negative transference) in her past. Miss Brown may look upon Nurse Jones as a loving or doting parent and her behaviour will be appropriate to this attitude. Nurse Jones will be expected by the patient to behave as a loving parent. If, in Nurse Jones, there is some great need to be a 'loving parent', she may respond to the patient's transference by falling into this role, and this may be unhelpful to Miss Brown by further fostering dependency needs in her. Age is no barrier to such a transference developing, and young nurses may feel acutely inadequate or embarrassed when older men or women cast them into a parental role through the mechanism of transference.

Considerable anxiety may develop in the nurse when a patient, on the basis of transference, sees her as a sexual partner. It is important in such circumstances to appreciate that the nurse is not the first to whom this has happened, and the matter should be discussed with her seniors or at a staff meeting. This is a load that does not have to be borne on one's own. It is in this area particularly that it is important for a nurse to be aware of her own inner needs or she may quite unconsciously, on the basis of countertransference, foster such attitudes in patients. It is very satisfying to feel that one is attractive and loved, but falling into this role to meet inner needs or drives may not be helpful to a patient, and it certainly won't be to the nurse, both in a personal and in an official sense.

Patients may see nurses as rival siblings and the behavioural reactions on both sides to this state of affairs may be many and varied. If a patient behaves towards you as towards a much disliked sibling you may feel strong emotions, for example, of resentment. Do not deny these to yourself nor for that matter to your fellow nurses (they have experienced the same). In general however, it is better not to let actions towards patients be determined by emotions aroused in you. In other words, don't *become* the jealous nasty sibling the patient sees you as. It is more helpful to point out to the patient what feelings his attitudes produce in other people (or in yourself for the matter) and how such attitudes affect his interpersonal relationships. Perhaps one could indicate that he behaves in this way because he feels insecure, unloved, or whatever you feel instinctively or on the basis of previous experience might be the reason for his behaviour. Emotions arising in the nurse frequently result from countertransference to the patient's transference, and it is on the basis of these countertransference emotions produced in the nurse, that she is able to make perceptive helpful comments. What of the nurse's countertransference to:

1. the patient's personality;
2. the material the patient presents (the conflicts presented); and
3. the treatment situation itself?

Most people treating psychiatric patients find that it is much easier to relate with and to be helpful to particular people. We are indeed exceedingly grandiose and best quality ostriches, if we deny this statement. It would be ideal if one could cope with all types of patients and all material presented equally competently. To achieve such a state of affairs, the nurse would need to be extremely well-adjusted, and have great self-knowledge and to be able to deal with her own needs and drives in acceptable healthy ways. This is one reason why the psychiatric nurse, in particular, requires the highest of personal attributes to be really effective in her work—something we should all aim at. Here are some examples of difficulties arising out of countertransference mechanisms in staff:

1. Unresolved conflicts with parents and siblings, which may be conscious or unconscious, may lead to unrealistic attitudes and behaviour on the part of nursing staff towards patients. 'She's just like my mother whose domination I never really learned to cope with.' 'He reminds me of my father who was weak and ineffectual, a despicable shadow of a man, who preferred his drink and horses to us children.' 'She's a demanding bitch, just like my sister.' 'He reminds me of my brother who was always mother's favourite.' Such thoughts may have their origin in actual qualities existing in patients, but certain minor characteristics may remind one of people in one's past, and such patients become the recipient of countertransference feelings. Obviously, if one sees patients as dominating, ineffectual, bitches, mother's favourite, etc., this could well colour one's attitude and behaviour towards such patients, to their detriment. On the other hand, on the basis of very strong positive feelings to one's father, inordinate care and attention may be lavished on the old dementing male to the partial exclusion of other patients.
2. Any material presented by a patient to a nurse in areas that the

nurse has not resolved within herself—possibly in areas such as aggression, sexuality or dependence—may produce resistances in the nurse, switching of the patient's conversation, or avoiding a subject about which the patient has a great need to talk.

3. In terms of the treatment situation itself it is natural to expect results, but expectations should be realistic. Just as the therapist may have narcissistic needs to be a wonderful healer, so too may the nurse. The nurse who does not have realistic expectations but whose expectations are based on her own needs to achieve something may, in order to maintain her illusion of herself as No. 1 healer, place blame on the patient, for example stating that 'he is not trying', or 'he is just using the place as a boarding house', 'he needs a swift kick', etc. There is no doubt that, in truth, some patients do fit into these rationalised categories, but one must not place them there merely to ameliorate one's injured narcissistic needs.

Pointers to a non-therapeutic relationship

The following are some indicators of the development of an unhelpful or non-therapeutic relationship with a patient, based generally on transference and countertransference mechanisms:

1. Excessive worry over the patient.
2. Feelings of intense hostility or love for him.
3. Preoccupation with one patient to the exclusion of others.
4. Inordinate feelings of pity for a patient.
5. A possessive attachment to a patient coupled with resentment of other nurses' attention to him.
6. The feeling that you are the only one who can nurse him adequately.
7. Feelings that other staff are jealous of one's relationship with a patient.
8. Inability to accept other opinions as to management of a patient.

Staff-staff relationships

The junior nurse may see her senior colleague in the same light as she sees her parents, and such a light is indeed variable. The senior may represent an authority figure towards whom extremely ambivalent feelings are held. The junior may be over-compliant with her wishes, may later test her out to see how much leeway she can achieve, or may even attempt to denigrate her in the eyes of other staff. Various rivalries for favours from the senior, the parental figure, may exist. These rivalries lead to increased efforts to please or to the minimising of one's peers' efforts.

In fact all types of transference reactions (both positive and negative) mentioned under staff-patient relationships may exist among members of staff. It would be well to re-read the previous comments on staff-patient relationships and draw parallels in the staff sphere.

Manipulation

Not all attitudes to and approaches by patients to nursing staff are on the basis of transference. A patient may attempt to manipulate a nurse into carrying out his various wishes. To manipulate means to handle, to deal skilfully with, or to manage craftily, and it is the latter aspect of this predominantly conscious manoeuvre of manipulation that concerns us most. Patients may engineer situations in order to derive particular satisfactions or to get their own way, be this the obtaining of a particular nurse's undivided interest or attention, or the causing of friction between members of the staff by playing one off against the other, thus deriving some unhealthy sort of satisfaction. The following are some of the common manipulative measures used by patients:

1. Trying to convince a nurse that she is the best of the bunch, the only one who really understands him;
2. Denigrating other nursing staff, especially if they have already seen through the patient's manoeuvres and have not permitted the assuagement of his unhealthy needs.
3. Blackmail in the form of suicidal threats may be used if a nurse does not comply with a patient's wishes. 'It will be your fault nurse if I kill myself' is the idea communicated in a variety of ways.

It becomes obvious that the nurse who is not conscious of her own needs and conflicts, may fall easy prey to such manipulations.

In actual fact (on the basis of transference feelings) a nurse may not really take to a colleague and she will be all too ready to agree with the patient that her colleague is, for example, incompetent and not of the same ability as her. If she feels somewhat inadequate in her sexual role, she may inappropriately welcome flattery from a manipulating patient.

In the modern psychiatric hospital, it is not necessary to bear the burdens of a patient's manipulations and of one's transference and countertransference feelings alone. In fact, it is possibly dangerous. Nurses should share such experiences with other staff members in an atmosphere of mutual understanding and acceptance. A number of nursing staff may have experienced the same feelings arising out of manipulations and transference phenomena. It is not a crime to admit to feelings of hostility, jealousy, love, rejection, etc., and it is often a relief to know that one is not alone in feelings engendered by patients. It is, however, unhelpful both to patients and nursing staff for the latter to 'act out' their emotions.

Acting out in this sense means not coping adequately with one's feelings and allowing them unbridled expression in action, the type of action engaged in obviously being dependent on the particular emotion experienced. To ask a nurse to refrain from 'acting out' emotions produced in her by patients is, in some instances asking a considerable amount, but in the management of our patients this ideal must always be aimed at if one is to use one's therapeutic relationship with patients to its fullest extent. The gratification of needs of any kind in psychiatric staff should be met outside the work situation.

The essential safeguard against acting out and against unhelpful emotional involvement both positive and negative lies in free communication between staff working together as a team.

Conclusion

Though this section has dealt mainly with possible pitfalls, it does not mean that work in a psychiatric ward or unit is necessarily as complicated as has been painted. Generally one's work is extremely rewarding, and staff-patient and staff-staff relationships are in most instances eminently satisfactory. We may appear to have strayed from the theme of the nurse as a person by concentrating more on the pitfalls inherent in her relationships. However, I feel that these require the emphasis given, for having dealt adequately with them, the nurse as a person using her mature personality attributes, can provide most satisfaction for her patients and herself.

From the above, it becomes apparent that in any treatment situation where a high standard of patient care is to be maintained, opportunities must exist for staff to speak freely with each other about the variety of relationships, both therapeutic and non-therapeutic, that arise at work. To this end, senior nursing staff should be receptive, sound leaders, and the place of staff meetings should be firmly established. In such a setting, the nurse as a person may develop greater self-understanding, will be helped to deal with the difficulties arising out of her current deficits, and will, in spite of the vagaries of nature common to us all, emerge as an effective therapeutic agent able to use her personality attributes to the full in the care of her patients.

5

PERSONALITY

Structure and measurement of personality

It is probably impossible to find two people who would act in precisely the same way in a variety of different situations, and each normal individual as he grows older, generally shows some alterations in behaviour under repeated similar circumstances. Such individual differences as are seen, result from what is termed the person's personality, which becomes manifest in the characteristic responses of the individual to his inner needs or drives and to his environment. The term personality is difficult to define. It refers to a quality or style of life demonstrated by an individual. Some authorities equate personality with the behavioural patterns exhibited, which, for all practical purposes, give the clue to this underlying quality. The characteristics of a person's personality include physical and intellectual qualities, a variety of traits and other capabilities or abilities. A trait may be regarded as the tendency of a certain mode of behaviour to appear constantly in a variety of situations, though particular traits or personality dispositions are more likely to show themselves in particular situations. The picture of an individual's personality is composed of the ability to form social relationships, intellectual activities and interests, characteristic moods, various standards relating to morals, religion, social and practical issues, the degree of energy and initiative displayed, and fantasy life. This list could be extended, but serves to demonstrate the complexity of personality structure.

Various attempts have been made to measure personality in terms of continua between differing, yet related, characteristics or traits such as introversion and extraversion. Is the person quiet, shy, not liking competition, absorbed in individual activities, or is he outgoing, a good mixer, highly competitive and gregarious, or where does he fall between these two extremes? Where does he fall on another continuum—normality-neuroticism? Such sliding scales are utilised in an attempt to measure this elusive quality. Both the definition of and the accurate measurement of personality are indeed complicated.

It has been inferred above that personality is not a static quality.

It undergoes changes either in the direction of more healthy development or retrogressive changes throughout life depending on various factors, some of which will now be mentioned. Before doing so however, it should be pointed out that personality, once developed under the influence of these factors, shows great resistance to change. This point is brought out in the definition of personality by one authority, Kimble, who sees personality as 'the unique organisation of fairly permanent characteristics which sets the individual apart from other individuals and, at the same time determines how others respond to him'. The point underlined in the present context is that the characteristics displayed by an individual are 'fairly permanent'.

Factors in personality development

1. Heredity

There is considerable evidence that the pattern of development of the personality is determined to an unknown degree by hereditary factors.

Let us look at personality as a building wherein the bricks are numbers of specific traits. With different bricks (or traits) the final structure (personalities) will obviously differ. Just as bricks can be used in different combinations and positions to produce a variety of final shapes, so the differing organisation and integration perhaps even of similar traits produce different personalities. Traits are measured along particular dimensions. Two dimensions, introversion-extraversion and normality-neuroticism, have already been mentioned. Other traits described include impulsivity and self-control, autonomy and passivity, dominance and submission, and the need for achievement. The task of defining and measuring particular traits (our bricks for building personality) is an extremely complex one and, until such traits can be accurately defined and measured, it is difficult to even start to measure the effects of heredity on personality. Hereditary factors however are not unimportant in the development of personality patterns.

The evidence for this statement will not be given here, but mention might be made of the relationship that exists between temperamental traits and bodily build, the latter known to be largely determined by hereditary factors in people under normal conditions of nutrition.

2. Environmental factors

Though heredity or genetic factors do play their part in personality structure and development, man is also flexible and adaptable, and his personality is influenced by the world in which he lives and grows.

(*a*) *Sociocultural.* In comparing parental attitudes in different social classes it has been found that marked differences occur in a number of areas, for example, in advice given to children regarding conformity to external standards as opposed to the development of self reliance and the acceptance of responsibility, and in the value placed on educational attainment. These class differences must surely be reflected in the developing personality. At another level Margaret Mead has shown that, in different cultures, human personality can develop along widely divergent lines, and quite fundamental attitudes, such as the relationship between a parent and child, whether males or females are 'dominant', whether a person is generally peaceful or belligerent, will vary in differing cultural climates.

(*b*) *Immediate Environment.* The attitudes of the infant's parents, and particularly mother, in the earlier years, the relationship of the child with his siblings, his experiences at school, during adolescence, early, middle and late adult years, all require adaptation in terms of attitude changes, and more fundamental changes in the individual's intrinsic qualities or personality may also occur.

Structural damage to the brain, due to pre-natal factors, may produce alterations in personality. Such factors include maternal infection during pregnancy, brain trauma, infections such as encephalitis and many conditions leading to cerebral degeneration to be mentioned in later sections. The original extensive leucotomy operation on the brain in some instances was followed by personality changes.

Theories of personality development

It is beyond the scope of this book to attempt even a cursory coverage of the work of all the clinicians and psychologists who have contributed to an understanding of personality development. Essentially in this current century there has been a large input and cross fertilization of ideas with each contributor adding something to a developing body of knowledge. Fundamental differences are seen to exist between theoretical orientations each of which probably contains a deal of truth. A few different viewpoints are presented briefly, and the interested student is referred to larger or more specific texts if he wishes to grasp the fundamental principles of these theories of personality development.

Psychoanalytic theory—Sigmund Freud

Psychoanalytic theory was initially developed by Sigmund Freud (1856-1939) and represents the first major attempt to develop a dynamic theory of personality development.

The study of the dynamics of behaviour and of the fairly permanent behaviour characteristics indicative of the individual personality is the study of the forces inside and outside the individual which have acted on him in the past, and which are acting on him in the present to produce particular behaviour or behaviour patterns. (See pages 48ff. for further description of 'dynamics'.)

The pioneering work of Freud was indeed outstanding and psychiatry owes a tremendous debt to this man who, against widespread opposition, developed the theory and practice of psychoanalysis.

Psychoanalytic theory, though important, does not give the full picture of factors relevant to personality development. Freud continued to modify his theories throughout his lifetime and had he lived longer would no doubt have incorporated into these, many of the things which he foreshadowed or which others, at a later stage, saw as important in the development of personality. It is interesting to note that, in discussing problems of aetiology, including what we would now term the dimension of neuroticism, he spoke of 'congenital pre-disposition', indicating his acceptance that heredity may be one of the determining elements in personality development and in the development of illness. Freud concentrated mainly on the individual. He did, in fact, enter the sociological field, but did not develop his ideas there to any extent.

Essentially Freud's theories stemmed out of his clinical study of the neuroses which, as we shall see later, comprise a major group of psychiatric disorders. His essential basic contribution to the understanding of personality may be summed up in the term *Instinct Theory*. In an individual, he considered the basic innate drives or instincts to be those of sex (libidinal drive) and aggression. Both of these basic drives Freud saw as arising from an unconscious function of the personality which he termed the *id*. Such basic drives require some outlet and the only way these instinctual drives can be gratified is by operating in some way through the conscious part of the mind, the *ego* or the 'self'. The ego selects objects in the environment which can form the basis for gratification of id impulses. Gratification of instincts leads to the relieving of unpleasant tensions. The individual has a basic urge to satisfy drives or instincts, thus lowering tension, and this mode of adjustment Freud referred to as the pleasure principle. The id may also accomplish its goal of tension reduction through primary process thinking such as occurs in dreams, *primary process thinking* being illogical, timeless, and not distinguishing between reality and unreality. The person who is motivated by self-interest, irrespective of the wishes of others, is said to have his life governed by the *pleasure principle*. The individual learns that the environment, or people in it, do not permit unlimited gratification of the instincts of sex and aggression. When, as usually happens in normal development, an individual learns to modify his own desires and adapts to the wishes or demands of others he is said to be living according to the *reality principle* as opposed to the pleasure principle. The ego which Freud saw as differentiating from the id is governed mainly by the reality principle and follows the rules of *secondary process thinking* which is characterised by logic, time orientation and a distinction between reality and unreality.

Limitations or strictures arising from other people, and particularly the parents of the growing infant and child, are taken into the individual (internalised) and become part of the structure of the ego or conscious mind in the form of what we might term a conscience. These internalised limitations, which mainly become part of the ego, constitute a superior ego which was called by Freud the *superego*. There then occurs within the individual a tussle between instincts or drives and the demands of the superego to conform to certain standards which may be reasonable or unreasonable, depending to a large extent on the early prevailing attitudes of parents and their effect on the developing self-esteem of the child.

Arising out of the innate or inborn strengths of drives, and on the degree of superego limitations on these drives, it becomes evident that a variety of behaviour patterns mediated through the ego can develop. Sometimes the ego is severely threatened by the drives or id impulses, and various unconscious mechanisms come into operation to defend the ego. These mechanisms are dealt with in a separate chapter (Chapter 6). At this point however, it may be stated that the habitual utilisation of such defence mechanisms can lead to certain personality characteristics.

Another important aspect of Freud's psychoanalytical theory as it effects personality development was his *libido theory*. This was an amplification of, or a closer study of the sex instinct. Though initially sex was very circumscribed for Freud, he later saw it as encompassing any pleasurable sensation relating to bodily functions. The word 'libido' is used interchangeably with 'sex'. Freud saw the individual as passing through certain stages of development. At each stage the libidinal drives were focused on different anatomical entities, namely the mouth, the anus and the genitals.

The most primitive stage of libido development is seen as a diffuse spread of libido energy throughout the body both internally and on the skin surface. This becomes focussed on the mouth area, introducing the *oral phase*, as evidenced by the young infant's interest in sucking and putting things into the mouth (early or passive oral phase). At about six months of age, active and aggressive oral tendencies come into being with the eruption of teeth (later or active oral phase and also referred to as the oral-sadistic stage), when biting as well as sucking occurs. The oral phase is present from birth until approximately the end of the first year, at about which time it is overlapped and superseded by the *anal phase.* This phase is characterised by an aim initially to expel and later to retain faeces, both acts being seen as pleasurable to the young infant, and occurring at about the time of central nervous system development when the infant gains voluntary control over the anal sphincter musculature.

Some parents, in an attempt to secure obedience from the young child, place him on the pot for extended periods until he conforms to their wishes. Their evident interest in, and concern over, this procedure inculcates in the child the fact that he has a powerful weapon at his disposal through which he may please parents by obliging thus gaining their praise. On the other hand if he feels angry towards them, the child may refuse to function in the expected fashion, thus showing resistance, hostility or 'independence'.

Depending on parental attitudes in terms of undue interest in, or disgust in the excretory functions, the young child is considered to develop personality characteristics in which he may develop an unusual interest in, or shame concerning, excretory functions. Such shame may lead to a personality characterised by scrupulousness, a too-well-organised or rigid pattern of living, or a preoccupation with cleanliness and avoidance of dirt. If all this be true, then it behoves parents and particularly mothers to be accepting, tolerant and exceedingly patient during the period of 'pot training'.

At about the age of four years, the young child develops an interest in the penis, leading into the so-called *phallic stage* (phallus: male sexual organ). His interest centres not only on his own phallus and body but in the physical characteristics of other people in his environment, and particularly in the differences between the sexes. It is presumed when the little boy sees an unclad girl without a penis such as he has, he assumes it has been taken away and wonders if the same thing will happen to him as some sort of punishment. This is referred to by Freud as *castration anxiety.* On the other hand the little girl is presumed to be envious of what the male has and she hasn't, and she becomes envious of male attributes. Such a feeling (sometimes referred to as *penis envy*) may persist into adulthood and be exemplified in the woman who cannot assume her truly feminine role and constantly envies and attempts to beat the male in his more masculine pursuits. The term *masculine protest* is given to this type of behaviour.

The oral and the anal stages are so-called prephallic stages of infantile sexuality and the pleasure derived in these stages does not require an external object. As such, they are referred to as autoerotic stages (autos: self; Eros: Greek god of love).

The phallic phase, or as it is sometimes called, the early genital phase, requires an external object for libidinal satisfaction and the child becomes greatly interested in, and possessive of the parent of the opposite sex. This situation leads to feelings of rivalry and resentment towards the same-sexed parent, together with feelings of guilt and the fear of punishment (castration anxiety). This situation was referred to by Freud as the Oedipus Complex, Oedipus being the king in Sophocles's play *Oedipus Rex* who fell in love with his mother and slew his father without knowing the identity of either, thereby bringing a plague upon Thebes. The oedipal situation is seen as the crown and culmination of infantile sexuality, and an unsatisfactory resolution of the oedipal complex was seen by Freud as leading to unsatisfactory personality development and to later development of certain psychiatric illnesses.

The *latency period* occurs from the fifth to the tenth years of life. This phase is latent, inasmuch as no qualitative changes occur in sexual or libido orientation. The child, during this period, has to adjust to the changes in his world relevant particularly to entering school, and he is faced with a multitude of new and absorbing stimuli. Sexual manifestations do, however, occur in this phase.

Prior to puberty, there may be a reinforcement of prephallic drives, seen when the child becomes more untidy and rebellious. This is followed at puberty by the commencement of adult sexuality.

The above phases and their implications are referred to as Freud's Theory of Psychosexual Development. Many of the characteristics of each stage are seen to linger even into adult life. Orality is seen in the persistence of thumb sucking and in such pursuits as kissing and smoking. Mention has been made of anal characteristics, such as extreme orderliness and avoidance of dirt. Added to this may be the tendency to collect and hoard (*cf.* anal retentive phase) or, on the other hand, some people may literally love to make a mess.

The problems of the phallic phase and oedipal complex may linger and become manifest in confusion of sexual role, inordinate dependence on the opposite-sexed parent or other persons, difficulties with people of the same sex, and so on.

Early breakaway group

A number of contemporaries and disciples of Sigmund Freud found themselves at variance with his viewpoints and developed alternative theories.

Among these were Alfred Adler, Carl Jung and Otto Rank. Brief mention will be made of the work of Alfred Adler whose concepts are equivalent to those of the later-developed ego psychology.

Individual psychology—Alfred Adler

Alfred Adler (1870-1937) was the first to embrace a holistic approach, meaning that he did not split off psychological processes as separate entities for study but saw man as a whole, with interwoven dynamic psychological, somatic and sociological processes operating in his struggle for self-realization and superiority.

To Adler, the motivating force behind all human activity stems initially from the infant's helplessness leading to feelings of inferiority (including insecurity and anxiety), which are compensated for by a striving for superiority. 'Superiority' is not used in the limited sense of 'I want to be better than you, Jack', but in the sense that each individual with his unique self concept strives to find meaning and significance in life and to achieve perfection and completeness.

Central to Adler's theory of personality development is the concept of *life style*, which means the way an individual actively adapts to the social milieu or environment. A person needs to be both part of society and yet maintain in his self-concept a sense of uniqueness, and so he develops a style of coping with living to satisfy both needs.

It is interesting that, although Adler termed his school of thought 'individual psychology' to emphasise his contention that the body and mind were indivisible and that the psyche did not consist of discrete sharply defined entities, the individual and the society in which he lives are equally important in his theory, for man cannot function in isolation.

The individual himself has the major part to play in the achievement of his life goals, which may change or evolve and which are subject to his degree of inventiveness or creativity. Such achievement is dependent on his self-concept, and on his ability to gain from past experience and to see himself functioning in the future. This active striving for the achievement of life goals is called *self-determination*.

Adler, initially described as a co-worker with Freud, could not ascribe to the latter's insistence that a person's inner psychological world was determined by past objective causes, that is, early experiences, and he also challenged the validity of Freud's concepts of basic drives and the assertion that repression is essential to the development of neurotic symptoms. Adler held the view that the person created his own inner psychological world and therefore did not see unconscious and conscious processes as being in conflict, but as representing two aspects of a single system. He did not see man or his conscious self as being under the control of the unconscious; he saw rather the individual as being directed by his subjective goals and values. And so Adler parted company with Freud and his followers and, in 1912, established his school of individual psychology which, with its emphasis on the whole man in society, anticipated many later developments in personality theory and in psychiatry.

A number of other lines of thinking emanated from the psychoanalysts. Groups described include the *Post-Freudians* such as Karl Abrahams, Melanie Klein, Anna Freud and Franz Alexander, who further developed Freud's ideas, and the *Neo-Freudians* for example, Karen Horney, Harry Stack Sullivan and Erich Fromm who while each making specific contributions, as a group put greater emphasis on social and cultural factors. Yet another group of clinicians who built upon Melanie Klein's ideas of the internalisation of object relations are the *Object-Relations theorists*, such as Michael Balint and Ronald Fairbairn.

There exists also, what is termed *Contemporary Psychoanalytic Ego Psychology*, which began with the work of Anna Freud (1895-) and Heinz Hartmann (1894-1970). Anna Freud completed the development of the concept of ego psychology begun by her father, Sigmund Freud, which views the ego as being the vehicle for the discharge of instinctive id impulses or drives, in the process of which the ego is formed by modification of the id, the reality principle gradually replacing the pleasure principle.

Hartmann modified Freud's concept of ego development postulating that both the ego and the id have a common undifferentiated precursor, and that there exists from birth primary autonomous ego functions namely, perception, mobility, memory and intellect. Through these rudimentary ego functions the infant relates to outside objects and the environment gaining satisfaction of instinctive needs and drives.

Hartmann asserted that there is an area of the ego which is 'conflict-free' and not derived from the instincts. This area includes capacities for perception, comprehension, thinking, intuition, language, learning, intelligence, and certain aspects of motor development. It is said that the conflict-free operation may be impeded if any of these functions become secondarily involved in conflict.

David Rapaport (1911-1960) developed Hartmann's ideas about the functioning of the ego particularly with respect to its cognitive functioning, which entails all aspects of knowing such as perceiving, imagining, and evaluating, as opposed to willing and feeling.

The work of Erik Erikson (1902-) has opened up fields for further study.

Psychoanalytic theory—Erik Erikson

Whereas Freud's Theory of Psychosexual Development deals with development up to puberty and therefore concerns itself essentially with interactions in the nuclear family, another psychoanalyst, Erik Erikson, took things further by studying the development of the child beyond puberty. In doing this he rejected the notion that personality development is fixed in early childhood. Erikson, indeed, sees development of personality or the ego as occurring from birth to death in eight stages which he designates: oral-sensory (first year of life), muscular-anal (second and third year), locomotor-genital (fourth and fifth year), latency (years six to eleven), puberty and adolescence (adolescent years), young adulthood (late adolescence through early middle age), adulthood (middle years), and maturity.

An important aspect of this extension of Freud's theory of personality development is that the individual himself, as he grows older, is seen to play a more responsible part in his own development, and the blame for faulty ego development cannot be placed entirely at the feet of parent or parent-substitutes as is possible if one adheres closely to Freud's theory of infantile sexuality.

Largely because he lived in a time and place where sexual taboos were rampant, Freud saw neurotic illnesses as arising out of sexual conflict, and he developed his theory from working with patients rendered sick as a result of repressed sexuality, the id playing a large part in his conceptual framework of personality development. Erikson on the other hand concentrated on the ego, it being the 'tool by which a person organises outside information, tests perception, selects memories, governs actions adaptively, and integrates the capacities of orientation and planning', and saw the ultimate in development as having a sense of identity or 'a sense of self in a state of heightened well-being'.

At each of Erikson's eight stages of ego development, the individual is faced with a fairly specific emotional crisis, the satisfactory resolution of which goes hand-in-hand with ego development. The particular crises related in order to the eight stages of development of the personality described by Erikson have been termed: trust versus mistrust, autonomy versus shame and doubt, initiative versus guilt, industry versus inferiority, ego identity versus role confusion, intimacy versus islolation, generativity versus stagnation, and lastly, ego integrity versus despair. The individual meets each subsequent emotional crisis armed with an ego or accumulated make-up shaped by resolution or otherwise of crises occurring at preceding stages. Should less than ideal resolution occur at a particular stage, all is not lost, as later experience may allow subsequent modification of attitudes and development pertinent to that particular stage.

Erikson's theory takes into account both cultural factors and the individual's interaction with the society in which he lives, and he sees deviations from normal development of the ego arising out of problems within the person, within his interpersonal relationships and within the society to which he is trying to adapt.

Erikson has added other dimensions to Freud's earlier theory of personality development and most important is his contention that personality continues to be moulded throughout life.

Apart from the above-mentioned theories of personality development gained through clinical experience there is a growing body of knowledge derived largely from psychological investigation which is subsumed under the heading of 'Psychological theories of personality'.

Psychological theories of personality

These approaches have not yet formed bases for independent theories of personality development. They are somewhat confined in their application but nevertheless are important because they have led to modifications of the more developed theories and in themselves have contributed towards the understanding of certain aspects of human development and behaviour. Also, from them certain forms of therapy have evolved.

Among the many involved in psychological approaches to the understanding of behaviour a few more names only will be mentioned.

Abraham Maslow (1908-1970) saw man as inherently good, with the capacity for love, and envisaged a theory of psychiatric health rather than of sickness. He postulated a hierarchy of needs underlying human motivation, these needs ranging from the lowest—namely physiological—through safety, love, esteem to self-actualisation; and he maintained that lower needs must be satisfied before the higher needs can seek expression. Maslow's theory was one of the *humanistic theories* which emphasise what is unique and distinctive about human behaviour and experience, and assert that each individual has the potential for self-actualisation. Kurt Goldstein (1878-1965) who is credited with the development of the construct self-actualisation, stated, 'The organism has definite potentialities, and because it has them it has the need to actualise and realise them.' Other proponents of humanistic psychology include Gordon Allport (1897-1967) and Carl Rogers (1902-), though the latter is associated mainly with phenomenological theory and an existential approach emphasising immediate experience, usually emotional, as opposed to the historical or developmental factors leading to the experience.

Other theories include: the *Field Theory* of Kurt Lewin (1890-1947) which has application in the areas of social psychology and group process; learning theories particularly the work of Jean Piaget (1896-) on the child's cognitive development; Gestalt theory; and stimulus-response theories.

There are many names associated with *stimulus-response theories* but perhaps the best known is that of B. F. Skinner (1904-) who became the leading advocate of so-called *behaviourist psychology.* Behaviourists such as Skinner see personality and behaviour as synonymous, in other words, 'one is what one does'. According to Skinner humans are controlled by their environment and therefore must arrange external conditions so that behaviours they desire are reinforced. Skinner and others developed one variety of behavioural learning theory; and subsequent workers applied learning theories to social learning, the basic theory being that children learn to become human beings only through contact with other people in society.

Neal Miller (1909-) and John Dollard (1900-) emphasised the importance of imitation (particularly of parents) in social learning.

The radical behaviourists see humans not as self-initiating actors but as mere machines dependent for any activity on outside stimuli; and their theories do not do justice to the higher symbolic and scientific activities of human beings.

There is as yet no integrated theory of personality development. There are many theories approaching the complex phenomena of personality from different viewpoints, some better formulated than others and some using differing terminology to describe similar concepts.

No simple theory gives the complete answer. Perhaps some day we shall come nearer the truth when proven aspects of all current and still-developing theories are combined.

6

ASPECTS OF HUMAN DYNAMICS

A dynamic person is one who is energetic and forceful. The derivation of the word dynamic is in fact the Greek *dunamis* meaning 'force'. When we speak of human dynamics, we are not referring to forceful people but are speaking of forces which operate on people and which become manifest in behaviour patterns. Particular forms of behaviour are not just haphazard or meaningless.

Behaviour is not static: it is a changing phenomemon, the direction it takes depending on the 'forces', both within and outside the person, which act on an individual at or around the time particular behaviour occurs.

The study of the dynamics of behaviour concerns itself with forces which result from a person's needs and drives, hence operate from within, and forces which impinge upon the individual from his environment. An important concept to grasp is that most behaviour can be understood in terms of the interplay between inner needs or drives and the influences of the environment. In dealing with the development of personality we have already seen how some of these forces operate. In this chapter, internal and external forces determining behaviour will also become apparent when we look at the concepts of adjustment and maladjustment, unconscious motivation, anxiety and defences against anxiety.

Before entering into fields dealing with forces and mechanisms which may lead to abnormal behaviour, we should look at what is meant by being mentally healthy, a state in which behaviour patterns are regarded as 'normal'.

MENTAL HEALTH

The World Health Organisation (1951) has defined mental health as '. . . a condition, subject to fluctuations due to biological and social factors, which enables the individual to achieve a satisfactory synthesis of his own potentially conflicting, instinctive drives; to form and maintain harmonious relations with others; and to participate in constructive changes in his social and physical environment'.

This definition refers to the possible fluctuations in a condition, to inborn drives or forces and to a person's relationships with his total environment. But let us look at the subject of mental health from a slightly different perspective.

It is not difficult to determine symptoms and signs indicative of gross mental ill-health, and even if these are absent, one is still able to hazard a reasonably close guess that certain behaviour in people is abnormal, after taking into consideration, of course, social pressures that may have a bearing on such behaviour.

A person's behaviour at first sight may appear abnormal, for example when aggressive behaviour is displayed, but on close examination it may become apparent that it is consciously determined and directed towards dealing with particular environmental pressures or circumstances. Behaviour which is not inconsistent with that demanded by a situation cannot be regarded as unhealthy.

Does the absence of symptoms and signs and of abnormal behaviour patterns indicate that a person is mentally healthy?

In a sheltered supporting environment, a person may show none of the abovementioned abnormalities; but if taken out of such an environment and placed in society with its multitudinous pressures and strains, such a person may show abnormalities and be quite unable to cope. Therefore, the absence of abnormal signs and symptoms and of abnormal behaviour in a sheltered supporting environment is not necessarily an indication that a person is mentally healthy. A mentally healthy person must exhibit an ability to deal with reasonable strain of all types.

As stresses imposed upon man vary in type and intensity, a degree of flexibility and adaptability are prerequisites for mental health.

While being flexible and adaptable, to overreact to pressures, even if the direction of the reaction is appropriate, cannot be regarded as a sign of mental health, and so a degree of stability is required.

Such stability is possible only if the individual has developed into what might be called a relatively mature or integrated personality, aspects of which will be touched upon in the next section dealing with adjustment and maladjustment.

Combining these factors which play a part in mental health we see that this concept implies the following:

1. The absence of gross psychiatric symptoms and signs.
2. The absence of behaviour patterns inconsistent with prevailing pressures.
3. An ability to deal with strain.
4. A degree of flexibility and adaptability.
5. The absence of a tendency to overreact to pressures.
6. A degree of stability such as is found in a mature or integrated personality.

When an individual displays these qualities to a high degree he may be said to be mentally healthy; will indeed be able 'to form and maintain harmonious relations with others; and to participate in constructive changes in his social and physical enviroment'.

This is certainly a worthwhile target both for ourselves and for our patients.

ADJUSTMENT AND MALADJUSTMENT

It has been pointed out that the mentally healthy person needs to adapt or adjust to physical and environmental changes. What precisely do we mean by adjustment and its converse, maladjustment?

Adjustment may be seen both as a process and a state. It has been described as the process through which an individual passes to enter into relationship of harmony or equilibrium with his environment. It refers also to the state or condition of having attained such a relationship.

There are many, however, who would say that a final state of equilibrium is never reached and that the individual as well as his environment are always in a constant state of change. If one takes this view, which to the author is a correct one, then the process of adjustment can never reach a static position.

Maladjustment indicates the absence of such a process of entering into a relationship of harmony or equilibrium with one's environment.

The above description of adjustment is concerned only with relationships of a person with his environment, the environment, of course, including relationships with other persons, or interpersonal relationships wherein adjustment may occur.

However, we can look at adjustment at intrapersonal levels as well as environmental and interpersonal levels. Adjustment within the person (intrapersonal adjustment) is necessary for satisfactory interpersonal adjustment; it is necessary for entering into a relationship of harmony or equilibrium with one's total environment, including other people. If we are not at peace within ourselves, this does in some way affect our relationship with our total environment.

Adjustment within the individual, or intrapersonal adjustment, has been called variously 'finding the self', self-realization, integration, individuation (Jung) and the like.

Seen in Freudian terms, such intrapersonal adjustment will concern itself with passing normally or eventually through the various stages of libidinal development, or at least being able to cope satisfactorily with the remnants of these stages of development in one's personality.

It is well to reiterate that there are many theories of the development of personality apart from that of Freud. We should not concern ourselves at present with these theories nor overmuch with psychoanalytical theory, but simply understand that all human beings have to pass through stages of development to reach a stage of relative adjustment.

To sum up, adjustment relates to the achievement of, or more realistically, the movements towards a state of harmony or equilibrium within the individual and between an individual and his total environment.

Intrapersonal adjustment involves the development of mature attitudes and behaviour in an individual and this intrapersonal adjustment goes hand in hand with interpersonal adjustment or the development of satisfactory relationships with other persons.

UNCONSCIOUS MOTIVATION

Motivation is the commodity that induces a person to act; it refers to any urge to satisfy a human need. Such an urge or motivation may arise out of fear, desire, hate, love, jealousy and numerous other emotions or personality characteristics. It arises out of 'built-in' or hereditary or instinctive drives as well as from learned relationships between individuals and between individuals and situations. The 'built-in' or intrapersonal factors and the learned or extrapersonal factors interact and the resultants are directed towards certain goals or incentives.

The concept of motivation based on feelings of which we are aware or conscious is not difficult to comprehend. It is a little more difficult, however, to grasp the fact that motivation is not always conscious, that we at times do or say things as a result of forces or feelings that are not in our conscious awareness.

It was Sigmund Freud who first highlighted the effects of unconscious motives in human behaviour. He described the mind as functioning in three layers, the superficial activity being *conscious*. Consciousness includes:

1. Awareness of one's own mental and bodily functions.
2. Awareness of objects in the external world.
3. The perception of oneself as an individual.
4. The perception of oneself as a member of a group.

The second mental activity Freud termed *preconscious*. This refers to the multitude of stored information in the mind which does not readily enter conscious awareness but can be drawn into conscious awareness virtually at will or as the result of certain associations. For example, my children's pet cat was run over by a car and I subsequently remembered in vivid detail the circumstances surrounding the death of a childhood pet, a dog, something that I had not thought about for years. This entry of preconscious material into consciousness occurs to us all continuously, and the act of remembering something involves drawing upon preconscious material.

The *unconscious* is the term used to denote the deepest layer of mental activity. This word 'unconscious' first appeared in the English language in 1712, when it indicated some vague background to consciousness. Herbart, in 1824, introduced the idea that a conflict existed between conscious and unconscious ideas. Freud later pointed to evidence for the existence of the unconscious and of its effects on human behaviour. Major pieces of evidence are seen in dreams which occur when we are far from conscious and which often portray drives and feelings of which we are not consciously aware, in slips of the tongue, forgetfulness and other errors in everyday life which, when examined carefully, will often reflect hidden attitudes and feelings, and in certain symptoms of psychiatric illness. For example, a patient developed a paralysis of the right arm for no apparent reason while she was making a basket for her daughter. It later became evident that she had mixed feelings towards her daughter. As a mother it was right and proper that she should do something for her daughter who was about to have a baby. On the other hand, as she had unloving feelings towards this daughter, which she would not or could not entertain consciously, why should she make a basket? The conflict was 'solved' in the production of a paralysed arm which would not permit her to carry on with her task. The point being made is that her hostility to her daughter was not at the time conscious but was quite unconscious, and through an unconscious mechanism, her arm became paralysed. She did not consciously or voluntarily beseech her arm to lose its function. It just happened and only after further exploration did it become evident that she harboured unconscious hostility towards her daughter.

Apart from such evidence, we see the result of unconscious mechanisms at work in our everyday life. Why, for example, do we sometimes take an instant liking or dislike to a person when we have insufficient evidence upon which to form a considered opinion of a person's worth? If we dislike a person, it may be due to the fact that we see in him things we do not like about ourselves—things very often that we are not initially consciously aware of.

It may be that the person's attitude strikes some deep hidden chord and produces emotions more relevant to someone in our past, of whom we may have no conscious awareness.

If we accept the fact of the unconscious mental mechanisms, and there appears to be ample proof of this, then the concept of unconscious motivation becomes a more readily understandable one.

In functioning as a nurse or functioning in any situation, be it a treatment situation or otherwise, it is necessary for us to recognise that certain motives in ourselves and in other people are unconsciously determined.

In terms of our patients and ourselves we are not always aware of why we or our patients behave in a particular way, because the activities or attitudes displayed arise out of forces or drives that are at the moment not conscious.

We become more effective and useful as therapists when we learn to know ourselves, when we gain some insight into our own mental mechanisms, which simply means becoming consciously aware of our own hitherto unconscious drives or needs.

ANXIETY

The Concise Oxford Dictionary describes anxiety as 'uneasiness or concern'.

It is a mood we have all experienced, though no doubt, find difficult to define. It may be our experience that situations which once produced a feeling of uneasiness, no longer do so. Other situations still make us feel anxious, and new experiences may, at times, be so productive of anxiety that we almost freeze up. What is anxiety, this feeling of uneasiness or concern which is experienced by most of us?

Firstly, anxiety does not mean precisely the same as fear. Fear is produced by a peripheral or objective threat by some situation outside a person, that can be assessed by the person, and to which the person may respond by attacking or facing the threatening situation, or by running away. The object or situation feared is a known and external one. In such a state of fear the individual is able to act. He is conscious of himself as a whole person. He knows his strengths and weaknesses and can accurately assess the dangers present in his surroundings. On the other hand, when one overreacts by a feeling of uneasiness or concern out of all proportion to the threatening object or situation, then we are not dealing with simple fear. It would seem that something is added to, or replaces, normal fear to produce an unwarranted apprehensive state. The name given to this something, is anxiety.

It may be fairly confidently stated that anxiety is one of the main motivating forces in much of human behaviour and provides a tremendous impetus to learning and adjusting throughout life. Many of our actions are seen, on close scrutiny, to be determined by the avoidance of anxiety. Some degree of anxiety appears to be necessary for healthy growth as well as for neurotic development.

What is anxiety really and what is its origin? The first part of this question has already been partially answered.

The Dictionary of Social Sciences defines anxiety as 'a reaction of apprehension ranging from uneasiness to complete panic, preceded by a real or symbolic condition of threat which the subject perceives diffusely and to which he reacts with an intensity that seems to be disproportionate'.

The emotion is preceded by a real threat or a symbolic one, symbolic in this sense indicating that objects or situations have a particular meaning for the individual concerned, often representing unacceptable impulses. The threat is perceived diffusely in contradistinction to fear wherein the threat can be accurately defined and assessed by the individual. Mention has been made earlier in this section that the emotions in anxiety are disproportionate to, or out of all proportion to, the apparent threat. This disproportion is the crux of the situation and if one can answer why the disproportion, then one is close to understanding the origins of anxiety.

Origins of anxiety

The theologian, Kierkegaard, regarded anxiety as resulting from separation from God and saw anxiety as an inevitable aspect of being alive. Presumably, the temptation in the Garden of Eden was essentially related to the first beings becoming independent of their Maker. Adam decided that, by eating the fruit of the tree of Knowledge, he and Eve would be as Gods knowing good and evil, a situation wherein man set himself up in some sort of competition with his all-knowing, all-powerful Maker. Whether we believe the story of the original sin to be factual or allegorical, it fits civilization in that man, in his quest for knowledge, sound and inevitable as this may be, places himself in a situation wherein he attempts to emancipate himself from God. Emancipation implies separation, and such separation produces similar emotions as are produced in a child when separated from parental figures. As man can never achieve a state of full emancipation from God along with absolute self-sufficiency, then anxiety is the inevitable lot of man.

Freud, who, as we know, pioneered explorations into man's inner life, discovered the role of inner conflicts or unconscious psychic processes and threats in the development of neurotic anxiety. He saw such neurotic anxiety as the basis for the development or other neurotic and psychotic symptoms which served as a defence against this neurotic anxiety or internal conflict. Some authorities do not agree that neurotic anxiety is the basis for the development of other symptoms and syndromes but see anxiety as parallel to other neurotic symptoms. Whatever view is taken, it is generally agreed that anxiety arises out of unconscious mental processes. For Freud, anxiety arose essentially out of an awareness of the ego (conscious part of the mind experienced by the individual as his 'self') of instinctual pressures from the id (an unconscious part of the mind made up of primitive or instinctual drives) and the person's inability, for one reason or another, to gratify these pressures. Freud later described superego anxiety (or moral anxiety) which arises out of guilt and fear of social disapproval, the superego containing a framework of moral standards derived in early life from parents and other figures of authority. As mentioned in the section on Development of Personality, Freud saw sexuality in its broad sense as the basis for this internal conflict.

Melanie Klein, while accepting unconscious conflict as the basis for anxiety, differs from Freud in seeing unconscious aggression as the core conflict rather than sexuality *per se.* This aggression directed towards parental figures produces anxiety and/or guilt in the child because the child unconsciously sees the parents as persecuting or punishing him for his aggression.

Goldstein, like Adler, took what is called a holistic view of the person, that is, he did not split the person into separate mental functions of id, ego and superego as did Freud, and pointed out that anxiety may be produced by a variety of events, the common element in all being a discrepancy between an individual's capability and the demands made upon him.

Cannon did pioneering work in the field of homeostasis, that is, the tendency for something when thrown out of balance, especially biochemical, to return to a state of equilibrium. He saw anxiety as an expression of threat to, a temporary failure of, and an attempt to restore balance at a new level.

Sullivan drew attention to the fact that human beings are an integral part of culture and he saw anxiety arising from a threat to an individual's security in interpersonal relationships. The infant or child who is accepted and approved, experiences a sense of well-being. Disapproval, on the other hand, produces a sense of discomfort different from pain or fear which Sullivan termed 'anxiety'. A person's development, referred to by Sullivan as the development of the 'self-system', is based on the avoidance of this 'anxiety'.

The views presented by these various authorities, give some clues as to the origins of anxiety as well as to the complexity of the problem. Unconscious conflicts, whether they concern separation, sexuality or aggression, lead to anxiety. This is essentially the view of analysts such as Freud and Melanie Klein. We have seen that Sullivan saw anxiety as 'anxiety of disapproval', brought about by conflict with the outer world. Sullivan and other so-called 'culture-pattern theorists' do not appear to go far enough. Conflict with the outer world merely mobilizes internal anxiety which is determined by unconscious conflicts, possibly by producing a sense of loss of one's external support and leaving one at the mercy of internal conflict and anxiety. If a person has but little internal conflict and is relatively well-adjusted or mentally healthy, even major losses or catastrophes in the outside world may be borne without crippling anxiety. On the other hand, when internal or unconscious conflict is powerful, it takes little external stress to mobilize anxiety, which may be felt as the emotion of anxiety with its accompanying physiological symptoms, or be productive of other symptoms, produced by the ego's defences against anxiety.

Before dealing with the defences against such anxiety, or as they are termed, the ego defence mechanisms, mention should be made of the physiological changes associated with anxiety, because these are the symptoms often complained of by the person who suffers from anxiety. Comment will also be made on normal anxiety.

Physical symptoms and signs associated with anxiety

A person may complain of the emotional state of anxiety but perhaps more frequently focusses on the physiological changes that occur in anxiety. Many of these bodily changes associated with anxiety, and with fear for that matter, may be seen as preparing the body for primitive 'fight or flight', that is, facing up to the situation squarely or running away from it as mentioned earlier in this chapter.

These changes take place throught the autonomic nervous system (the involuntary sympathetic and parasympathetic systems) and through the actions of the endocrine or ductless glands. It was these aspects of anxiety that interested Cannon mostly. Sympathetic nervous system activity is largely responsible for:

1. Increase in heart rate and cardiac output, often amounting to palpitations wherein a person becomes aware of a rapid forceful beating of the heart.
2. Contraction of the blood vessels of the skin and intestines so that more blood can be diverted to the heart, lungs and muscles. This leads to pallor of the skin and may be partly responsible for the lack of appetite for food which often occurs when anxiety or fear persists.
3. Increase in muscle tone which may be experienced as tension in the muscles or may lead to tremors.
4. Mobilization of blood sugar or glucose from the liver, which provides readily available energy.
5. Dilatation of the pupils.
6. Goose flesh, produced also by cold weather, and due to contraction of tiny muscles, the arrectores pilorum, attached to hair follicles which, when shortened, cause the hair to stand upright. This is seen in some animals when they are disturbed and it is the same mechanism that causes a tingling at the back of the neck and scalp in humans who experience fear or anxiety.

The parasympathetic nervous system is concerned with:

1. Sweat secretion. In states of anxiety this is often quite marked from the palms, soles and axillae.
2. Contraction of bladder and bowels with relaxation of their

sphincter mechanisms. No doubt we have all experienced frequency of micturition before anxiety-provoking events, such as examinations.

Prominent in states of anxiety is a respiratory discomfort often described as a suffocating feeling, which leads to hyperventilation, and sometimes to the end result of this, namely tetany (see page 215).

Normal anxiety

So far, we have discussed what might be termed neurotic anxiety. The term normal anxiety, or reality anxiety is used to describe the emotion due to real threats to the individual from the external world. However, if one sees anxiety as being a disproportionate response to a real or symbolic condition of threat, then it follows that there must always be something abnormal about anxiety; and 'normal anxiety' cannot be equated with fear, which is specific and is directed proportionately towards the threatening situation.

As pointed out by Weinberg, the term normal anxiety has been applied to:

1. Anxiety shared by a group and resulting essentially from beliefs held rather than from actual dangers present.
2. A reaction resulting from a genuine outside danger where the response, though disproportionate, is minimal.
3. A reaction of mild apprehension and uncertainty related to the achievement of a vital but somewhat vague goal. An example of this is the striving for success in a highly competitive middle-class society, and for success to be achieved, some degree of anxiety is necessary as the motivating force.

Defences against anxiety

We have seen that the unconscious component of mental life often contains conflicting material that can lead to anxiety. Among such material are painful memories and unacceptable or dangerous drives or urges. These phenomena are frequently quite illogical and contradictory to the predominant conscious trends in a person's mental life and do not become crystallised until they are dealt with consciously. When such memories or urges threaten to enter consciousness, a person feels a diffuse threat which leads to anxiety. If one is unable to cope at the time with the unconscious and consciously unacceptable material emerging into consciousness, certain mental mechanisms automatically come into play as a protective measure.

These protective measures, themselves unconscious with the exception of two occurring at conscious level, are known as mental defence mechanisms or ego defence mechanisms. They occur in everyone and must be considered as part of normal mental functioning. When, however, a person never or hardly ever faces inner reality and these unconscious mechanisms habitually come into play inappropriately or to excess, normal development and functioning do not occur. Such an individual does not develop the full range of potential personality attributes and mental functioning may become abnormal.

Conscious mechanisms

Before examining the unconscious mental mechanisms, mention will be made of the two conscious ways of dealing with anxiety. The first of these is *suppression* or a conscious pushing back or aside of feelings or impulses. If a player is illegally mistreated in a football scrum, his initial justifiable reaction may be to punch his opponent. On brief reflection he knows that if the referee, who may have missed the initial insult, sees him throwing punches, he may be sent off the field. So he consciously holds himself in check or suppresses his hostility for the moment. Maybe he will tackle his opponent hard at a later stage of the match to relieve his aggrieved feelings, but, for the time being, the process of suppression is involved. This example does not deal with suppression of anxiety but of aggressive feelings, though it serves to highlight that suppression is a conscious deliberate process. Suppression is also operating when, being faced with memories or other unacceptable thoughts or feelings of anxiety, we try to forget or push them out of our minds. We may try to aid this process of 'forgetting' by throwing ourselves into work or other activities. This conscious and deliberate method of dealing with our thoughts and their associated feelings usually offers only temporary relief.

Intellectual control as it is called, affords a second method of dealing with unwished for feelings.

In terms of anxiety, the basis of which is unconscious (and therefore the anxiety may seem quite irrational and completely out of proportion to external circumstances), we might say to ourselves 'Don't be silly, you are not acting like a grown up; it is not logical to feel like this'.

The same type of conscious control may be exercised over the many thoughts and emotions experienced. Many people consciously strive to fit the roles their families or society demand of them or to behave in the way they feel is most fitting to their particular occupation or sphere of activity.

One would not deny the benefits, even the necessity for intellectual controls, but if they become the only way of dealing with one's emotions or of relating to others then a fairly rigid, restricted, often colourless personality will be the result.

We shall now look briefly at the unconscious mental defence mechanisms which, it must be remembered, are simply attempts to explain clinical material in 'psychological' terms.

Unconscious mechanisms

The following will be described:

1. Sublimation—the most healthy mechanism.
2. Rationalisation.
3. Negation.
4. Repression—a key mechanism.
5. Reaction formation.
6. Counterphobia.
7. Undoing.

8. Dissociation (and isolation)
9. Displacement
10. Conversion

—operate particularly in development of hysterical neurosis.

(The mechanisms below, though present in normal persons, are frequently found to be associated with the development of a severe degree of disorder and hence may be regarded as more pathogenic mechanisms.)

11. Regression.
12. Denial
13. Projection

—operate in the development of paranoid delusions.

14. Introjection
15. Identification

—associated with early stage of psychosexual development

Before looking at this rather imposing list it is worth stressing again that these mechanisms occur to some extent in all human beings, though some are more prevalent at particular stages of development than others.

1. Sublimation consists in the transformation of consciously unacceptable drives or urges, which may previously have been repressed, into personally and socially acceptable activities. This mechanism is regarded as the most healthy and acceptable of the ego defence mechanisms. Numerous examples can be cited. The youthful sporting enthusiast may be sublimating aggressive impulses. Spinsters unable to express sexuality and creativeness in childbirth may become avid gardeners, take a consuming interest in animal breeding and care, or engage in other creative pastimes. Much satisfying and socially acceptable behaviour and endeavour may be determined largely by unacceptable drives or frustrations transformed by the mechanism of sublimation.

2. Rationalisation is the process whereby one constructs rational and logical reasons to account for actions. The reasons given may have little or no connection with underlying motives. This mechanism enables a person to maintain self-esteem by selecting personally and socially acceptable reasons for behaviour rather than accepting actual reasons which may show one in an unfavourable light. It also helps to give peace of mind by giving an acceptable reason for unexplainable actions.

Failures in examinations, job situations and in interpersonal relationships, are explained in any way that will save face. Nurses, doctors and other people caring for psychiatric patients often rationalise patients' reactions in terms of the patients 'illness' when they themselves may be instrumental in evoking certain reactions in patients. This is something we must watch in ourselves if we are to be effective in our roles. Extensive use of rationalisation hampers the development of personality as one never looks squarely at one's real motives.

If a rationalisation is challenged there is usually a strong emotional response, as challenging it threatens to expose the true and unacceptable motive behind an action which is being hidden through the operation of this mechanism.

3. Negation consists of describing an underlying drive or emotion in terms opposite to what is unconsciously felt and really meant. For example, the person who says, 'I don't envy him his job,' may, in some instances, be negating an unconscious envy of the person in a job which may carry more power and prestige than his own.

4. *Repression* consists in the removal from consciousness of unacceptable ideas, memories, feelings, drives and unresolved conflicts, and the thrusting of them back into the unconscious realms of the mind. What is seen by a person as being unacceptable is largely determined by parental and social education and by the moral ideals and rules operating in the particular culture in which the person lives.

Though removed from or denied admission to consciousness, such repressed ideas or feelings still operate in the unconscious, giving rise to dreams, slips of the tongue, irrational attitudes or neurotic symptoms, particularly at times of stress. To give an example of an irrational attitude, a person with repressed hostility towards parents may find difficulty in relating satisfactorily to figures representing authority in his day to day living.

5. *Reaction formation* consists in presenting the opposite emotion or behaviour to that which is entertained by and which is unacceptable to the person. The main areas wherein conflict arises in our culture appear to be concerned with hostility, sexuality and dependency. Reaction formation may become an habitual way of dealing with unacceptable ideas, emotions and drives and may greatly influence personality development.

A person filled with unconscious anxiety-producing aggressive impulses may compensate or overcompensate by habitually displaying submissive character traits.

The belligerent aggressive person, on the other hand, who is always throwing his weight around may be employing the mechanism of reaction formation to hide from himself the unacceptable fact that he is basically insecure and dependent.

The pacifist may be protecting himself against inner aggression. In some cases however, the militant pacifist may be utilising the mechanism of sublimation described earlier by directing aggressive energies into a more socially acceptable channel. Over-concern for one's children or spouse may be a reaction formation against unconscious or barely conscious desires to have them out of the way.

The defence of reaction formation may break down and the person may show genuine surprise at the result, because, as well as fooling other people, he has come to fool himself and really believes his apparent personality, shaped to some extent through reaction formation, to be the real person. The man who suddenly finds himself almost killing through physical violence, somebody who has offended him or a person close to him may later utilize reaction formation and other defences to an even greater degree to cope with his aggression. He now has proof of his boundless hostility and it becomes even more difficult for him to accept his aggression as a normal, not necessarily destructive, part of his personality.

6. *Counterphobia* may be regarded as a special form of reaction formation, the counterphobic defense being aimed specifically at anxiety associated with phobias (page 73). It is seen as an attempt by an individual to

gain mastery over and derive some pleasure from situations or activities that cause discomfort or fear.

Following a tour of duty in South Vietnam a young soldier would not board the plane that would fly him home to Australia, so marked was his flight or plane phobia. The author acceded to a request to escort the young man home in a subsequent plane. The trip was not uneventful as the soldier, initially agitated, had to be persuaded with some difficulty not to tell the pilot how to fly the plane. In conversation it came out that he held a pilot's licence and had no difficulty in flying as long as he was at the controls. It appears that he had in the past attempted to overcome his phobic fear of flying through a counterphobic defense namely, learning to fly himself.

7. Undoing is a defense mechanism which eliminates the conscious or unconscious feeling of remorse usually associated with aggressive impulses or fantasies, through a retraction of them by thought or action. The mechanism is generally associated with obsessive compulsive disorders (page 224). People with these disorders appear to confuse aggressive wishes with actions and there is some magical or omnipotent quality about such wishes as if they themselves could cause injury. A person who entertains an obsessional aggressive thought may immediately say to himself, 'I take that back', in order to annul (or undo) the harm he believes the thought will produce. The undoing is also a form of magical thinking.

8. Dissociation may be regarded as a partial repression wherein a portion of the personality, intolerable to conscious awareness (or sometimes referred to as ego-alien), is split off.

In such a way, there may be loss of memory for certain painful events. Emotion too difficult to bear may be split off and not felt, even though the person remembers the event. This may occur, when, on the death of a loved one, grief is not felt at the time, but may be experienced later. This mechanism whereby a person can dissociate feelings from the rest of the personality and thus face grossly traumatic experiences with outward calm is sometimes referred to as *isolation*. The term isolation however, is used by some authorities to cover the whole concept of dissociation wherein, as indicated above, unfavourable or ego-alien experiences are 'blocked' from full conscious awareness.

9. Displacement is the attachment of the emotion provoked by one object to another more convenient object. Once again it is prone to appear when repression is failing. Anxiety is reduced by this process of displacing or transferring frightening feelings from dangerous objects or situations on to objects or situations more acceptable to the person or to society. At one level, if we are hostile to our superiors for any reason and if we think our well-being in our job may be jeopardized if we express our anger directly, we may take out our feelings on subordinates or even kick the proverbial cat.

10. Conversion is the mechanism operating when a conflict or a repressed idea or drive expresses itself in bodily symptons. A partial failure of repression of painful truths about the person often leads to this mechanism being invoked. The bodily functions affected are those normally under the control of the central nervous system, that is voluntary functions.

The mechanism of conversion may be the basis for paralysis, abnormal motor movements including convulsions, sensory abnormalities such as anaesthesia, lack of speech (aphonia), deafness or blindness (amaurosis). Any of these symptoms may be seen in hysteria and it is obvious that abnormal physical conditions can be mimicked when this mechanism operates.

Examples of this mechanism are legion. A person entering a dangerous situation may have anxiety mobilised, leading to the development of paralysed legs. The physical symptom replaces the anxiety and also saves the person from facing the dangerous situation. The woman weaving a basket for her pregnant daughter towards whom she had unconscious hostile feelings, and who developed a paralysis of her arm (mentioned in section dealing with unconscious motivation) was exhibiting the mechanism of conversion. Women with sexual conflicts may develop vaginismus (spasm of vaginal muscles) rendering sexual intercourse impossible.

Such symptoms as mentioned above provide only a temporary solution to problems.

11. Regression implies functioning at a level of feeling, thinking and behaviour appropriate to an earlier stage of development. It is an ego defence mechanism in the sense that the individual avoids failure and responsibility by reverting to a less mature mode of adjustment. All of us may, under stress, behave immaturely or childishly, becoming dependent and demanding. Most mental illnesses involve regressive behaviour to a greater or lesser degree. It is seen particularly in patients suffering from schizophrenic reactions and in many suffering from severe depressive illnesses. People looking after psychiatric patients must be aware of the increased tendency of such folk to regress. As important as early support of many patients is, it is equally important to withdraw support as early as possible in order not to further foster dependency needs in such patients.

12. Denial is the mechanism whereby emotions, thoughts and drives which would be unacceptable to the conscious mind are simply denied. Their existence is not acknowledged. The mechanism may be regarded as 'normal' in childhood. An example frequently quoted is that of the child, extremely sleepy but perhaps not wishing to face the uncertainty of a lonely bed, insisting he is not tired. Denial in adulthood has more serious implications than in childhood. Gross physical disability or even a state of normal pregnancy may not be acknowledged. Severe personal loss may be completely ignored; a person who would normally be expected to respond by being depressed may show no evidence of this and, in fact, may present a happy or unconcerned facade. At its worst, denial represents a complete break with reality in which state a person may be regarded as psychotic.

13. Projection is the mechanism whereby unacceptable wishes and impulses, the recognition of which in the self might cause discomfort, are ascribed to others. People often criticise in others, qualities and faults that they themselves possess, being unaware that they are a true reflection of aspects of their own personalities.

At a simple level, projection may involve placing the blame on circumstances, for example, projecting one's own inadequacies on to the equipment one is using to perform some task.

Much more serious is the part projection may play in the development of hallucinations and delusions.

The person with deeply repressed homosexual tendencies may at some stage ascribe these tendencies to others with whom he comes into contact, believing that they are making homosexual overtures to him. Fundamentally, and quite unconsciously, it is he who wishes for the gratification of such drives in himself.

A person may see other people as hostile towards him on the basis of attributing to them, through the mechanism of projection, the hostility present in himself. Hallucinatory voices emanate not from the outside world, but are aspects of a person's own thoughts projected externally.

14. Introjection. To start with, a clear-cut definition of this mechanism would be to oversimplify, probably erroneously, a concept that is difficult to understand, and which, being so loosely applied by many authorities in the past, leaves most of us wondering what it is really all about.

Introjection has been described as the opposite of projection, involving taking into the person something of the outside world, while, as we have seen, projection involves throwing out part of the person. Melanie Klein gives the process of introjection an important place in her theory of personality development. She points out that, from the beginning, the infant's poorly developed ego introjects or phantasises the incorporation of either of the two parents or parts of them. What is introjected are referred to as 'objects', the mother's breast being the prototype of these objects. These introjected (internal) objects, whether whole of part, are felt to be either 'good' or 'bad' depending on the projection of the child's feelings into them. For example, the breast is good when it satisfies, bad when it doesn't. The love objects of infancy and early childhood are major sources of frustration and tend to be hated as well as loved, that is, they tend to be loved ambivalently. It is possible that, whether the breast or other objects of love are providing satisfaction or not, the infant, in striving to cope with his aggressive impulses, imputes to them or projects on to them these aggressive feelings. When the object of love or desire is withdrawn or lost, or when withdrawal or loss seems imminent, the object may be set up imaginatively inside the infant's personality in order that he might have it for all time. This incorporation of objects into the infant is the process of introjection. The danger of losing something is extremely distressing in the infant who is totally dependent on its environment, so introjection is probably very common if not universal in infancy, being utilised to maintain love objects even though feelings towards the love objects be ambivalent.

In infancy therefore, one can see introjection as a defence against anxiety set up by a situation, or threatened situation, of loss. Introjection is also said to play a part in the development of the superego, presumably by the incorporation of standards and ideals set by parents and society.

Introjection, though characteristically a phenomenon of infancy, may occur in adult crises where there is frustration in love, a loss or deprivation of love or a real or imagined threat of such a loss. The object that is introjected is always one that has been loved ambivalently. The utilisation of introjection in adulthood is usually in association with the development of the severer forms of mental illness.

Introjection has been described as the defence mechanism by which a person directs towards himself emotions really felt towards other people. It is conceivable that the aggressive component of ambivalent feelings towards another person may produce anxiety that such a person will be driven away or harmed, in short, lost in some way. In order to prevent such an occurrence the totality of emotion directed to the person, both loving and hating elements, is taken in or incorporated into the person entertaining the ambivalent feelings, by the process of introjection. Such incorporation prevents loss. However, introjected feelings or ideas become part of one's own personality, and if aspects of these are disturbing in their degree of hatefulness, a person will hate himself, or even destroy himself by suicide in an attempt to destroy the introjected mental image of a partially hated person.

I am doubtful whether this description has aided in the understanding of the concept of introjection, but before leaving the defence mechanisms mention should be made of *identification*, a word that is also used too loosely and which has been used interchangeably with introjection as if to further confuse an already clouded topic.

15. Identification is the unconscious or more or less unconscious process whereby an individual responds to the behaviour of other people or objects by initiating, in phantasy or in reality, the same behaviour in himself.

Threats to self-esteem or physical threats, may lead to identification. It is frequently the unfavourable discrepancy felt between one's own powers or abilities and those of another person that lead to identification. This is why heroic or sensational figures elicit identification in almost anyone.

Identification is not lasting and disappears when it is no longer needed as a temporary prop. Children normally model themselves on their parents and other adults while they gradually develop their own distinctive personalities. When this happens, identification ceases. Identification can be the basis of certain delusional ideas in some psychotic illnesses.

Psychiatry owes a debt to Sigmund Freud* for the development of many of the above concepts. As inferred earlier, the labels and descriptions of the defence mechanisms constitute Freud's explanations of events noted by him in his clinical work and study. They were attempts to explain why a particular symptom or why certain behaviour occurs.

These mechanisms are seen to be operating in the normal individual as well as in sufferers from overt psychiatric disorders. As we shall see in

* Freud's daughter, Anna, refined and expanded her father's earlier concepts of mental mechanisms in her work *The Ego and the Mechanisms of Defense* (1937).

Chapter 8, they in no way explain fully the basis of many symptoms and signs.

7

PSYCHIATRIC SYMPTOMS AND SIGNS

In a psychiatric hospital, one sees patients presenting with a variety of symptoms and signs, and at an early stage of one's training it is important to learn to recognise these. They may be seen as the building blocks of the variety of psychiatric disorders that are encountered, and each disorder has its own fairly characteristic behaviour patterns which the nurse must be aware of, and must be able to anticipate. With a sound basic knowledge of symptoms and signs, leading to a better understanding of likely behaviour patterns, the nurse will be in a better position to provide the most rational and helpful management. A general overview will therefore be given of symptoms and signs occurring in psychiatric disorders.

At this point it will be worthwhile to indicate some method of presenting the facts that we observe about patients, and to this end we shall look at a number of headings under which we can place the information gathered from observations of patients. These headings will subsequently constitute the basis for the description of various psychiatric syndromes.

They are:

1. General appearance;
2. Behaviour patterns;
3. Form of speech;
4. Content of speech;
5. Mood;
6. Intelligence;
7. Insight and judgment.

We shall examine these headings separately, looking at the symptoms and signs embraced by each. Symptoms classically refer to what is experienced by the patient and signs refer to what is observed by someone else to be occurring in the patient.

General appearance

Under this heading are included the following:

1. Facial expression: alert, responsive, anxious, hostile, apathetic.
2. Posture: tense, 'depressed', strange postures as in catatonia, flexibilitas cerea.
3. Gait: stilted walk as in catatonic schizophrenia; gait may suggest hysterical neurosis or some neurological condition.
4. Mannerisms, tics.

5. Mode of dress.
6. Personal care: neglected looking or suggestive of narcissism.
7. Physical deformities and abnormalities, suggesting mental retardation, neurological conditions or hysterical neurosis.
8. General physical condition and nutrition.

Catatonia is the term used to describe a peculiar state of muscular rigidity present in some schizophrenic patients. Abnormal postures, stilted gait, complete lack of any movement and muteness may form part of the picture of catatonia. The catatonic patient's limbs may remain for a considerable time in positions in which they are placed, a condition described as *Flexibilitas Cerea* (Waxy Flexibility).

The term *Catalepsy* is sometimes used to describe any form of sustained immobility and, as such, it describes a component of catatonia. Some confusion is caused by the descriptions of catatonic schizophrenia, a psychotic illness to be dealt with later, in which depression, stupor and excitement may all form part of the symptomatology of the catatonic type of schizophrenia. Catatonic symptoms may also occur in certain organic brain diseases.

Mannerisms are repeated small movements of an habitual kind frequently characteristic of the personality of the person exhibiting them. They often consist of movements of the hands or face. In themselves they are not abnormal but may feature in rather bizarre fashion in certain psychotic disorders. An old school-master of mine, before speaking, habitually stroked, with his left ring and little fingers, the place where his moustache should have been, providing us with an example of a mannerism.

Tics are habitual spasmodic contractions of muscles usually involving the face, mouth, eyelids or neck. Under conditions of stress or tension tics may become more marked and frequent.

Narcissism is the name given to excessive love of self seen especially in immature personalities. It is derived from the Greek, Narkissos, a youth who fell in love with his reflection in the water.

Behaviour patterns

General

Is the patient in touch with his surroundings, cooperative or uncooperative, sociable or suspicious, conventional or eccentric, consistent or unpredictable, industrious or idle, passive and dependent or showing initiative? Note also should be taken of appetite and sleep.

Specific abnormalities

Under this heading one looks for evidence of:

1. Overactivity;
2. Violence;
3. Destructiveness;
4. Retardation;
5. Stupor;

6. Inertia;
7. Stereotypy;
8. Negativism;
9. Echopraxia (and echolalia);
10. Compulsions.

Retardation is the term applied to a general slowing down of mental and bodily functions. It involves a slowing down of thought and of action. There may be a diminution of initiative and slowness in carrying out any activity. This is also seen in the realm of speech, even amounting to mutism, as will be mentioned in the relevant section of our mental state examination.

When retardation reaches such a degree that a patient is completely motionless and relatively or completely unresponsive to stimuli he is said to be in a state of *stupor*. Stupor used in this sense does not imply, as it does in general medicine, a state between full consciousness and coma where a patient still responds to painful stimuli.

Retardation is not infrequently seen in psychotic disorders such as severe depressive illnesses. Stupor may be seen in such psychotic disorders as severe depression, catatonic schizophrenia, and in hysteria.

Inertia . In physics, this term is used to describe the phenomenon whereby matter if at rest remains at rest, or if in motion remains in motion in a particular direction unless this is altered by external forces. Its use in psychiatry is not so specific and it describes a state of inactivity or apparent lifelessness. It may be associated with apathy or indifference.

Stereotypy. Though dealt with in this section on behaviour patterns, stereotypy also involves speech. A suitable definition is as follows: An action or group of actions or words monotonously repeated, or a posture maintained long after fatigue would ordinarily have caused relaxation. This pattern of activity occurs in some patients with schizophrenia, and is exemplified by patients who follow a set course in pacing the ward or courtyard of traditional mental hospitals which, fortunately, are fast disappearing.

Negativism consists in responses exactly opposite to those normally elicited by a given stimulus. Schizophrenic patients may do the exact opposite of what is asked of them. For example, when asked to open his mouth a patient may shut it firmly.

Echopraxia is the repetition of actions seen. This phenomenon, the opposite of negativism, and also occuring in schizophrenia, is referred to by some as automatic obedience. Such automatic obedience is also seen in *Echolalia* in which patients repeat words or statements spoken to them.

Compulsion is the term applied to an impulse or movement which a person feels he must carry out and yet has a desire to resist, knowing it is quite unnecessary and even absurd. The person is uneasy until the particular act or movement is carried out. Examples of compulsions are the frequent washing of hands, repeated checking that the gas is turned off, that something hasn't fallen from the table into the waste paper basket, and so forth. The compulsion as indicated in the above examples, usually has a recurrent or persistent nature and is seen in obsessive-compulsive disorders. The term *ritual* is sometimes applied to compulsive actions. Acts which appear to be compulsive but which the patient does not attempt to resist are probably part of a psychotic illness.

Form of speech (abnormalities in thought processes)

In speech, there are two main elements to be considered, the form or structure of speech and the content. We are dealing here with form and, under this heading, the following are looked for:

1. Acceleration, which apart from pressure of talk, may involve flight of ideas and clang associations.
2. Retardation.
3. Mutism; Aphonia.
4. Blocking; pressure of thoughts (often subjective only).
5. Disordered association of ideas—erratic thought sequence, apparent irrelevancy, incoherence.
6. Aphasia.
7. Circumstantiality.
8. Perseveration.
9. Condensation.

It is important to note how the form of talk varies with the subject under discussion. For example, a patient may be able to speak relatively freely about topics such as his garden or some other non-emotionally charged topic, but as soon as one touches upon the way he feels or something in which he is emotionally involved, some of the above features may become more apparent. This is noticed particularly in respect to blocking in schizophrenic patients.

Pressure of talk refers to accelerated speech found in states of excitement and overactivity. If overactivity is marked, the person speaking may jump from one topic to another, the stream of thought being altered by chance associations between the fragments of conversation. This state of affairs is referred to as *flight of ideas.* Flight of ideas may be determined by *clang associations* in which rhymes or puns form the associating link between ideas. As an example of punning, a patient may refer to the light (electric light), switch over immediately to speaking about the Light of the world, then refer to some object being light (not heavy).

Retardation refers to a slowing in the stream of thought and hence in speech. At its extreme, this may amount to *mutism* when the patient does not speak at all. Gross acceleration of talk and retardation are associated with psychotic disorders.

Aphonia means simply absence of speech but is not related to retardation. The term is usually restricted to describing lack of function of the vocal chords which may occur as a symptom of hysteria, the mental mechanisms of conversion being implicated.

In *Blocking or thought blocking,* there occurs a sudden stoppage in the stream of thought (and consequently of talk) occurring apart from any environmental influences and without the patient being able to account for the stoppage. The patient, who is most likely to be suffering from schizophrenia, may after a considerable pause, continue on the same topic or on a completely unrelated topic. Even though the observer may sometimes have difficulty in picking up this symptom, patients are often subjectively aware of the difficulty.

A mild degree of blocking is probably not uncommon in normal individuals under conditions of emotional stress, for example, answering questions in examination vivas, especially if one is not properly prepared.

Also found in schizophrenia is *'pressure of thoughts'*. Here the patient is aware of a multitude of different ideas racing through his mind, ideas over which he has little or no control.

Disordered association of ideas. When we think, our ideas usually flow logically towards a particular goal, and we have what is termed a determinative goal in thinking. Along the fringe, as it were, of our mainstream of ideas which start at one point and finish logically at another, are associated thoughts which do not normally interfere with our determinative idea. In certain schizophrenic patients, the associations at the fringe seem to impinge upon the mainstream of thought, leading to woolliness in thinking. In speaking with these patients, one gets the feeling that a common 'wavelength' is not achieved. It has been described rather as if a pane of glass exists between the interviewer and the patient. Where a greater degree of disturbance exists, normal logical associations become quite bizarre and one is completely unable to follow a schizophrenic patient's conversation. The term 'knight's move' thinking is sometimes applied to such disordered thinking. An extreme degree of disturbance of association of ideas in which little or no sense can be extracted from speech is termed *incoherence.* Such patients may repeat a word or phrase over and over again (*verbigeration*). When the degree of thought and speech disorganisation is so great that a string of disconnected words, often nouns, is poured out, the term *word salad* is applied.

Condensation is the fusion of two or more ideas or concepts into one.

Aphasia should not be confused with aphonia. Aphasia is a term applied to the inability of a person to express ideas. It is due to organic cerebral conditions such as 'strokes'. A person may be aware of what they wish to say but be unable to use words properly to express these thoughts. (This is really a 'motor aphasia'. 'Sensory aphasia' refers to the inability to understand what is spoken.)

Circumstantiality refers to speech where there is much unnecessary detail and great spontaneity, but the object in view at the beginning is ultimately reached. It frequently occurs in states of organic damage to the brain.

Perseveration is the abnormally persistent repetition of a word, phrase or sentence. A person with organic brain damage may be asked 'What is your name?'—'John Smith' he may reply. The next question may be 'How old are you?', the answer again being 'John Smith', the initial train of thought being followed despite a change in topic.

The term perseveration may also be applied to the repetition of a recent movement or action as well as to speech.

The term *thought disorder* was commonly limited to abnormal thought processes occurring in schizophrenia but today it would appear to be applied to all abnormal thought processes.

Content of speech

The patient's conversation can provide a wealth of information in terms of particular preoccupations and may demonstrate very well a number of psychiatric abnormalities. Evidence of the following must be sought:—

1. Delusions

   Types of delusions:

   (a) Persecutory delusions—do people or forces influence him bodily or mentally; do people laugh at him, avoid him, try to kill him, etc.?

   (b) Delusions of grandeur—does he claim to be related to royalty, immensely wealthy, extremely influential, the Son of God Himself, etc.?

   (c) Delusions of guilt—does he denigrate himself, blame himself unnecessarily, express ideas of unworthiness?

   (d) Nihilistic delusions—does he believe his bowels are not there, his brain has gone, he is dead or his relatives (actually alive) are dead, etc.?

   (e) Hypochondriacal delusions—are there false fixed beliefs concerning bodily abnormalities?

   (f) Delusions of reference—does he feel that people, things or events have a special reference to him; do strangers look at him in the street or talk about him; do newspapers, radio or television items refer especially to him?

   (g) Delusions of influence—does the patient believe his thoughts, feelings, actions are controlled or affected by outside agencies via radio waves, electricity, mental telepathy, hypnotism, radio active substances; do people read his mind?

   (h) Somatic delusions—does the person believe his appearance has changed, that he is turning into a woman, etc.?
2. Overvalued Ideas.
3. Obsessions.
4. Hallucinations—auditory, visual, olfactory, gustatory, tactile, visceral.
5. Illusions.
6. Phobias.
7. Hypochondriasis.
8. Neologisms.

A *delusion* is a belief which is:

(a) not true to fact;

(b) cannot be corrected by an appeal to the reason of the person entertaining it;

(c) is out of harmony with the individual's educational and cultural background.

The first two points in the definition require no explanation. Perhaps the reference to educational and cultural background does. If a rustic Irishman believes in 'the little men', or leprechauns, he may hold a false belief which cannot be altered by reasoning, but in terms of his particular culture and teaching the belief cannot be regarded as a delusion. If I, as an Australian, believed in 'little men' this would cast grave doubts on my sanity.

Delusions are indicative of a break with reality and, as such, are symptomatic of psychotic conditions. They are present in a number of psychotic illnesses which will be described later in their relevant sections.

The origin of delusions will be dealt with in a subsequent chapter. At this stage we shall look briefly at the types of delusions, but before doing so the terms 'unsystematised' and 'systematised' will be clarified. Some patients may show delusions which are fleeting in nature, changeable and unconnected with each other. Such delusions are referred to as *unsystematised delusions.* When delusions are built up in a logical manner into a complex more fixed system they are referred to as *systematised delusions.*

I call to mind the example of a labourer from Northern Ireland who was under the impression that a well-dressed woman in a Rolls Royce smiled and spoke to him in London some years before. Perhaps logically he felt that this would produce jealousy in her husband or male acquaintances. As she was well-dressed and in a Rolls Royce, this meant that she moved in high society, in fact, in the political sphere. Politics somehow is involved in the administration of the country and entails the activities of at least the Police Force and the Customs Department. This man built up a delusional system whereby there was a large-scale governmental plot to 'get him' in some way, and any newspaper reference to the Police or Customs had some sinister implications for him. What commenced probably as a misinterpretation and perhaps an hallucinatory experience, developed in his case, the hallmarks of a systematised delusion in which the whole government of a country came to be the persecuting agent.

Persecutory delusions or *Paranoid delusions*, as the terms imply, are delusions wherein the person wrongly believes he will be affected in some harmful or persecutory way. The man quoted as an example under 'Systematised Delusions' suffered delusions of persecution.

Persecutory delusions may occur in a variety of psychotic illnesses, namely schizophrenia, paranoid states, psychoses of organic origin and the affective psychoses. In affective psychoses the persecution is part of the picture of guilt and self blame. It is not inconsistent for the guilt-ridden unworthy person to believe that people are outside digging his grave or that the Police will take action against him.

Delusions of grandeur are delusions where the patient holds exaggerated false beliefs with respect to his status, power and so forth. Such delusions occur in schizophrenia, manic depressive psychosis, and general paralysis due to syphilitic infection.

Delusions of guilt, self-reproach and *unworthiness* require no further definition. They occur in psychotic depressive illnesses and more rarely in those cases of schizophrenia in which a strong depressive element is present.

Nihilistic delusions are literally delusions pertaining to nothingness, the term nihilistic being derived from the Latin *nihil* meaning 'nothing'. They occur particularly in psychotic depressive illnesses.

Hypochondriacal delusions, also referred to as delusions of bodily disease, are present when a person holds fixed false beliefs concerning bodily disease or abnormalities in the face of evidence to the contrary. He may believe he has cancer, venereal disease, tuberculosis, bowel obstructions, etc. Such delusions are found in schizophrenia and psychotic depression illnesses.

Ideas of reference is a term which may be used synonymously with delusions of reference and, as indicated above, relate to the belief that people, things and events refer to the patient in a special way. They occur in schizophrenia, affective psychoses and in some non-psychotic people who have abnormally sensitive personalities.

Delusions of influence or, as they are also called, passivity feelings, occur in schizophrenia, and refer to a patient's false belief that he is being influenced or driven by forces outside himself, or that he or his thoughts are controlled by someone or something in his external environment.

Somatic delusions and hypochondriacal delusions may be difficult to differentiate. However, the term somatic (pertaining to the body) delusion is usually applied when there is a fixed false belief regarding anatomical alterations as opposed to the presence of disease or other abnormality. Somatic delusions may arise out of abnormal bodily sensations occurring in schizophrenia but these are not necessary as precursors.

The woman who wrongly believes that she has a cancer in the nose is suffering from a hypochondriacal delusion. The woman who quite wrongly and irrationally believes that her nose is too large or is misshapen entertains a somatic delusion.

Overvalued ideas (or *overdetermined ideas*). These fall somewhere along the continuum, normal—delusional, and refer to preoccupations with some aspect of a person's life, appearance or personality, often to the complete exclusion of other possible competing ideas. There is usually a factual basis for the concern or preoccupation shown, but being determined by some tremendous need or unconscious drive in the patient, such ideas assume apparently unnecessarily gigantic proportions in the person's thinking.

Obsessions. An obsession is a recurrent or persistent thought or idea accompanied by a sense of subjective compulsion, and a desire to resist it. In plain language one seems obliged to formulate an idea while appreciating that it is unnecessary and even absurd, and tries to resist it. Not infrequently, obsessional thoughts revolve around topics quite foreign to the person's usual conscious mode of thinking. The young mother may be obsessed with thoughts of killing her offspring. The religious person may find that some blasphemous phrase or sentence looms into consciousness no matter how hard he tries to check it. In common everyday usage, the term 'obsession' does not really parallel its usage in psychiatry. In everyday usage, to be obsessed with something means to be preoccupied by it, there being no effort to resist the thought, nor are such thoughts foreign to the personality. Thus the term 'obsession' is used in common parlance to denote what we would regard as an overvalued idea.

Obsessions, as defined, mainly occur in obsessive-compulsive disorders. Some apparently obsessional thoughts are not in any way resisted by the patient. In these instances, such thoughts (as with compulsions) probably form part of a psychotic illness.

Hallucinations. An hallucination is a mental impression of sensory vividness occurring without an external stimulus.

Hallucinations may involve all senses, namely, hearing (auditory), sight (visual), touch (tactile), smell (olfactory), taste (gustatory), and internal organs (visceral). Two other forms of hallucination are the kinesthetic hallucination involving a false perception of movement or sensation, and the Lilliputian hallucination in which the falsely perceived object is seen as diminished in size.

Hallucinations signify a break with reality and when present, in general, are indicative of a psychotic state. Mention might be made of what are termed hypnagogic hallucinations which occur at a time between sleep and wakefulness. At such times, a person may, for example, hear his name called. These hallucinations are not necessarily indicative of psychosis. Also, if a normal person is placed in a situation of sensory deprivation—no sound, no light, etc.—then the boundaries between the self and the outside (ego boundaries) may become blurred, the person's thoughts may seem to come from outside himself, that is, are projected out, and hallucinations may occur.

Illusions. An illusion is a mental impression of sensory vividness arising out of the misinterpretation of an external stimulus.

The person walking in fear along a dark country lane may mistake the sight of a tree stump for a person or animal, or on hearing the rustle of leaves in the wind, may misinterpret this as someone approaching to attack him.

The ball of wool seen out of the corner of the eye or in poor light may be mistaken for a mouse.

In anxious children and in normal adults under stress, such experiences may be frightening enough. They are, perhaps, more so in acute organic psychotic states such as one sees in the alcoholic suffering from delirium tremens.

Phobias. The term phobia is derived from the Greek word *phobos* meaning 'flight, dread, panic or fear'.

When a fear becomes attached to objects or situations which are known by the individual not to be a source of danger, then the term phobia is used for this irrational fear. A classification of phobias is given in Chapter 14.

Hypochondriasis. This consists of a morbid preoccupation with or fear of physical disease. The symptom may occur in conjunction with psychotic illnesses such as schizophrenia and depressive states, and is seen at times in certain of the neuroses.

There are some people who show no features of psychosis or neurosis and whose sole symptom is hypochondriasis. They talk incessantly about their state of bodily health, see their doctor or doctors frequently, take any pills prescribed and return to the doctor for further expositions of their unfounded complaints, having in the meantime belaboured their long-suffering friends and neighbours with their story. These people are termed hypochondriacs. Hypochondriasis, as mentioned earlier may assume delusional proportions when false fixed beliefs of bodily disease are present.

Neologism is a term which describes a word of the patient's own making, that is, invented by the patient, possibly to express what to him is a complex idea. A neologism may be a condensation of several words and as such may be classified under the abnormal thought processes (for example, sarrible=sad and terrible).

NOTE—It is perhaps rather artificial to place delusions, overvalued ideas, obsessions, hallucinations, illusions, phobias and hypochondriasis under 'Content of Speech'. It is obvious that some of these symptoms may be apparent apart from through a patient's speech. For example, the auditorily hallucinated patient may adopt listening attitudes, phobias may become obvious through a patient's behaviour. However, it is convenient to group them together as the experiences may all be determined through the expression of ideas held by patients.

Some mental status examination schemata use a separate heading for hallucinatory and illusory experiences, namely *disorders of perception.*

Mood (or affect)

In the assessment of any patient, one should note his appearance insofar as it is indicative of his mood. Simple though it may be, one should ask questions such as, 'How do you feel in yourself?', or 'How about your mood?'. The following should be noted:

1. Depression.
2. Elation; euphoria; ecstasy; exultation.
3. Anxiety.
4. Panic.
5. Hostility.
6. Inappropriate (incongruous) affect.
7. 'la belle indifference'.
8. Apathy.
9. Labile or shallow affect.
10. Suspicion.

Mood, or *affect,* is difficult to define. The terms are used interchangeably and refer to a person's feeling or emotional state.

Our mood changes in response to circumstance. In some situations we feel happy, in others we may feel depressed or hostile. One cannot say that it is more normal to feel happy than it is to feel depressed or hostile or even suspicious. It is normal under certain situations to feel and display such emotions and the affect or mood is then said to be appropriate. Abnormality can be assumed when the mood is not consistent with, or is out of all proportion to precipitating circumstances, or when it persists for an undue length of time.

Depression indicates a mood state ranging from minor degrees of sadness or unhappiness to feelings of complete dejection or hopelessness, the extreme state usually being accompanied by a gross degree of pessimism with lack of hope for the future.

The symptom occurs in 'normal' people, in the neuroses and in psychotic illnesses, the degree in general differing in these situations. In psychotic depressive illnesses where the future seems to hold nothing, where the feeling of complete uselessness and lowered self-esteem are marked, the risk of suicide is great. Some of the features associated with depression in psychotic depressive illnesses may include retardation in action and speech, agitation and delusions of guilt, poverty, nihilism.

In the neuroses, depression may be the only marked sympton, or other neurotic symptions such as anxiety, phobias, obsessions and compulsions may be present as well.

In many patients you will observe that there appears to be no, or minimal, external precipitating events leading to depression. Such depression appears to have some constitutional basis or to arise out of hidden mental processes, and is referred to as *endogenous*. On the other hand the term *exogenous* is used by some to indicate that external factors are responsible for the mood.

Elation refers to an elevation of mood wherein the patient is happy, optimistic, and self-confident. It may be regarded as pathological when it reaches a degree not justified by external events. Such a person may make unrealistic plans for his future and be unable to carry them out as he over-reaches his capabilities. Elation may be associated with pressure of activity and thought.

Euphoria is the term given to a lesser degree of elation in which the person experiences an increased sense of well-being, confidence and enthusiasm.

More rare is the symptom of *ecstasy* which is an extreme degree of elation and is usually associated with an element of mysticism. Elation is infectious; not so ecstasy, which is a very personal state of rapture and bliss not able to be shared with others. In terms of the well person, a state of ecstasy may be present fleetingly at times of some religious or sexual experience.

Exulation is the term used to describe a state of elation wherein there are overtones of grandeur and pomposity.

All the above mood elevations occur most frequently in psychotic states, namely, the affective psychoses, some cases of schizophrenia and in some psychoses of organic origin.

As has been pointed out such mood changes may occur temporarily in normal persons.

We have considered *anxiety* at length in an earlier chapter. It consists of a blend of fear and uncertainty, and may be present in both neurotic and psychotic disorders; in fact, it is the most common of all psychiatric symptoms. Mention will again be made of physical symptoms and signs associated with anxiety, namely, tachycardia, sweating, pallor, muscular tension, dryness of the mouth.

The severest form of anxiety is referred to as *panic*, in which state the sufferer may freeze of flee, or react in a variety of ways indicating a state of gross emotional disequilibrium.

The combination of anxiety plus restlessness is known as *agitation.*

Hostility refers to feelings and thoughts of opposition, as well as describing angry or aggressive behaviour.

Hostility may be a perfectly normal reaction in appropriate circumstances. It may be regarded as abnormal when it persists for an undue length of time or is out of all proportion to the stimulus which excites it. Hostility which is felt may not be expressed directly in hostile acts or words. Instead, the person may become irritable, sulky, uncooperative, stubborn or negative. This veiled type of hostility is known as *passive aggression.*

The symptom of hostility may occur in both neurotic and psychotic disorders as well as in normal people. In children, hostility may become evident in transient outbursts of violence occurring with little or no provocation. Such outbursts are called *temper tantrums.*

Inappropriate (incongruous) affect, though not present in all cases of schizophrenia, is pathognomonic of the illness, that is, its presence means that the person is suffering from schizophrenia. Inappropriate affect or mood is a mood which is not consistent with ideas held at the same time. A patient who laughs or shows unconcern while expressing ideas that he is about to be killed or undergo some normally terrifying ordeal shows inappropriate or incongruous affect. The same may be said of the patient who, while complaining to the staff of being detained wrongfully in hospital, accepts hospitalisation without demur and even good humouredly.

Inappropriate affect should not be confused with *la belle indifference* which is a bland unconcern shown in the presence of distressing complaints or symptoms and which occurs in hysteria.

Apathy is the state in which a person shows lack of emotional response. We all feel apathetic or disinterested at times but when the term is applied to psychiatric patients, it is indicative of a more severe and long-lasting flatness of mood. The symptom is common in schizophrenia and in the later stages of organic conditions leading to dementia (that is, permanent loss of some intellectual functions).

Labile affect. Mood is said to be labile when there are quick changes from one feeling to another. Lability of mood is frequently present in patients suffering from the organic psychoses. Such patients may be laughing one minute and weeping the next.

In dementing processes such as senile dementia, mood may be *shallow*, as the progressive emotional deterioration that occurs leads to a failure in normal emotional response.

Suspicion. It is disputed whether suspicion is a mood. Some authorities see it as an intellectual rather than as an emotional condition. As an abnormal mood, it occurs most frequently in paranoid personalities and in psychoses with paranoid features.

Before leaving this section of mental state examination comment should be made on the fact that one's mood has a great bearing on one's ideation or on what one thinks about. When depressed for example, we are inclined to look on the gloomy side of things, concentrating on morbid situations and tending to be pessimistic. On the other hand, when in good spirits morbid topics are rarely mentioned and topics indicative of optimism fill our minds.

Intellectual functions

1. Memory disturbances.
   (a) Amnesia—is this for recent, intermediate or remote events; is there selective impairment of memory for special incidents or periods; what is the patient's attitude to his forgetfulness?
   (b) Hypermnesia.
   (c) Confabulation.
   (d) Déjà vu.
   (e) Retention and recall—test by giving an address, name or number, or 'Cowboy Story', and ask patient to repeat these. Ask patient to repeat digits forwards and then backwards. An intelligent normal person should be able to repeat 8-9 digits forwards and 6-7 backwards.
   (N.B. Results of these tests may be vitiated by lack of attention and concentration.)
2. Attention, concentration and consciousness.
   (a) Failure of attention and concentration and distractibility. To test concentration, ask patient to tell the days of the week or months of the year in reverse order, to do simple arithmetical problems requiring 'carrying over' (112–25), or subtract serial 7s from 100 (give answers and time taken—allow 2 minutes and 2 mistakes), to estimate the cost of 3 eggs at 60 cents per dozen.
   (b) Orientation for time, place and person. Record the patient's answers to such questions as the time of day and the date, the place where he is and his own name. Is there anything unusual to him in the way in which time seems to pass?
   (c) Confusion (subjective or objective).
   (d) Stupor, coma.
   (e) Depersonalisation.
3. Abstract thought. Request the meaning of proverbs. Ascertain the patient's ability to differentiate between items that have some similar properties or features, e.g. glass and ice, river and sea, child and dwarf. Note whether patient's replies reveal ability for abstract thought or whether thinking is concrete.
4. General information. Vary tests according to patient's educational

level, his experiences and interests. Answers to the following should be recorded in all instances:

(a) Name of sovereign and immediate predecessors.
(b) Name of Prime Minister.
(c) Capitals of France, Japan, Italy, Spain, England.
(d) Years of beginning and end of World Wars I and II.
(e) Six cities in Australia.

5. Intelligence. In assessing basic intelligence, use patient's history of educational and occupational attainments and his current approach to situations requiring some degree of intelligent appraisal.

Amnesia is a loss or absence of memory which may be complete or partial. In organic cerebral conditions where there is a diffuse impairment of brain tissue function leading to dementia, recent memory first becomes affected. Later, memory of remote events is also lost.

Following severe head injury, there may remain loss of memory for a period of time following the trauma (*post traumatic amnesia*) or in more severe injury, memory for events for a short time prior to trauma may also be impaired (*retrograde amnesia*). Apart from the time surrounding the injury, memory is unimpaired unless there are other factors present. Such amnesia, where memory before and after is satisfactory, is known as *circumscribed amnesia*. This may also occur following epileptic seizures and in hysteria. In the latter case, when anxiety is mobilised, for example by a conflicting or threatening situation, a process of dissociation or splitting off of some mental content may occur in such a way that the disturbing thoughts and memories are forgotten. The circumscribed amnesias present in both epilepsy and hysteria may be associated with a *fugue*, which is a state of altered consciousness in which the person makes a short or a long and sometimes complicated journey.

Patients who appreciate that their memory is failing, generally show some concern over this or try to cover up in various ways. In an hysteria, there is a lack of concern shown—the 'la belle indifference' mentioned under the section on mood.

Hypermnesia is the excessive retention of memories, especially of detail. It is found in certain prodigies and in disorders such as paranoid states and in the manic type of manic-depressive psychosis.

In *confabulation* the patient fabricates memories. This is one of the methods of covering up for memory impairment. It is seen most frequently in conditions leading to dementia, a state in which amnesia is usually the most outstanding symptom.

The French words *déjà vu* (already seen) refer to false memories. In this condition, a person believes that events or situations which he is experiencing for the first time have been experienced by him before. Out of any class of normal students a proportion will have experienced déjà vu phenomena. As a symptom of psychiatric disorder, it occurs in epilepsy where the temporal lobes are affected by the abnormal neuronal discharges, and in schizophrenia.

Retention. In order to remember something it must be taken in through the senses, particularly those of sight, hearing and touch, registered and then stored away. The ability to store away impressions is termed *retention.* To be able to utilise stored impressions or experiences, one has to be able to *recall* them. Both these functions of retention and recall may be deficient. Without the faculties of registering, retaining and recalling experiences, one would be hampered in learning new things and in modifying behaviour in the light of one's past successes and failures, as memory would be deficient.

The student may understand material presented: he may not take it in properly due to lack of attention: he may not take it in, in a suitable form for retention; and even if it is retained, he may have difficulty in recalling it. It often happens that we cannot recall something until we are given a clue or unless we have some well-learned framework about which we can pin our thoughts. For this reason, the major headings of the Mental State Examination should be known thoroughly as they will aid recall of associated facts.

Excessive anxiety in a situation may impair recall. We have seen in the section on ego defence mechanisms how some anxiety-producing memories are repressed and not allowed to enter consciousness—hence are not remembered.

It is interesting to see that a deep trance hypnotic subject, when regressed to childhood, may recall vividly details of some early experiences, many of which are not recalled once he is out of the trance state.

The main psychiatric disorders associated with failure in retention and recall are those in which there is a diffuse impairment of brain tissue function, that is, the organic brain syndromes.

Concentration. If we are keenly interested in reading something in our psychiatric text books we are able to direct our attention to the subject in hand without being diverted by a concurrent television programme. This faculty of attending to something in hand in spite of competing distractions is known as concentration.

Sustained attention or concentration can be impaired in numerous ways. One may simply not be interested in a subject or may deliberately shut it out. This latter may be a manifestation of negativism.

It is a fact that the more we are concerned with or preoccupied with our own problems the less we attend to things outside ourselves. So, in any psychiatric illness where mood is lowered and one becomes self-absorbed, attention and hence concentration are diminished. At the other end of the scale, when the mood is elevated, as occurs in the manic type of manic-depressive psychosis or in the excitement seen in some cases of catatonic schizophrenia, the attention moves quickly from one thing to another, giving rise to failure in concentration. When lack of concentration reaches an extreme degree and the patient cannot help switching his attention rapidly from one stimulus to another, the term *distractibility* is used.

Attention and concentration are also impaired in organic brain conditions where diffuse impairment of brain tissue function occurs.

Orientation. The normal person is said to be correctly oriented for time, place and person. This means that he knows the approximate time of day, the day of the week and the date; he knows where he is and does not readily become lost, as he can work out what are known as spatial relationships; he knows who he is and is able to name or correctly classify people in his environment. *Disorientation* is the term applied to the state wherein a person is defective in any of these areas, and it occurs in organic diseases of the brain. In such conditions, disorientation for time and place usually precede disorientation for person.

Confusion is the term applied to a state of perplexity, muddled thought processes, lack of awareness of one's surroundings, and disorientation. A confused person will answer irrelevantly or maybe not at all. Such a state, which occurs in many conditions where there is diffuse impairment of brain tissue function, may or may not be associated with obvious impairment of the state of consciousness of the patient. In confused patients, memory and judgement are also impaired to a varying extent.

When such a state of confusion is obvious to an outsider, the term *objective confusion* is applied.

Very often, if we are tired or worried about something, we say we feel confused. This feeling of confusion is probably due to lack of attention with consequent failure to grasp things and to our inability to decide on a particular course of action. If we are talking with a colleague and, in spite of our state of inner concern and tiredness and feeling of confusion, we can bring ourselves to concentrate on the subject in hand, then our state of mind is not apparent to our colleague. The term *subjective confusion* is given to this state, wherein we, the subjects of the confused emotions or feelings, are the only ones who know about them. Subjective confusion occurs in many anxious and depressed patients and in sufferers from schizophrenia. If we can form some sort of relationship with such a patient who feels this confusion and can hold their attention for long enough in conversation, it becomes apparent that there is really no permanent objective confusion.

A common mistake is to assume that an elderly depressed patient is confused and dementing (that is, has permanently lost some intellectual functions) when, in fact, it is only lack of attention and concentration and gross self-preoccupation that leads one to feel they are confused. It is remarkable to see how frequently 'lost' intellectual functions and 'confusion' clear after the depression is treated.

The term *stupor*, referring to a degree of retardation so great that a patient is completely unresponsive to stimuli, has been described in an earlier section on specific abnormalties of behaviour. Stupor, in the present context, refers to that state wherein consciousness is impaired due to organic damage to the brain or to a diffuse impairment of brain tissue function. In stupor, the patient's level of awareness is greatly diminished and contact with surroundings is consequently grossly deficient. The patient is mute and motionless. He responds to painful stimuli, but not in any purposeful way.

The final state wherein the patient is unresponsive to anything including painful stimuli is *coma*. This progressive loss of consciousness through stupor to coma may occur in many kinds of illnesses affecting only the brain or may arise from other more general physical conditions which also affect brain function. Among such states are included acute generalised infection, meningitis, encephalitis, diabetes mellitus in which coma can supervene in a hyperglycaemic state (high blood sugar) or in a hypoglycaemic state (low blood sugar) due, for example, to failure to eat when receiving insulin or similar acting drugs, or to the insulin dosage being too high. Barbiturates and alcohol are examples of drugs that may produce stupor and coma.

Depersonalization refers to the state where a person feels different or unreal or may lose his sense of identity. He may express this as feeling odd, peculiar, as if in a dream, as if he were outside himself looking at himself doing things. *Derealization* refers to the experience of things or events outside the person seeming different or unreal. Both depersonalization and derealization may occur together.

Mild transient depersonalization and derealization are not uncommon in normal individuals when they are fatigued. It may occur in association with practically any psychiatric illness, but perhaps more commonly in schizophrenia, depressive illnesses, epilepsy and hysteria. In passing, it might be mentioned that some authorities see depersonalization as essentially an emotional disturbance, rather than one of intellectual function.

Abstract thought. Normal people of average intelligence are able to generalise from concrete facts. If one asked an intelligent normal person what is the meaning of the proverb, 'Too many cooks spoil the broth' he will be able to give a concrete reply, such as 'Too many cooks over the same cooking pot or in the same kitchen will spoil the soup'. He will also, however, be able to abstract from the statement ideas or thoughts that can be applied to other situations as well, for example, 'If there are too many people engaged in some project they will get in each others way and achieve little of value', or 'If too many people tackle some project they may have such divergent and conflicting ideas about the project that no definitive plan can be put into operation'.

The latter two statements are manifestations of abstract thought as opposed to concrete thought shown in the first description of the meaning of this proverb.

Abstract thinking may also be determined by asking a person to differentiate between objects which differ but have some properties in common. For example, an intelligent well person would be expected to be able to see that a child and a dwarf may be the same size and yet differ in age.

Failure in abstract thought and a tendency towards concrete thinking is seen in schizophrenia and organic brain syndromes. People of low intelligence may be deficient in the ability to think in abstract terms and this, of course, does not necessarily mean they are schizophrenic or suffering from an organic brain syndrome.

General Information. Questions on general information are fairly non-specific in terms of eliciting particular mental state aberrations.

However, such questions often throw light on things such as interest, attention and concentration, memory and intelligence.

Intelligence. The assessment of a person's intelligence at interview or in conversation with him can be nothing but an approximation. Numbers of short tests may be applied to determine a little more accurately a person's intelligence quotient (IQ). Longer and more precise tests are the province of the clinical psychologist.

In spite of the difficulties in assessing intelligence, it is worthwhile to attempt to gauge our patient's intelligence, as this has some practical applications in their day-to-day management. More realistic activities and rehabilitation programmes for a patient can be planned while he is in hospital if something of his intellectual capabilities is known. Intelligence also has a great bearing on one's expectations of a patient in group psychotherapy programmes. As well as being helpful in patient management, an assessment of current intelligence as compared with a patient's educational and vocational history may provide some indication as to whether or not *intellectual deterioration* has occurred. Such intellectual deterioration is seen particularly in organic brain syndromes.

Mental retardation is the name given to a defect in general intellectual functioning existing from birth or before full development of the brain. This subject will be dealt with more fully later (Chapters 8 and 24).

Insight and judgment

The types of areas touched upon here are: What is the patient's attitude to his illness; does he regard his illness as 'mental' or 'nervous' in origin; does he think he needs treatment; what is his attitude towards social, financial and ethical problems; what does he intend to do when he leaves hospital?

No examination of a patient is complete without assessing his degree of insight and whether he displays good or defective judgment.

Insight has various levels of meaning in psychiatry. In a more general sense, it is the term applied to the recognition by a patient that he is ill. He is then said to have insight which may be complete, partial or absent. The degree of insight is not a satisfactory criterion for distinguishing neurotic from psychotic illnesses. Many markedly psychotic patients show complete insight in the sense that they know they are ill. Also, while insight may appear to be completely lacking in the florid stages of a psychotic illness, a patient, during recovery, may develop partial or complete insight into the fact that he was indeed ill and that his delusions and hallucinations formed part of his illness. At a second level, a patient may freely admit to being sick but will attribute the illness to physical factors, ignoring completely the contribution of intrapersonal and interpersonal difficulties in the genesis of his present state. This partial or spurious insight may occur in both neurotic and psychotic illnesses.

At what may be called a deeper level by psychotherapists, insight refers to the acceptance and understanding by patients of the part that more dynamic or emotional factors play in the production of symptons. The aim of many forms of psychotherapy is to develop this insight in a patient.

Judgment. A person's judgment is impaired under emotional stress, in organic brain syndromes and in many psychotic illnesses. If one asks a dementing old man what he intends to do when he leaves hospital and his reply is that he is going to undertake a University course it would be reasonable to conclude that his judgment is impaired.

The meaning of symptoms

Before closing this section, brief mention should be made of the possible meanings of symptoms.

Many cannot be accepted entirely on their face value. We must always remember that psychiatric symptoms may be the result of a number of things:

1. They may arise directly from some lesion or have been learned during stressful situations.
2. They may also be efforts to compensate for the effects produced by lesions or stressful situations, as in the happy front (manic defence) put on by people who are inwardly depressed; and
3. Psychiatric symptoms may represent efforts to counteract the actual lesion or stress.

It requires careful evaluation and constant practice to be able to determine whether one, two or all three of these factors are operating in the production of a particular patient's symptoms.

Difference between a psychosis and a neurosis

The terms 'psychotic' and 'neurotic' and 'psychosis' and 'neurosis' have been used freely in this chapter. These types of disorders will be looked at more closely in subsequent sections.

At this point however, a general distinction will be made between these two categories of illness.* In a psychotic illness the patient is unable to test and evaluate external reality in various spheres and he shows some degree of personality deterioration or disintegration. That is, there is some break with reality, and usually a fairly gross defect in ego-functioning or ego-strength. In neurotic illnesses, on the other hand, there is minimal loss of contact with reality and the patient does not show the same degree of personality deterioration. The I.C.D. states:

> Neurotic disorders are mental disorders without any demonstrable organic basis in which the patient may have considerable insight and has unimpaired reality testing, in that he usually does not confuse his morbid subjective experiences and fantasies with external reality. Behaviour may be greatly affected although usually remaining within socially acceptable limits, but personality is not disorganised. The principal manifestations include excessive anxiety, hysterical symptoms, phobias, obsessional and compulsive symptoms, and depression.

Both the neurotic and the psychotic patient may be greatly incapacitated in their ability to work and carry out everyday functions, and work

* The 9th Revision of the World Health Organisation International Classification of Diseases (I.C.D.) gives the following definition of psychoses: 'Mental disorders in which impairment of mental function has developed to a degree that interferes grossly with insight, ability to meet some ordinary demands of life or to maintain adequate contact with reality. It is not an exact or well defined term. Mental retardation is excluded.'

ability does not necessarily constitute a point of difference between these two groups of disorders.

In practice, it may sometimes be a difficult task to conclude whether the clinical picture presented by a particular patient is psychotic or neurotic.*

---

* The concept of psychosis has been broadened during the past several decades. Classically the term psychotic indicated a loss of reality testing or an impairment of mental functioning manifest by delusions, hallucinations, confusion and impaired memory, emphasis being on the loss of reality testing. To this concept has been added severe impairment of social and personal functioning manifest by social withdrawal and inability to carry out normal daily activities, and ego regression, which has come to be synonymous with severe impairment of social and ego functions.

8

THE BASIS OF THE MAJOR SYMPTOMS AND SIGNS OF PSYCHIATRIC DISORDERS

In a psychiatric hospital, one sees patients presenting with a variety of symptoms and signs such as we have discussed in Chapter 7. Certain symptoms or signs may be found grouped in particular patients. These groupings form particular syndromes or clinical entities.

A number of clinical entities or syndromes* have certain symptomatic features in common and together form separate or broad groups of conditions, each group having characteristic features with regard to the symptoms and signs presented by patients. In this section, rather than dealing with symptoms and signs singly and somewhat indiscriminately, we shall study four major groupings, the psychoses, the neurotic disorders, organic brain conditions and mental retardation, looking particularly at what is known of the causation of the oustanding symptoms and signs occurring in each grouping.

In large general psychiatric hospitals, one sees more patients suffering from psychotic disorders than patients suffering from the other three categories of illness mentioned, with perhaps organic brain conditions in second place. There are probably a number of reasons for this:

1. Mental retardation usually requires special programmes with an emphasis on education in its broad sense and special hospitals are usually set aside to deal with such a special problem. Also, many mentally retarded people remain within their family circle.
2. The organic conditions may be acute and reversible or chronic and irreversible in nature. Acute organic conditions usually clear up relatively rapidly with proper management. A large number of the chronic organic conditions occur in an older age group in which the cardiovascular system is frequently deteriorating and the life expectancy of most of this group is not great. This, of course, is a generalisation and younger patients may suffer from chronic or irreversible organic conditions, and with modern medical care, their life expectancy is but little shortened. Large numbers of

* A *syndrome* refers to a group of symptoms and/or signs that are recognised as frequently occurring together, and for descriptive purposes such a constellation of symptoms or signs is given a particular name or label.

ageing people with organic brain conditions are managed at home or in nursing homes and private hospitals.

3. Many psychiatric hospitals have sections where patients suffering from neurotic disorders are managed in a special programme. Other hospitals may specialise predominantly in dealing with such patients. In general however, admissions of patients suffering from a neurotic disorder to hospital inpatient care constitute but a small proportion of total admissions to psychiatric hospitals. This is because the majority of these patients can be treated as outpatients, or day or night patients, in community psychiatric facilities, in general hospital units or in doctor's consulting rooms.
4. People suffering from a psychotic illness with its more bizarre presentation are less readily tolerated by the general population than are people with neurotic symptoms. Also, perhaps, a more realistic reason for the presence of larger numbers of psychotic patients in hospitals is that psychotic disturbance frequently leads to behaviour which warrants at least some temporary segregation from the population at large.

The various clinical entities falling within these major subgroups will receive attention in the next chapter dealing with psychiatric classification. A description of most of the symptoms and signs occurring in psychiatric illness has already been given. We shall look now at the causes, where they are known, of a number of symptoms or signs, attempting to place them in the major subgroups. It will become obvious that, in many instances, a particular symptom or sign occurs in more than one subgroup. The *Ninth Revision of the International Classification of Diseases* will serve as the basis for our groupings.

The psychoses, neurotic disorders, organic brain conditions and mental retardation are not the complete range of disorders met with in psychiatry. Other groupings include: the personality disorders, sexual deviations, alcholism, drug dependence, physiological malfunction arising from mental factors, special symptoms or syndromes not elsewhere classified, acute reaction to stress, adjustment reaction, disturbance of emotions specific to childhood and adolescence. This sounds an imposing list, but a large proportion of patients will be found to be suffering from conditions falling within the four major groupings already mentioned and which will now be discussed.

Psychoses

The psychoses are severe emotional illnesses where varying degrees of personality disintegration are found. They are commonly characterised by loss of contact with reality, distortion of perception, regressive behaviour and attitudes, and abnormal mental content, including delusions and hallucinations.

Using our mental state examination headings as a basis, we find that the major symptoms and signs fairly specific to psychotic disorders fall under the following headings:

GENERAL APPEARANCE—catatonic features, neglect of personal appearance.

BEHAVIOUR PATTERNS—retardation, stupor, stereotypy, echopraxia (and echolalia).

FORM OF SPEECH—acceleration, retardation, mutism, thought blocking, pressure of thoughts, disordered association of ideas, incoherence, neologisms.

CONTENT OF SPEECH—delusions, hallucinations.

MOOD—depression (severe), elation, inappropriate affect.

INTELLECTUAL FUNCTIONS—impairment of intellectual functions does not feature greatly in the psychoses except in those of organic origin. Failure in abstract thought, i.e. concrete thinking does occur in some psychotic illnesses.

INSIGHT AND JUDGMENT—both frequently affected.

Catatonia

The features of catatonia may be said to be due to the peculiar generalised rigidity of muscles that exists. This state is not a neurological one, nor a motor paralysis, but arises out of the patient's inability to will or want to move. Without this will or drive patients may be remarkably suggestible or compliant to the will of others to the extent of leaving their limbs in bizarre postures imposed (flexibilitas cerea), or even poking their tongues out when asked to after you have made it clear you wish to stick a pin in it. Echopraxia (and echolalia), examples of automatic obedience, probably have their origins in this compliance and abnormal suggestibility. The reverse of this compliance to the will of others occurs in many patients however, in which state they resist orders or do the opposite (negativism). Why this happens is little understood.

One theory relating to the presence of catatonic features is that people who show these have never really developed confidence in their own decisions. This may have been brought about by parents or parent substitutes insisting that the child follow decisions that were made for him. If the child acted independently, he was made to feel that he had acted wrongly and thus felt guilty. Such a child may well fail to develop confidence in his actions and never develop reliance in what is termed his 'capacity to will'. Later in life, this anxiety produced by making decisions and carrying out actions, persists. Such a person may find some relief in obsessive compulsiveness or by being compliant, or he may show swings from being compliant to exerting his own will, a form of ambivalence.

When anxiety is excessive, and the defences of compliance and obsessive compulsiveness break down, being insufficient to deal with the anxiety, then the patient virtually freezes and undertakes no action. Any action would imply willing something. To will, in such patients, is to create anxiety or even panic, and the development of catatonia is the ultimate defence against such panic. There are all degrees of the state and the ambivalence mentioned may be marked in some patients. For example, if you proffer your hand for a handshake the patient may begin to extend his (a willed action), then suddenly withdraw it.

The catatonic patient may be in a state of stupor at one time and be extremely overactive or manic at another, even to the extent of being violent or homicidal (catatonic excitement). At such times it is as if the catatonic patient loses his fears and guilt and defies his previous fear, presenting symptoms and signs quite opposite to those seen in catatonic stupor.

Patients with the symptoms described above are suffering from a form of schizophrenia. As mentioned earlier, catatonic features may also be present in certain organic brain syndromes. The theory of the development of catatonia described above should not be stretched to the point where it is seen as a cause of schizophrenia. Theories relating to the aetiology of schizophrenia will be mentioned in Chapter 13.

Retardation and stupor

In the same way as a patient suffering from catatonic schizophrenia may enter a phase of stupor, so the sufferer from psychotic depression may first show retardation, which, at its most extreme degree, renders a patient completely motionless and relatively or completely unresponsive to stimuli, a condition referred to as depressive stupor. Stupor occurring in severe depression is not associated with the peculiar muscular rigidity that occurs in catatonia and catatonic stupor.

Retardation, as it occurs in affective or mood disorders presenting with severe depression, is an all pervasive condition evidenced by a slowing of thought, speech, action and physiological mechanisms. Thus lachrymal glands (tear glands), salivary glands and other digestive glands in the alimentary canal produce less secretions, giving rise to inability to cry, dry mouth and symptoms relating to the alimentary canal in many patients suffering from psychotic depression. It would appear that the actions of the parts of the brain associated with mood and vegetative functions are in some way deficient, giving rise to retardation and other symptoms found in psychotic depression and other psychiatric conditions where depressive mood changes form part of the clinical picture.

Abnormalities in thought processes

To describe what is known and conjectured about the basis of thought disorder would occupy several volumes. Here we shall look briefly at some of the factors that are probably implicated.

1. Thinking undergoes development from infancy to adulthood. The young child's thoughts revolve around himself (*egocentric thought*). Up until 3 or 4 years of age he is unable to differentiate satisfactorily between himself and the outside world and, in varying degrees, between different objects in the outside world; he tends to invest inanimate objects with the qualities of life (*animism*). There is a tendency to attribute qualities of an object to part of the object or to something associated with the object. For example, a spider's web may be endowed with the same fearsome qualities as the spider itself. To a child, there are magical properties in thought (*magical thinking*). To think 'good things' may protect the child from harm. On the other hand, a child who has destructive wishes towards parents may become extremely anxious lest they really die as a result of his thought. Again, up until the time the child is able to discriminate between himself and the outside world, concrete rather than abstract thought predominates. Thoughts are seen as a material part of the young child, something that can be touched or even taken away. The same thing applies to thoughts which are drawn or written down.

Many of the above characteristics of a child's thinking processes form part of what is known as *primary process thinking.*

The mature and normal adult on the other hand, uses little of this mode of thinking and instead, his thinking is more realistic, logical and practical and indicates that he has a sound grasp of who he is and what his correct relationship with his total environment is, that is, his so-called *ego boundaries* are intact. Such normal adult thinking where conscious rational ideas predominate is termed *secondary process thinking.*

The schizophrenic patient undergoes some degree of personality disintegration, his concept of himself as a person becomes unclear (that is, his ego boundaries become blurred) and he reverts or regresses to primary process or infantile thinking. However, even in the most regressed patient suffering from schizophrenia, there is always some residual ego function or realistic portion of the personality remaining. This can lead to the situation where, at one time, thinking is rational and understandable and, at another time, it may show the hallmarks of primary process thought. Both realistic or secondary process thinking and primary process thinking may occur in the same conversation with a patient, making the conversation extremely difficult to follow and giving rise to the phenomenon of thought disorder.

2. Seen in young children and also occurring in some sufferers from schizophrenia is what has been called *paralogic thinking.* In this type of thinking, a person identifies subjects on the basis of similar or identical predicates. As an example of this, a male patient for whom I was caring once wrote a letter to the British Government. At about this time, Kruschev's letters to the British Government made headlines in the local newspapers. The common or similar predicate was the writing of a letter(s), the subjects were the patient and Mr Kruschev. This young man came to believe that he was Mr Kruschev, or at least was related to him.

Since many different objects or people can form the subject of an identical predicate and the observer is not to know which of the subjects a patient will identify, the patient's communication may appear quite bizarre, unpredictable and completely incomprehensible.

3. Apart from the effects of primary process thinking and paralogic thinking in the production of thought disorder, there is the idea put forward by Schilder, in 1920, that conscious thinking is guided by a *determinative idea.* Conscious thinking has a goal towards which clear and relevant thoughts move. Along the fringe of this determinative idea or main theme are numerous less clearly defined thoughts or associations running parallel to the main theme. The schizophrenic patient is said to be unable to stick to the determinative idea, and associated ideas from the fringe insinuate themselves into the main stream of thought producing a disjointed communication which may or may not be understood. This may be represented diagrammatically (Fig. 1). In (a) the determinative idea starts at S and finishes at G (the goal). In (b) a topic starts at S, follows a number of associations unpredictable to the listener, and the final goal is not reached.

In mild form such erratic thought processes may lead to 'woolly', vague conversation. When more marked, 'knight's move' thinking and gross

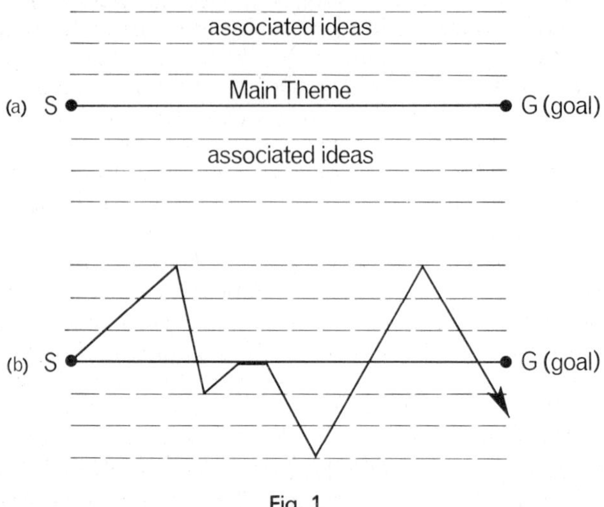

Fig. 1

disorders of association, even incoherence, may become apparent. Negative symptoms in schizophrenia such as *poverty of ideation* with gaps or little or no free-flowing speech may also arise out of a patient's inability to follow a determinative idea. It may be that in thought blocking, a patient loses the main theme, is aware of this and tries often unsuccessfully to find his way back. (This comment on thought blocking is rather speculative and other mechanisms may be involved.)

A *neologism* is a word of the patient's own making. We are dealing with this term under form of speech, as a neologism is not infrequently a condensation of whole or parts of numbers of words. One theory of their origin is that neologisms are invented by schizophrenic patients because their experiences both perceptual and emotional may be so bizarre that words in everyday use are inadequate to describe them.

Delusions

Delusions are superficial indications of the presence of gross mental disorder. What is the basis of these ideational symptoms, consisting of false fixed beliefs not in keeping with a person's educational or cultural background? The content of a delusion is largely determined by the patient's past and present experiences. Without some religious background or knowledge of religion, it would be impossible, for example, to entertain delusions pertaining to religion. Likewise, before the discovery of electricity and wireless waves, such forces could not form part of a delusional belief. It is relatively simple to explain the content of a delusion but it is more difficult to explain the form of this symptom, and why it occurs. In fact, there has never really been a satisfactory explanation of this phenomenon.

In looking at dynamic theories, we find that most authorities agree that the defence mechanisms of denial and projection are paramount in delusional development. Regression also occurs, and ego boundaries become extremely tenuous with the development of such regression. Ego boundaries being deficient, internal drives or instincts which are denied by the patient are more readily projected on to the environment, that is, the denied instincts are generally attributed to other people or other objects or situations in the environment. In this context, delusions may be seen as justification of something the patient cannot accept in himself. He denies ideas or feelings, and blames someone or something in his environment for them. Thus, delusions may be seen to have some protective value to an ego about to be overcome by unacceptable impulses of the id. To give an example, one may quote the development of delusions of jealousy. Freud sees such delusions as arising out of unconscious homoerotic trends, or homosexual impulses present in the id. Such homosexual impulses are unacceptable to the conscious mind and, through the defence mechanism of denial, a male patient with homoerotic trends would say, 'I don't love him'. He projects his erotic feelings on to a woman whom he also feels affection for, and the situation becomes 'I don't love him, *she* does'. The belief that the woman loves the male whom he unconsciously 'loves', forms the basis of delusional jealousy. It can be seen that such a patient is denying unacceptable impulses, and the delusion in some way protects him from accepting these impulses in himself.

One view developed by Freeman, Cameron and McGhie regarding the aetiology of schizophrenic illness and manifestations of some other illnesses, and one that is gaining wider acceptance, is that schizophrenia is essentially an illness of the ego, the outcome of which is a loss of what is termed 'ego-feeling' or 'self experience' necessary for a person to see himself as an entity, separate from his environment. That is, 'ego boundaries' are deficient. The basic ego pathology does not allow the patient to perceive the world realistically nor does it allow his total personality or ego to develop satisfactory attitudes or relationships. If a person does not perceive or see things as they really are, that is, realistically, due to this breakdown of ego boundaries, delusions may develop to justify or make more meaningful the state he or she experiences subjectively. It is as if the remaining healthy portion of the ego or personality is acting in a rational way to give an explanation of the person's inner feelings. In this sense, delusions are again seen as an attempt to repair a break with reality arising out of the basic disintegration or fragmenting of the ego.

Whether one is born with a sick ego or whether this develops due to early experiences, forms part of another question which will be looked at later. It is extremely difficult to tie these theories in with the sudden onset of what are known as *primary delusions*, in which quite suddenly there is some disturbance of symbolic meaning. Usually following emotional stress of some kind, the patient, for example, suddenly knows that the street lights on the hill have a special message or meaning for him, that all the people in the room are hostile to him, that they are there to judge him; on reading a passage in the newspaper about a train disaster in another state, he may immediately feel that he is responsible for it, and even responsible for all the world's calamities.

These delusions are sudden and fully developed, and are immediately believed by the person who experiences them. They are similar to some of the 'insights' experienced by people who have been given lysergic acid or mescaline.

Once the primary delusion occurs, further rationalisations of delusional intensity usually follow to explain the experience. These delusions are termed *secondary delusions*, and the term is also applied to delusions following hallucinations or emotional experiences wherein the symptoms are interpreted in a delusional fashion.

There is no end to the development of such secondary delusions, as seen in the example quoted on page 71.

One young male schizophrenic patient who was incontinent could not be convinced that he was not in the ocean where fish were biting him. The discomfort of wet urine on his skin was delusionally interpreted as his being in the ocean with fish biting him. One could say that it was an *illusion* inasmuch as here occurred a misinterpretation of an external stimulus (a prickling sensation from wet urine) but the idea assumed the proportions of a delusion, as it was held in spite of the efforts of the therapist to alter this false belief.

Hallucinations

There are a number of psychiatric conditions in which hallucinations may occur. Included among these are schizophrenia, organic brain syndromes including epilepsy, psychoses associated with physical conditions and sometimes the affective psychoses.

As with other psychiatric symptoms and disorders, there are a large number of theories relating to their origin.

Psychoanalytic theory for example, stressed regression in psychotic states, and just as a small child does, the adult patient is seen to project outside himself his wishes and complexes, replacing reality by imagining that certain things are actually happening.

As with delusions, the content of hallucinations may be understandable in terms of the patient's drives and life experiences, but such a theory does little to elucidate the actual phenomenon of an hallucination. Why does it happen? After all, many people have similar drives and life situations and yet never hallucinate.

Again, following the concept developed by Freeman, Cameron and McGhie, a basic ego weakness may be seen as the central factor. If the inherent or developed ego structure is weak, we see that a person has a diminished sense of personal identity, that is, has blurring of ego boundaries, including both mental processes and the sense of body image. In such a situation, where the patient's bodily sensations, special senses and thoughts, have no definite boundaries within the person, all types of sensations and mental impressions, though occurring in the individual, may appear to be derived from outside. This could account for all forms of hallucinations, auditory, visual, olfactory, gustatory, visceral and tactile, and as mentioned earlier, delusional interpretation of such phenomena may occur. The voices heard are from people persecuting the patient, the tactile sensations are caused by people directing electricity at him, and so forth. The essential feature in the development of most hallucinations is some blurring of ego boundaries from whatever cause, whether it be the type of ego fragmentation that occurs in schizophrenia, or whether it is produced by altered states of consciousness and by any other factors that may reduce awareness of the mental and bodily ego.

Normal individuals, if placed in a situation where stimuli such as light, sound and touch are reduced to a minimum (*sensory deprivation*), will experience this lack of personal identity or lack of mental and bodily awareness to such an extent that they feel disembodied and may even experience auditory and visual hallucinations.

In that state between wakefulness and sleep, normal people may experience *hypnagogic hallucinations.* For example, they may hear their name called. Hallucinations may be produced by direct electrical stimulation of parts of the cortex of the brain and depending, for example, on whether it is a visual or auditory area that is stimulated, the person will experience visual or auditory hallucinatory phenomena.

The abnormal electrical discharge occurring in epilepsy may have a similar effect in producing hallucinatory phenomena, the type of course, depending on the site of the abnormal neuronal discharge.

Drugs such as mescaline, through their effects on the brain may produce hallucinations in normal people.

Depression

Though in this section we are interested essentially with depression of psychotic intensity, comments will be made on depression as a normal component of living, as it is seen in neurotic illness, and finally as a psychotic symptom. It is perhaps more satisfactory to view depression as a continuum, having different levels of intensity, than to talk in some arbitrary fashion of different types of depression in the major subgroupings of psychiatric disorders.

Fluctuations of mood are common to us all, and indeed it is perfectly normal to react with feelings of depression or elation to appropriate stimuli. A change in either direction becomes abnormal when it is of an intensity or duration out of all proportion to the precipitating event.

There are some people who, as a feature of their personality, appear to have a consistently low mood level; others appear to have a consistent mild elevation of mood with its accompanying increase in activity. These people are said to have an affective personality. Some in this category of affective personality disorders, show alternating moods of elation and sadness (cyclothymia) quite independent of external circumstances, which suggests that the mood changes are stimulated by internal factors of some sort.

The symptom of depression, apart perhaps from anxiety, is the commonest symptom occurring as part of the clinical picture in psychiatric disorders. It may be associated with all types of functional disorders (Chapter 13), with organic brain conditions, and with a host of abnormal physical conditions.

From a dynamic point of view, the essential precipitant of depression is a loss of some valued object, that is, of someone or something important to the individual.

The loss of a valued object may occur in :

1. The death of a person important to the patient.
2. The realisation by the patient that a failure of an important interpersonal relationship exists (frequently with the spouse).
3. A severe disappointment in relation to an institution or occupation to which the patient has devoted the best part of his life.

The loss of anything naturally produces sadness. Depression supervenes when the quality of the sadness changes, or when the duration of the sadness persists for an inordinate length of time.

In neurotic depression (page 227), there is an element of pessimism added to the sadness caused by a situation of loss. The patient is convinced that what has happened must happen again, or that things will never improve. Such depression occurring in a neurotic depression, frequently responds to environmental changes such as diversionary bright company or activity.

When a depression reaches such intensity that the person experiencing it can only see things in terms of the way he feels and not as they really are, then the depression is of psychotic depth. Environmental situations or external reality, which may be essentially bright and satisfactory, are seen by the patient as being quite hopeless and unsatisfactory. Such a patient may indeed be said to be out of touch with reality and to be suffering from depression of psychotic intensity.

Having seen that loss precipitates depression, we shall look further into the psychodynamic mechanisms in psychotic depression. Knowledge of these mechanisms is rather fragmentary. One theory emanating from psychoanalysis is that the following are prerequisites for the development of psychotic depression:

1. A constitutional and inherited over-accentuation of oral eroticism.
2. A special fixation of the libido at the oral level.
3. A severe injury to infantile narcissism brought about by disappointments in love such as loss of the breast, or mother having to attend to the new-born babe.
4. The occurrence of this disappointment before resolution of the oedipal complex.
5. The repetition of this primary disappointment in later life.

As already mentioned, a major precipitating factor is a loss in later life, which mobilises the same sort of feelings that occurred in infancy when the individual felt abandoned by his mother.

The loss might appear quite trivial to an outsider, for example, the death of a pet canary, but the reaction to the loss depends to a large extent on the loving emotion the person has invested in the lost object.

Paradoxically, apparently pleasant events may precipitate depression. For example, the marriage of a son or daughter or a promotion in a job. In the first example, the marriage of one's child may be seen as the end of a satisfying or need-fulfilling parent-child relationship; in the second, promotion means a new position and added responsibility which removes security, and which may be seen as jeopardising previous friendships with workmates.

An added factor in the development of depression appears to be that such sufferers are basically aggressive, and rather than turn their aggression on to the appropriate persons who may in consequence reject them, they turn their aggression in on themselves by the unconscious mechanism of introjection.

The seat of emotions is considered to be the hypothalamus and adjacent interconnected portions of the brain. There are some cases of depressive illness where depression of suicidal intensity descends extremely rapidly, suggesting perhaps that some sudden biochemical change may be a factor in the genesis of depression. In many cases, this is borne out by a patient's good responses to antidepressant drugs, and sudden relapses when drugs are reduced or stopped.

Depression in these patients frequently lifts on the reintroduction of appropriate drug therapy, without any effort to deal with the possible psychodynamic factors.

This does not do away with the possibility that both dynamic and biochemical factors have a part to play, perhaps to a different extent in different people.

The following comments, though conjecture, are food for thought.

If, in psychosomatic disorders (Chapter 18), emotions are associated with biochemical changes, it is conceivable that dynamic factors leading to depression may concurrently alter the body's biochemistry.

Elation

Just as, within limits, depression and sadness occur in the normal individual, so does the reverse emotional state. This has been mentioned already when speaking of the affective or cyclothymic personality. Once again, this state of heightened mood is not considered abnormal unless its intensity or duration is out of all portion to the precipitating event, and again one may postulate dynamic or biochemical factors or both, as casual.

In looking at the psychodynamic mechanisms of elation or mania, it is very likely that a patient with this symptom has the same problems as the patient with depression but reacts by denial of these problems, and not only does he act as if the problems were not there, but he goes to the opposite extreme.

Inappropriate affect

No adequate explanation exists for this fundamental of psychotic symptoms.

Inappropriate or incongruous affect or mood consists of a lack of coordination between mood and thought processes occurring in schizophrenia.

It may be seen as a splitting of the personality wherein ideas expressed (a person's ideation) are out of step with, or not in keeping with simultaneous mood.

Intellectual functions

As a broad generalisation, intellectual impairment does not figure largely in functional psychotic disorders. Where psychotic manifestations are associated with organic brain impairment however, a major fall-off in intellectual functions may occur.

If we look at the various capacities subsumed under our heading of intellectual functions it will become apparent that they are affected in varying degrees.

In terms of memory, which involves registering, retaining and recalling facts, there will be a disturbance if the patient is preoccupied, hallucinated or has other disorders of perception. Attention and concentration will also be impaired, as will the ability to use abstract thought.

When one looks at intelligence, which is something measurable to a fair degree of accuracy, it may appear to be quite markedly impaired. Such impairment, however, is only apparent when the psychotic patient is unable to use his intelligence properly because of such symptoms as thought disorder, lack of drive or volition, preoccupation with hallucinatory phenomena and delusions.

Many patients with long-standing schizophrenia may appear to be mentally retarded, but at certain times, particularly if overcome by an intercurrent physical illness, they regain their grasp of reality and show nothing of the supposed diminution of intelligence.

If psychotic disorders are present in young children, their ability to learn will be greatly affected and quite obviously, while the psychotic process predominates, they will always function poorly in intelligence tests. Intelligence however, is not 'damaged' *per se* and the potential for learning and further intellectual development remains.

Insight and judgment

The loss of insight and judgment appears to be related essentially to the degree of personality deterioration and to the extent of the loss of contact with reality.

With respect to judgment, patients who are living in a fantasy world bearing little relationship to real situations are unable to make decisions appropriate to the existing eternal circumstances.

The degree of insight varies in psychotic patients and there is a general tendency towards loss of insight. Some quite deluded and hallucinated folk however, may have complete insight into the abnormality of such experiences from the outset, while others show increased insight as their condition improves. Still others maintain a delusional system in such a way that it does not interfere with day-to-day living. Though holding fixed false beliefs, they are able to keep these to themselves, except under great stress, frequently knowing that, although they do not regard such beliefs as abnormal, other people do—a form of pseudo insight. When a patient's unreal world is kept apart from the real world, his delusions are said to be *encapsulated.*

Neurotic disorders

Neuroses are emotional maladaptations due to conflicts within the personality.

The conflicts within the personality about dependence, aggression or sexuality lead to the state of unconscious anxiety, which is felt directly as anxiety or which, through the utilisation of the ego defence mechanisms (Chapter 6), are unconsciously and automatically controlled, giving rise to a number of different clinical types of neuroses.

It is not known precisely why different people develop different neurotic syndromes as a result of the common precursor, anxiety.

Within the framework of our mental state examination headings, we shall look at the more common symptoms and signs found in the neuroses, throwing some light on to the origin of a number of these.

GENERAL APPEARANCE—anxious facial expression, symptoms and signs suggestive of hysterical neuroses involving gait and physical abnormalities, tics.

BEHAVIOUR PATTERNS—overactivity, compulsions.

FORM OF SPEECH—acceleration.

CONTENT OF SPEECH—obsessions, phobias, hypochondriasis.

MOOD—depression, anxiety, panic, agitation, 'la belle indifference'.

INTELLECTUAL FUNCTIONS—failure of attention and concentration, amnesia and depersonalisation as they occur in hysteria.

INSIGHT AND JUDGMENT—insight in the sense that a person knows his reactions are abnormal is not impaired; judgment may be minimally impaired.

Abnormal gait, physical abnormalities, amnesia, and 'la belle indifference'

These may all feature in hysteria and, as the basis of these symptoms and signs is similar, will be dealt with together.

In hysteria, anxiety is converted into physical symptoms or leads to a state of mental dissociation.

Janet proposed that the manifestations of hysteria were due to one series of ideas becoming isolated from consciousness in the process of dissociation, which is one of the ego's defences against anxiety.

Freud produced evidence that a disurbance of sexuality gives rise to the anxiety in such cases. He maintained that hysteria in all its forms is related to the climax of infantile sexuality, the oedipus situation, wherein occur incestuous wishes towards the opposite-sexed parent and hostile or destructive feelings towards the same-sexed parent. Having destructive feelings towards the same-sexed parent produces fear of retaliation or, in Freudian terminology, castration anxiety. Freud suggested that the personality of people liable to exhibit hysterical symptoms was one with fixation at the phallic or early genital phase. An emotionally charged situation which cannot be faced leads to a regression to this point of fixation with reactivation of emotions relevant to the oedipus situation. These emotions are intolerable and are excluded from consciousness by the mechanism of dissociation or conversion.

Dissociation leads to the symptoms of fugue and/or amnesia, double or multiple personality and depersonalisation. Through the mechanism of conversion, physical abnormalities and disturbances of gait occur along with complacency in the presence of gross objective disability produced through this mechanism ('la belle indifference'). Examples of physical disabilities ensuing include convulsions, paralysis, involuntary movements, bizarre gait and sensory disturbances such as pain or partial or complete anaesthesia.

An interesting manifestation is *astasia abasia* which describes the condition where movements may be carried out when lying or sitting down, though standing and walking cannot be performed.

Obsessions, compulsions

These two symptoms are usually found together and are said to have a common origin. They are essentially neurotic symptoms; the patient has insight into the fact that they are unnecessary and tries to resist them. Most commonly, they are found in obsessive-compulsive disorders, but as with other neurotic symptoms, they may also be found in association with affective psychoses, schizophrenic reactions and psychoses of organic origin, in particular following encephalitis lethargica.

The symptoms are most likely to appear in people who suffer from *anankastic* (obsessive-compulsive) *personality disorder.* These people are rigid, inflexible and conscientious, they love order and discipline and are punctual and precise. These are but some of the easily-seen personality traits and they represent an over-compensation for feelings of internal insecurity.

Underneath the prim and correct demeanor of these people, there is often found a crude, turbulent sexualism occasionally expressed in perversions.

Stresses of various kinds lead to the appearance of obsessional and/or compulsive symptoms which reflect the basic weakness in the personality structure. Obsessional ideas and fears arise out of a sense of insecurity and compulsive actions are said to represent expiation for failure and inadequacy.

In psychoanalytical theory the anankastic or obsessive-compulsive personality is regarded as having an overdeveloped and savagely critical superego, this being associated with anal-erotic tendencies and a sadistic quality of personality.

We must not delude ourselves into thinking that an adequate explanation of the basis of obsessions and compulsions has been presented. It would occupy many pages of print to present a coherent picture of the dynamic theories relating to these symptoms, and this will not be attempted.

Phobias

Phobias occur in patients in whom anxiety has been displaced on to some symbolic idea, object or situation. The main ego defence mechanism involved is displacement. By avoiding the object or situation on to which anxiety has been displaced, the person attempts to control his anxiety.

Phobias principally occur in the condition called phobic state, but the symptom may also be seen in association with other psychiatric conditions.

Psychoanalytical theory of phobias

In Freud's classical case of Little Hans, who was a child who refused to go into the street for fear that a horse might bite him, the root of the phobia was a conflict between the boy's instinctual strivings and his ego demands.

A reconstruction of the case is as follows:

1. Hans had a sexual desire for his mother.
2. He feared and hated his father and wanted to kill him.

(The foregoing are the basis for the oedipal complex with fear of retaliation from father—castration anxiety.)

3. His sexual excitement and desire for his mother were transformed into anxiety.
4. Displacement occurred and fear of horses became symbolic for fear of father.
5. Hans' illness also kept him at home near mother where he wanted to be.

Various mental mechanisms may be involved in the development of phobias, namely, repression, displacement, projection, indentification and regression.

At this stage one should point out that there are many authorities who feel that the available evidence in the case of Little Hans does little to validate certain psychoanalytic principles that Freud drew from it. It is now recognised that not only genital sexuality but pregenital drives as well (e.g. aggression and dependency) are a source of anxiety leading to the development of phobias.

Dollard and Miller, who are experts in learning theory, describe phobias as learned responses to painful experiences.

'Separation anxiety' also appears to play an important part in the development of certain phobias, for example, 'school phobia', which will be described in a later section.

Organic brain conditions (or syndromes)

Except for a few discrete syndromes, the I.C.D. groups all brain syndromes of organic aetiology under the rubric 'Organic Psychotic Conditions'. It is arguable whether a person suffering, for example, from simple senile dementia should be regarded as psychotic without an overlay of more florid symptoms, but the broadening of the definition of psychoses (Footnote, page 84) would appear to allow the encompassing of this group of disorders which in the past has tended to occupy its own nosological compartment.

In order not to confuse the issue this section will deal with symptoms and signs emanating specifically from organic brain disorder and which are present whether or not there is a greater or lesser degree of those symptoms and signs described under the heading 'psychoses'. In other words psychotic features such as loss of contact with reality, and abnormal mental content, for example delusions and hallucinations, will not be described again in this section.

General appearance—in some instances, personal care neglected, neurological conditions may be present, poor nutrition.

Behaviour patterns—there may occur lowering of ethical standards and exaggeration or emergence of personality traits leading to particular behavioural manifestations.

Form of speech—incoherence in severe cases, aphasia, circumstantiality, perseveration.

Mood—shallow or labile.

INTELLECTUAL FUNCTIONS—amnesia, confabulation, poor retention and recall, and lessening of attention and concentration, leading to impairment of comprehension, calculation and learning capacity, disorientation, 'Frontal lobe syndrome', a fall-off in General information and Intelligence levels.

INSIGHT AND JUDGMENT—both impaired.

Neurological conditions may form the basis of the organic psychotic conditions and be well in evidence, for example, Huntington's chorea (page 158).

Old and dementing patients in particular *neglect personal hygiene* and stick not infrequently to a diet of tea and biscuits leading to gross *nutritional deficiencies.*

We have seen that *incoherence* occurs as an extreme degree of thought disorder in schizophrenic patients. It may also be present in organic psychotic conditions arising from impairment of brain tissue function.

Aphasia is essentially a neurological symptom due to organic damage to, or disturbance of function of, areas of the cerebral cortex that are concerned with speech. The brain lesions which produce aphasia are located in the left hemisphere in patients who are right-handed and vice versa. Two types of aphasia are described, *motor aphasia* in which the patient cannot express ideas properly, and *sensory aphasia* in which he cannot satisfactorily comprehend what is said to him. Areas of dysfunction situated anteriorly lead to motor aphasia and lesions posteriorly lead to sensory aphasia. There is frequently a mixture of both types of aphasia present in the one patient.

If a patient is severely aphasic it is difficult, if not impossible, to elicit other facts sought in mental state examination.

Circumstantiality occurs especially in people suffering from mental retardation or organic psychoses. It is also seen in normal people. The disturbance of logical associations seen in schizophrenic thought disorder is not present however. Either through an inability to distinguish between what is trivial and what is not, or through a high degree of distractibility, departures are made from the determinative idea or main theme, and masses of irrelevant detail are communicated. The essential difference between schizophrenic thought disorder and circumstantiality is that in the former the goal is not reached (Fig. 1), whereas the person who is circumstantial in speech eventually reaches the goal. The process may be shown diagrammatically (Fig. 2).

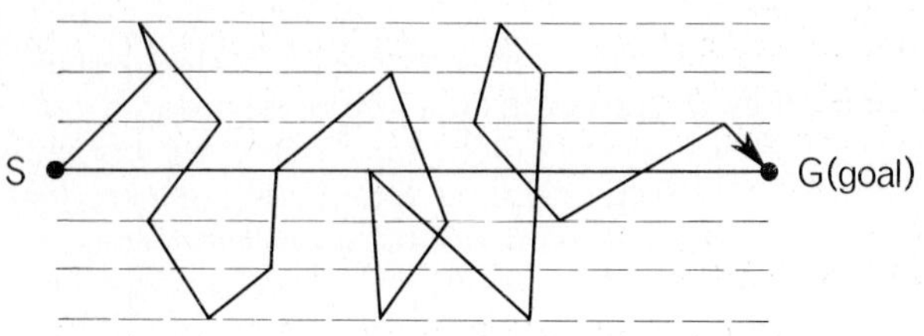

Fig. 2

The idea being presented starts at S. Conversation meanders through unnecessary detail but finally reaches the intended goal G. This type of speech is referred to colloquially as 'beating about the bush'. Patients with organic psychoses or severe mental retardation, sometimes demonstrate what might be seen as the opposite of circumstantiality. They have difficulty in getting off a particular topic and repeat words, phrases or a single theme. This phenomenon is known as *perseveration.* The inability to register new impressions and elaborate on these and the loss of the capacity to think quickly and accurately lead a patient to cling to the already elaborated or tried words and themes.

Egocentricity probably has the same basis inasmuch as a person who cannot take in new impressions concentrates on the thing he knows best—himself.

Such symptoms as *shallowness* and *lability of affect, amnesia, poor retention and recall, lessening of attention and concentration, disorientation, fall-off in intelligence* and the features of *frontal lobe syndrome,* may be accounted for by a decrease in the number of functioning cerebral neurones. This lack of functioning may be temporary or permanent depending on the cause, and the areas of grey matter affected determine to a large extent, the particular symptom displayed. For example, the temporal lobes play an important part in memory function, and lesions of the parietal and temporal lobes are associated with spatial disorientation.

Confabulation arises out of the patient's endeavours to fill in gaps in memory. A full description of an entirely fictitious day's activities, including working, shopping, etc., may be given when a patient is asked what he did yesterday, whereas in fact, he was in a hospital ward the whole time.

There are some who regard *insight* and *judgment* as being functions largely of the frontal lobes of the brain; however, the evidence for this appears inconclusive. Many patients after leucotomy show quite good insight and judgment, but this again may depend on the number of association fibres cut at operation. Many patients show sound judgment when speaking of events happening in the distant past, while judgment in recent matters is poor.

We have looked at the basis of some symptoms and signs found principally in organic psychoses. Much has been discovered about the more specific functions of various areas of grey matter in the brain, the impairment of which leads to fairly specific symptoms and signs. The complete delineation of specific functional areas is extremely complicated however, as these areas of the brain are connected together by multitudinous fibre tracts, and poor function in one part may produce distortion of function in another. As a generalisation, therefore, it seems reasonable to state that the basic symptoms and signs described under organic psychoses are due to impairment of brain tissue function from a wide variety of causes.

Mental retardation

The term mental retardation refers to a condition of arrested or incomplete development of mind which is especially characterised by subnormality of intelligence. In many instances, mental retardation may be associated with some other mental disorder.

Symptoms and signs will vary greatly according to the conditions leading to mental retardation.

GENERAL APPEARANCE—physical abnormalities and characteristic appearance are present in many conditions associated with mental retardation.

BEHAVIOUR PATTERNS—these again encompass a wide range and depend to a large extent on the condition leading to mental retardation, or on the associated brain condition, and on the degree of mental retardation. With gross mental retardation the patient may be dirty in habits. He may be quiet and apathetic, or overactive, violent and destructive. So-called tension habits are found, consisting in nail-biting, rocking to and fro, head banging and self-mutilation. Many of the behaviour patterns may be contributed to by the programme of management of these patients or to the lack of suitable management programmes.

CONTENT OF SPEECH—generally there is apparent poverty of ideation, this being govered by the inadequate vocabulary mastered by the mentally defective patient. As mentioned earlier, the patient with severe mental retardation may be unable to formulate words, much less sentences.

MOOD—often normal; may be extremely labile or shallow if there is associated brain damage. Low frustration tolerance may lead to explosive outbursts of rage.

INTELLECTUAL FUNCTIONS—unless some concomitant mental disorder of an organic or psychotic nature is present, registration, retention and recall are unimpaired. Apparent loss of memory may be due to lack of understanding of what is communicated to the patient or to his inability to apply himself to the task of recall.

Mentally defective patients are able to concentrate on simple tasks that interest them. The ability to formulate abstract thought is dependent on the person's linguistic tools or vocabulary. General information is deficient.

INSIGHT AND JUDGMENT—are dependent upon the level of intelligence, lack of which is the fundamental symptom or sign in uncomplicated mental deficiency.

What are the reasons for this arrested or incomplete development of mind characterised by subnormality of intelligence? We shall answer this question in general terms, leaving the description of more specific aetiological factors to a later section.

Intelligence

Most naturally occurring measurements such as height and weight are ranged under what is called a normal distribution curve. The majority of people are at or near average height. There are many fewer people who are very short or very tall.

Over the years, a number of tests have been devised to determine the level of a person's intelligence. Among these are the Wechsler Adult Intelligence Scale (W.A.I.S.), and the Wechsler Intelligence Scale for Children (W.I.S.C.), both used in individual test situations. Two other less time-consuming and less reliable tests which can be used with individuals or with groups are the 'Mill-Hill' Vocabulary Scale which tests verbal ability and the 'Progressive Matrices' test which gives an estimate of non-verbal ability.

From the application of such tests a measure of the function of intelligence or Intellegence Quotient (IQ) is determined.

If the IQ of a very large number of people is assessed, this measurement is found to follow a normal distribution curve in the same way as physical characteristics such as height and weight. This is shown in Fig. 3.

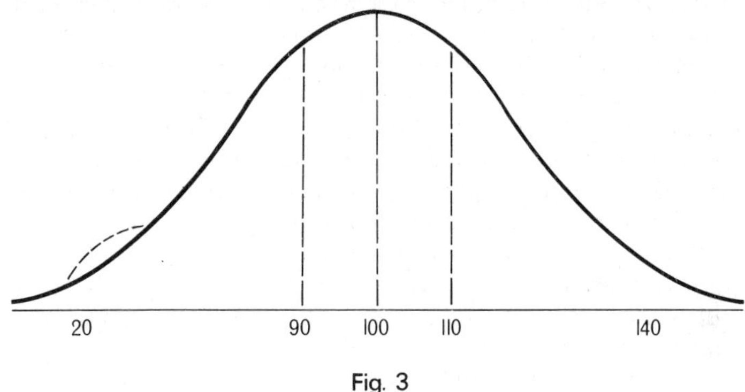

Fig. 3

IQs between 90-110 are considered average and the large bulk of the population fall within this range, represented by the area under the curve between these figures. It will be seen for example, that the areas under the curve at either end of the scale, between 20-40 and 120-140 respectively, are much less than between 90-110, which means that more people have IQs near the average than at either end of the intelligence scale.

Such variation in intelligence as portrayed by the normal distribution curve is largely due to multiple inherited factors. Most authorities agree that intelligence level is determined by approximately 75% hereditary factors and 25% environmental and accidental factors. In short, this means that some are born 'brighter' than others. Obviously, however, opportunity, singleness of purpose and sound application to learning and to one's occupation may to some extent outweigh the limits apparently set by an inherited level of intelligence.

We are speaking of mental retardation, and therefore are concerned with those people whose intelligence falls towards the lower end of the normal distribution curve for intelligence. The interrupted line superimposed on the normal distribution curve in Fig. 3 is produced by a population of people suffering from severe grades of mental retardation brought about by factors other than multiple hereditary factors. This severely retarded population produces the 'hump' at the lower end of the distribution-curve for intelligence.

Factors which usually cause a marked lowering of intelligence and hence the hump at the lower end of the intelligence scale include:

1. Specific hereditary factors leading to specific physical conditions affecting the brain.
2. Factors affecting the mother during pregnancy such as virus infections, for example rubella (German measles).
3. Factors during the birth of the child such as asphyxia and other brain damage.
4. Factors after birth, for example, severe brain trauma and infections of the brain.

Apart from these four groups of factors, early segregation into institutions and 'homes' leading to lack of educational opportunity, defective vision or hearing, reading disabilities, emotional disturbances, epilepsy, etc., may affect learning ability and lead to diminution of performance in intelligence tests.

In summary, the basis of the essential symptoms and signs in mental retardation consist of:

1. Multiple genetic or hereditary factors, operating in the same way as multiple genetic factors produce variation in height.
2. Factors such as specific genetic abnormalities and other factors operating before, during and after birth, all of which produce some abnormality or inadequate development of brain function.

9

CLASSIFICATION OF PSYCHIATRIC DISORDERS

We have studied the principal psychiatric symptoms and signs (Chapter 7) and have looked at the basis of some symptoms and signs occurring in four of the major subgroupings of psychiatric disorders (Chapter 8). It would indeed be most convenient to be able to say that particular symptoms and signs occur only in particular conditions, and to be able to place 'conditions' in water tight compartments. Nothing could be further from the real state of affairs however.

Psychiatric disorders are not 'diseases' in the way one tends to look upon conditions seen in general medicine. For example, sufferers from diabetes mellitus may have various symptoms arising out of an alteration in the level of blood sugar. It is known that such alterations in the level of blood sugar are due to a deficiency in the production of insulin in the Islets of Langerhans, and the specific lack may be corrected by administering appropriate doses of insulin or similar-acting substances. A patient with a stricture of the pylorus may see a doctor because he is unable to keep food down and because he has had symptoms relating to his gastro-intestinal tract for some time. The clinical picture plus a barium meal examination may reveal the presence of a peptic ulcer with scarring in the surrounding tissues, and a slow emptying time of the stomach. Removal of the obstruction at operation will both relieve the symptoms and confirm the presence of an ulcer with scarring. A peptic ulcer is perhaps not an ideal example as there may be other factors present, including psychological ones, in the production of the ulcer, and removal of part of the stomach may not have dealt with the true aetiological factors, but may simply be a cure for the current symptoms. The point being made however, is that, in general medicine, it is easier to delineate a cause, name a condition and deal with it by appropriate action. In psychiatry on the other hand, the delineation of causes is not so straightforward and great variations can arise in clinical states, as, in most instances, the presenting clinical picture of a patient is the outcome of a multitude of factors. In some conditions there may be constitutional factors, for example, specific metabolic disturbances. There may also be definable organic conditions leading to psychiatric symptoms and signs largely amenable to direct treatment measures. However, in the majority of cases, there are other less well-defined, quite elusive factors at work. The patient's personality may be a factor in an unhappy adaptation to life.

His efforts to adjust, to deal with conscious and unconscious motivations, and his tendency to utilise particular ego defense mechanisms may lead to particular behaviour patterns.

Apart from the difficulty in delineating treatable causes of mental disorders, there is a vast difference in people's attitudes to so-called medical disorders and mental disorders. Medical disorders are often associated with physical pain, disability and death, and therefore there is a ready acceptance of these conditions as being undesirable and warranting treatment. On the other hand, the majority of mental disorders do not lead to physical pain, disability and death but to particular symptoms and signs which may broadly be called behavioural manifestations. There are vast differences both transculturally and even within a particular culture in attitudes towards these behavioural manifestations, ranging from a high degree of acceptance to non-acceptance, the latter signifying their undesirability. If certain behaviour is acceptable or not undesirable are we correct in classifying its progenitor as a mental disorder? One may put another question: At what stage of severity do psychiatric symptoms and signs indicate the presence of mental disorder?

Defining mental disorder is as difficult as defining mental health. Mental disorders may be said to be manifest by behaviour which deviates from an acceptable concept of normality, and hence is regarded as undesirable. However, how does one decide upon a concept of normality or desirable behaviour and upon what is undesirable? Should preferred homosexuality for example be regarded as undesirable? How deviant or undesirable do personality traits have to be before they can be said to constitute disorders? Is the behaviour of certain antisocial personalitites to be regarded as emanating from mental disorder, or are these people to be seen as bad and not the proper concern of mental health professionals? Doubtless there will always be differences of opinion on these questions.

In all endeavours to understand man and his environment, man has reduced the complexity of phenomena into categories, in other words classified them. This has occurred in medicine, the classification of disease entities being called a *nosology* (Gk. *nosos* = disease, *logos* = science). In general medicine there appears to be little argument as to what should or should not be classified as a physical dysfunction or disease, but, as indicated above, there are still some differences of opinion about including certain groups of symptoms and signs or conditions in a classification of mental disorders. This fact can be highlighted by looking at two groups of conditions. In the first, the person experiencing the condition suffers and regards it as undesirable, and people without the condition would also regard it as undesirable. Such conditions include schizophrenia, anxiety neurosis and severe affective illnesses. There is little difficulty in classifying these conditions as mental disorders and rightly the concern of mental health professionals. A second group exists in which those with the condition may or may not find their state undesirable depending on the degree of distress it causes them, while most people without the condition would regard it as undesirable. Here one might include, for example, exclusive homosexuality and schizoid personality traits.

If mental health professionals take the view that any deviation from an ideal state of positive mental health is abnormal they will be tempted to label the deviant as suffering from a mental disorder and try to treat him. If indeed his condition is causing him distress, or in other words he finds it undesirable, then therapeutic interference is commendable. If, on the other hand, his deviance from what is considered the ideal state of positive mental health is causing him no distress, then any diagnostic labelling or attempted treatment is regarded by many as being highly questionable. It is at this point that psychiatry has been accused of acting as an agent of social control by designating as mentally ill someone who does not feel sick or ill and who does not seek help. On the other hand, there are some glaring exceptions where a person may not believe himself to be ill yet cause untold suffering to others. A person exhibiting catatonic excitement (page 189) or manic depressive psychosis, manic type (page 206) are two examples. It is the author's view that a number of psychiatry's most outspoken critics have never experienced or even seen such severe disturbance which does warrant some form of intervention, even when the patient does not conceive of himself as being ill.

In spite of the difficulties mentioned above, there have been many classifications of psychiatric disorders put forward over the years, some on a purely descriptive basis, that is, essentially in terms of presenting symptoms and signs, and others on an aetiological (causal factors) basis. One method of categorising disorders is into *functional* and *organic*, functional indicating that there is no demonstrable physical basis for psychiatric disorders, and organic meaning that there is a physical cause for the condition. The depressive illnesses and schizophrenia would formerly have been placed unhestitatingly into the category of functional disorders. With more refined techniques of investigation however, it is possible that specific biochemical abnormalities may be found to account for these 'illnesses'. Indeed there are many authorities today who, on the basis of current investigations, are convinced that a metabolic or biochemical basis will be found for some of these reactions. If this proves to be so, then such disorders should probably more correctly be defined as organic rather than functional.

Another method of categorising the more common psychiatric disorders is into psychoses and neuroses, and on page 83 the major classical differences between these two groups of disorders have been touched upon. In practice however, it is not always easy to place the total picture presented by a patient into one or other clear cut compartment. Some symptoms and signs are found to occur in both these major subgroups. Also, other major subgroups of disorders or syndromes have either neurotic or psychotic manifestations accompanying their own basic symptoms and signs. In some instances, even more difficulty is experienced in being precise about disorders falling within the same major subgroups. For example, is the patient essentially suffering from an affective psychosis and showing some schizophrenic features, or is the picture presented essentially a schizophrenic reaction with some superimposed affective element? In such a situation, a clinician has to exercise expert judgment in order to decide which of the presenting features predominate or are more fundamental in the disorder presented by the patient.

International Classification of Diseases

The classification of mental disorders followed in this book is contained in the 9th Revision of the International Classification of Diseases (World Health Organisation). Of Section V, entitled 'Mental Disorders', the Manual of the International Statistical Classification of Diseases, Injuries, and Causes of Death, states:

> This section of the Classification differs from the others in that it includes a glossary, prepared after consultation with experts from many different countries, defining the contents of the rubrics. This difference is considered to be justified because of the special problems posed for psychiatrists by the relative lack of independent laboratory information, upon which to base their diagnoses. The diagnosis of many of the most important mental disorders still relies largely on descriptions of abnormal experience and behaviour, and without some guidance in the form of a glossary that can serve as a common frame of reference, psychiatric communications easily become unsatisfactory at both clinical and statistical levels.

The value of a classification

The first useful feature of a classification that provides descriptive guidelines is that it clarifies communication. It allows people to communicate more readily with each other about phenomena they deal with in common. The application of a particular name to a particular cluster of symptoms and signs becomes a convenient shorthand way of describing a state that would otherwise require the use of a multitude of words. A standard nomenclature, that is the specific terms used to identify categories and disorders, should lead to more precision in diagnosis and the knowledge that different workers are speaking about the same condition. A common world-wide classification makes it more possible to compare relative incidences of different disorders in different countries and locations, under different social, economic and cultural conditions. In other words, a common classification has statistical value and serves as a basis for comparison.

The giving of a correct diagnostic label to a patient after a sound appraisal of his symptoms and signs and of factors leading to their production will, to the initiated, give some indication of the probable course or outcome of the illness and suggest broad guidelines for management. It is known, for example, that psychotically depressed patients are at a high risk of suicide, and steps can be taken to prevent such an unhappy occurrence and initiate appropriate treatment.

Patients suffering from hebephrenic schizophrenia are usually more unpredictable than those with typical paranoid schizophrenia. One may perhaps, give only minimal support to some manipulative patients suffering from certain types of personality disorder.

It has been pointed out above, that a diagnostic label provides only a board general guide and one must not slip into the bad habit of lumping all schizophrenic patients into a single stereotype and treating all alike. Patients have individual personalities, and a schizophrenic illness for example, is the end result of a multiplicity of factors, and many differing factors may require attention. Each patient must be seen as an individual and treated as such. While on this topic of the error of casting into the one mould as far as management is concerned, all patients in a particular diagnostic category, I would point out that people working in psychiatry should never use terms like, 'He's a schiz'. Apart from subtracting from the patient's individual or unique personality, this shows extremely imprecise thinking as it is not made clear whether the patient is suffering from a schizoid personality disorder or from one of the group of schizophrenic illnesses.

In the interests of clarity, the I.C.D. glossary is quoted freely throughout this text and the 9th Revision of the I.C.D. (W.H.O.) is included as Appendix I to this volume. It is sound practice to refer to the classification when particular conditions are described in later chapters, and also as you meet with patients falling under various sub-categories during your working day. In this way you will gradually familiarise yourself with the names of conditions described under each major category.

10

FACTORS IN CAUSATION OF PSYCHIATRIC ILLNESS

Comment on some early beliefs about the causation of mental illness was made in our first chapter. Usually a single factor was implicated and this may have been sin, some demon, a punishing god or a wandering uterus.

With the advance of knowledge, it has become apparent that one cannot attribute normal or abnormal behaviour of man to any single cause. We and our patients undoubtedly wish things were simple and easily explained, which could both tend to make us accept some simple and spurious dogma about causation, and our patients to demand a single cause for their present emotional state. As workers in psychiatry, sometimes placed in the position of being expected to know all the answers, how often have we been tempted to give a concrete answer, a god-like pronouncement, that 'your problems are the result of your parents' poor relationship', that 'getting locked in the cupboard as a young child is definitely the cause' or that 'the trouble may be placed at the feet of heredity'?

Such factors may be blameworthy to differing degrees but ex cathedra pronouncements may close the door to further delineation of problem areas and to their understanding and eventual acceptance and 'working through' by patients.

To be realistic, sometimes we all need some sort of rationalisation to explain our actions, and in the same way a patient may require, for the time being, some face-saving explanation in terms of a definitive cause until his ego resources are sufficient to look squarely at himself.

The above two paragraphs may seem like having 'six this way and half-a-dozen the other' but they highlight the need to be sensitive to the needs of our patients as well as being cautious in our decisions and comments about causation. If this chapter does nothing more than make us wary of dogmatic statements regarding causation of psychiatric illness, then it may have some value.

Let us visit for a moment, a busy casualty ward in a general hospital. In one cubicle is a middle-aged woman with a deformity above the right wrist joint resulting from a fall onto the outstretched hand, and by coincidence a middle-aged man is in an adjoining cubicle with a similar injury.

Clinical and X-ray examinations in both cases reveal a fracture of the right radius with a typical dinner fork deformity at the lower end of the right upper extremity; there is no evidence of any other bone pathology. It is fair to assume that in both patients the fractures (Colles fractures) have resulted from undue stress being placed on the bone, the stress of trauma being the necessary and sufficient cause of the fracture and deformity.

Knowing the cause of such a deformity, rational remedial steps may be undertaken, consisting of reduction of the fracture under general anaesthesia and the application of suitable splinting to keep the bone ends in close proximity until union occurs.

When we ask the resident doctor or casualty sister how the fractures occurred, we are told that the woman, on her way to water her garden at night, fell over a toy wheelbarrow left on the side path by a grandchild, whereas the man stumbled and fell as he has done often in the past. Now why should a man often stumble and fall? In this instance, we learn that this man has foot-drop due to peripheral neuritis, arising from a long-standing dependence on alcohol, associated with neglect of proper nourishment.

Many people with peripheral neuritis and foot-drop do not sustain Colles fractures, therefore peripheral neuritis with foot-drop cannot be regarded as a necessary and sufficient cause of a Colles fracture. We are still left with the feeling, however, that the man's chances of sustaining a fracture would have been much less if he had not been dependent on alcohol.

One could go back further into this man's history and discover the following possible factors. His drinking may have commenced during frequent and painful attacks of gout, a disorder determined largely by hereditary factors. On the other hand, a high intake of alcohol may have arisen through our patient being unable to cope with certain life stresses arising out of either a constitutional or developed inability to deal with a stress, or perhaps he had to face repeated immense stresses intolerable to the 'average' person. Again, the stress may be multiple in origin, connected with employment, family, financial, social or cultural difficulties, to give just a few examples.

Being faced with such a problem as our male patient presents, a good doctor would probably see the correction of the painful deformity as the number one priority, and then would make it his business to institute treatment or some management programme for the multiple contributory factors. The patient requires help with these associated factors and their correction will obviously lessen the chance of his sustaining other fractures.

If we look at both our patients, we may say that in each case a fall was the precipitating event leading to a fracture. In the case of the man, we find a multitude of obvious predisposing factors present in his background.

In psychiatry, it is relatively rare to find a simple cause and effect relationship or a single necessary and sufficient cause for the development of symptoms (e.g. female patient). This is partly due to our lack of knowledge of aetiologies, but largely due to the fact that psychiatric illnesses generally have many factors in their causation (e.g. male patient).

Also, the aetiology of a particular psychiatric illness frequently does not involve a simple chain of events, but there may be present at conception, in the distant past or early enviroment, and currently, a variety of factors all contributing to the behaviour of a patient before us.

Before dealing with the various factors or groups of factors in turn, it would be well to clarify some of the terminology and arguments surrounding the area of aetiology. Brief comment will be made on heredity versus environment, organic versus psychological, essential and contributing factors, predisposing and precipitating factors.

Heredity versus environment

Controversy, fortunately diminishing, has raged for years over the relative influence of heredity and environment. Protagonists for heredity claim that psychiatric illness is due essentially to the particular genetic structure inherited from one's ancestors, while the environmentalists say that the genes do not matter, and claim that psychiatric illness is due entirely to environmental factors. These statements are, of course, at the extreme poles of both contentions.

It is foolish to maintain such a clear cut dichotomy in the light of present knowledge. The basic symptomatology of a few illnesses can be attributed solely to hereditary factors, some illnesses can be attributed essentially to environmental factors, but the vast majority are probably the result of both hereditary and environmental factors interwoven in varying degrees.

Organic versus psychological

Another argument which, in some instances, may be a variation on the heredity-environment theme is the split between organic as opposed to psychological causes, especially in the development of what are termed functional disorders. The term 'functional' is applied to an illness in which there is no demonstrable basis or cause in terms of altered structure or even in altered biochemistry.

Most psychiatric disorders currently fall into the functional category as, for most, no specific organic or biochemical cause has been demonstrated. A person adhering to the organic theory holds that psychiatric illness will be found to have an organic or biochemical cause which may be hereditary or genetic in origin. People holding essentially to the psychological viewpoint believe that psychiatric illnesses, in the main, arise out of a person's psychological development, his total life experiences, and his environment both in the home and in the broader social setting.

The argument does not exist in those psychiatric illnesses with a known organic cause, such as cerebral arteriosclerosis or other brain pathology leading to mental symptoms, or in the case of folk who, owing to structural and/or biochemical abnormality of the central nervous system, are mentally retarded. However, even with similar brain pathology, different patients may exhibit a variety of superimposed psychotic, neurotic or behavioural symptoms which are, to a large extent, determined by pre-existing personality characteristics or previous life experiences—an example of both organic and psychological factors operating in the same patient.

Psychiatry cannot yet state whether mainly organic or psychological factors are operating in the large group of functional illnesses. It may be that some will be found to have a basis in altered biochemistry or physiology which is genetically determined. However, in the same way that emotional changes provide measurable alterations in levels of various chemical substances in the body, psychological factors may lie behind such biochemical changes as may be found associated with psychiatric illness. So, which would come first—biochemical (or organic) or emotional (i.e. psychological) changes? As yet there is no real answer to this question.

Essential and contributory factors

In the case of our male patient with the Colles fracture, the essential cause of the deformity or fracture was trauma resulting from a fall. Contributory factors to this injury were foot-drop due to peripheral neuritis arising out of alcoholism and poor food intake. Other contributory factors were those leading to his drinking habit.

When we focus upon psychiatric illnesses, it becomes clear from our previous discussion that few essential causes are known, though as we shall see later, there are a variety of possible contributory factors in the genesis of psychiatric disorders.

Predisposing and precipitating factors

Another way of describing certain causal factors in psychiatric illness is to speak of pre-disposing and precipitating factors. It is rare for one event or circumstance to be the sole determinant of a psychiatric illness: certain factors such as heredity and learned ways of adapting to life, as indicated in an earlier section on personality development (dynamic factors), in many instances may be said to predispose an individual to succumb later to some disturbing event or precipitating stress. A person not so predisposed would most likely be able to adjust to life's stresses without developing psychiatric symptoms.

As similar factors may, in different circumstances, be seen as essential, contributing, predisposing, or precipitating, in terms of differing orientations to psychiatry, no attempt will be made to organise causal factors under any of these headings. Instead, the outline given in Fig. 4 will be followed.

Heredity

As certain perhaps unfamiliar terms will be used in this section, an outline of the development of genetic principles will be given first.

In the Abbey of Brunn, an Austrian Monk, Gregor Mendel, experimented with garden peas during the years 1856-1863 and published his findings in 1866. The importance of his work was not recognised until 1900, sixteen years after his death. Part of Mendel's experiments consisted in cross-pollinating pea plants. He studied, in particular, the attributes of tallness, shortness and colour of peas and pods, and conceived

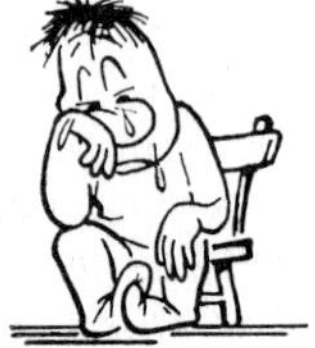

Fig. 4. **Factors in causation of psychiatric illness**

the idea, after counting the different types of plants resulting from hundreds of cross-pollinations, that single characteristics such as tallness behave as if determined by paired particles. An Englishman, William Bateson, developed Mendel's theory, and a Danish botanist, Wilhelm Johannsen, in 1909, introduced the term 'genes' to describe the 'particles' which he referred to as 'determinants', refusing to identify them in a material sense.

Improvements in the microscope throughout the nineteenth century in Germany, and study of individual cells confirmed the presence in cell nuclei, of bodies later known as chromosomes, and a German zoologist, August Weismann, in the 1870s, saw the chromosomes as the basis of heredity and postulated their role in sexual reproduction.

The elementary factors in heredity, the genes, were at first considered to be minute invisible protein particles or large molecules situated along a chromosome like beads on a string. This concept has changed, and a gene with the basic chemical structure of deoxyribonucleic acid (DNA) is seen as a clearly defined functional region (locus) which maintains its identity, has a specific action, is capable of reproducing itself, and provides a code for the production of proteins which are often enzymes which speed chemical processes in cells. Chromosomes are simply chains of genes, and are long, fine filaments which, at certain times, assume a form like that of a tightly coiled spring.

In normal growth, cells multiply by a process called mitosis and each newly formed cell or daughter cell is an exact replica of the adult cell, carrying the same number of chromosomes which are composed of exactly similar gene material. These chromosomes are paired, one member of the pair having been derived from the male, and one from the female 'parent'.

Before an organism produces offspring, germ cells are formed, the germ cell from the male containing half the number of chromosomes normally present in cells of the organism and that from the female also containing half the number of chromosomes normally present. At fertilisation, germ cells from the male and female organism come together in a single cell, thus reconstituting the number of chromosomes found in the nuclei of the cells of the adult of the species.

Consider a pea plant with gene T (for tallness) on one chromosome, and the allele (alternate form) t of that gene on another chromosome. Chromosomes bearing sets of identical or allelic genes are present in the plant in pairs known as homologous pairs. The pea plant may produce both male and female germ cells, and Figure 5 shows what can happen to T and t in the process of germ cell formation, and fertilisation, which produces a zygote, a single cell which may grow into a new plant.

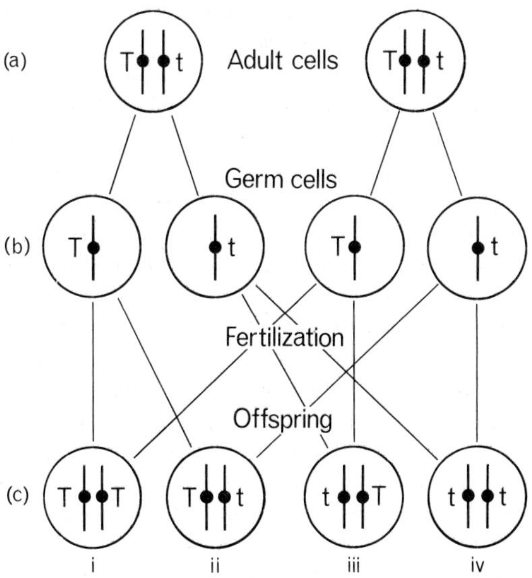

Fig. 5. The formation of germ cells and mode of transmission of single hereditary characteristics

Of the four possible plants formed from the four zygotes, three are tall (TT, Tt, tT) and one short (tt). Since T and t occur at corresponding places (loci) on paired chromosomes and give rise to tall plants if one of each is present (Figure 5c, ii and iii), T (for tallness) is said to be dominant to t (for shortness). t is then said to be recessive, and two recessive genes must be present before the characteristic they determine is expressed (in this case, shortness).*

The above serves to demonstrate the transmission of a single characteristic in a plant, such as tallness, and fits Mendel's original concepts that single characteristics behave as if determined by paired particles.

The process is, however, not always as straightforward as postulated by Mendel and other workers. Genes on the same chromosome may be separated by 'crossing over' due to the formation of chiasmata during germ cell formation. The process of chiasma formation is shown in Fig. 6, which is a representation illustrating the formation of germ cells. Without going into details of meiosis or reduction division, it may be stated that when germ cells are formed there are two divisions of the nuclei and but one division of the chromosomes. It is this operation that gives rise to half the chromosome number in a germ cell (male or female). During this process the crossing over occurs in one or more places in each chromosome, so that genes originally on one chromosome may be trans-

FIRST STAGE OF MEIOSIS

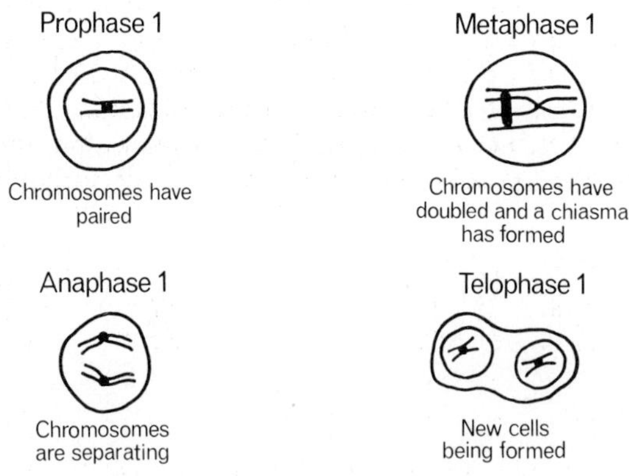

SECOND STAGE OF MEIOSIS

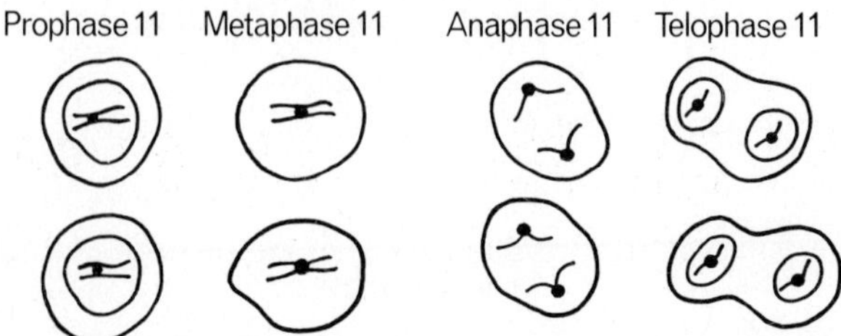

Fig. 6. The formation of germ cells (meiosis) and chiasmata

* When considering genetic transmission in humans, a person receiving the same gene from both parents is said to be a homozygote for that particular gene, cf. homologous pairs TT and tt. If different genes appear on corresponding loci of paired chromosomes, one from each parent, the person is said to be a heterozygote, cf. Tt.

ferred to another chromosome, and so a chromosome may undergo an alteration in its genetic structure, the genes as mentioned above having specific activity in terms of contributing hereditary characteristics.

The formation of chiasmata or crossing over leads to the possibility of great variation in transmitted hereditary characteristics.

As well as this feat of 'crossing over', variation may arise through suppression of a particular gene by its opposite number (its allele) or by other genes present in the cell nucleus.

In every human cell there are forty-six chromosomes or twenty-three pairs, one member of each pair being derived from the female parent through the ovum, the other from the male parent through the sperm. One pair of chromosomes are called sex chromosomes as they are responsible for the definitive sex of an individual; namely XX (female) and XY (male), and the remaining twenty-two matching pairs are called autosomes.

Using tissue cultures of skin biopsies or blood cells (lymphocytes are used mainly), it is possible with special techniques to observe chromosomes in the cell nucleus under a microscope at a stage when they are just beginning to divide. Such chromosomes, still joined together at a point called the centromere, can be divided into twenty-three pairs which are numbered according to their size and the position of the centromere. Pairs 1-22 are autosomes, pair 23 are the sex chromosomes. Figure 7 is copied from an enlargement of a photograph taken through a microscope and shows the chromosome complement (karyotype) of a normal male.

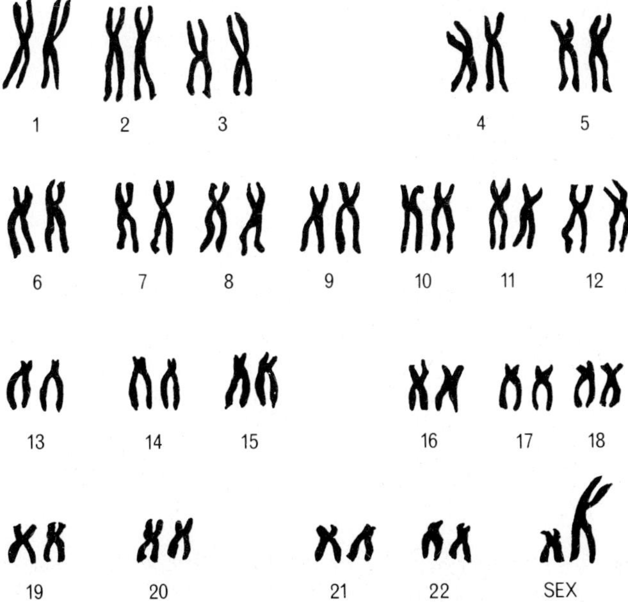

Fig. 7. Karyotype of a normal male. Drawn from a photograph provided by Dr Brian Turner, former Director of the Oliver Latham Laboratory, Psychiatric Centre, North Ryde

What we are looking at are paired chromosomes from a human nucleus, arranged for counting and the study of morphology (shape). With this large number of chromosomes, each composed of multitudinous genes, the possible variation in characteristics displayed is enormous through the effects of single genes or a number of genes and through the massed effects of many genes, the latter being referred to as multifactorial or polygenic inheritance.

In human beings, it would seem that the measurable effects of heredity are greatest in determining physical characteristics, somewhat less in the determination of intelligence and much less still in the determination of other aspects of personality.

We have seen that physical characteristics, intelligence, and other aspects of personality may have a bearing on the development of psychiatric illness, but when we look at heredity as an essential cause, we find but few illnesses where hereditary factors are definitely implicated. It must be pointed out however, that it may be many decades before the role of heredity in the abovementioned characteristics and in illness is fully worked out.

Some disorders due essentially to hereditary factors

Gene abnormalities may arise through mutations, that is, deleterious changes which alter the previous genetic structure. These mutations may be sub-microscopic and are referred to as point mutations.

Huntington's Chorea arises from such a point mutation and is due to a single abnormal dominant mutant gene.

The transmission of the dominant mutant gene is represented schematically in Fig. 8, in which only one pair of chromosomes from each parent is shown, the abnormal gene H being carried in this instance by the mother.

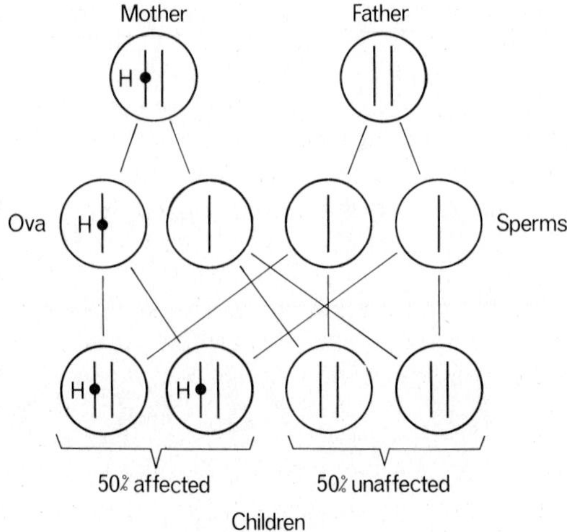

Fig. 8. Mode of transmission of Huntington's chorea

It is apparent from Fig. 8 that the chances are that 50% of the children of such a union will be affected and 50% unaffected. (The illness manifests itself most frequently in middle life.)

Tuberous Sclerosis (or Epiloia), is another condition due to a dominant mutant gene. A patient with this condition classically displays mental retardation, epilepsy, adenoma sebaceum and other skin lesions, and frequently tumour formation in the heart and kidneys.

Phenylketonuria, usually associated with mental retardation, is considered to be due to recessive mutant genes. The transmission of such a recessive disorder is represented schematically in Fig. 9.

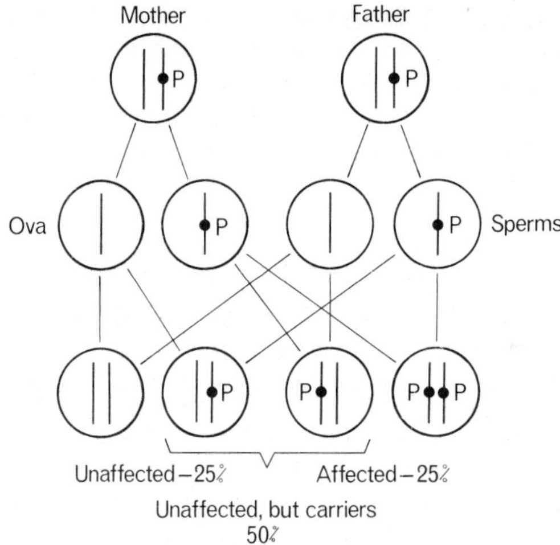

Fig. 9. **Mode of transmission of a recessive disorder phenylketonuria**

We know that two recessive genes are necessary to produce the particular characteristics they determine, in this instance a metabolic disorder called phenylketonuria (page 365). Two new terms will be introduced at this point, namely, genotype, which refers to genetic make up or constitution, and phenotype, which refers to physical characteristics, or in this example, metabolic characteristics.

Of the possible genetic combinations arising from such a union, it will be seen from Fig. 9 that the chances are that one offspring (25%) with an abnormal genotype will also have an abnormal phenotype, or, in other words, will suffer from the clinical condition. Two offspring (50%) will have an abnormal genotype, being carriers of the recessive trait, but phenotypically they will be normal, showing none of the characteristics of phenylketonuria. The offspring (25%) resulting from the remaining possible combination will be both genotypically and phenotypically normal.

Certain other forms of mental retardation are known to have a genetic basis and are due either to abnormalities in chromosome number or in chromosome morphology (shape). Such abnormalities can be detected under the microscope.

Mongolism (Down's syndrome), in its common form, is associated with the presence of an extra autosomal chromosome. The chromosome concerned is chromosome No. 21, and instead of there being two paired chromosomes, there are three, giving rise to the term 'trisomy 21' to describe the mongol child genetically. Such children are usually born of older mothers. A less common form of mongolism known as familial mongolism is associated with an abnormality of chromosome morphology.

Another morphological defect is the presence of a ring-shaped chromosome which gives rise to physical abnormality and mental retardation.

These defects of chromosome number and morphology are 'chromosome mistakes', or genetic in nature, rather than hereditary in the popular sense. A few women of mongol type have borne children, 50% of whom have been similarly affected. Defects in such children could strictly be regarded as hereditary.

These are but some examples of the many forms of mental retardation now known to be caused by genetic or hereditary factors. Certain conditions which may also be associated with mental retardation and which may lead to psychological stress are due to abnormalities of the sex chromosome number. Examples of these are *Turner's syndrome*, in which an apparent female has only forty-five chromosomes (deficient in one X chromosome), and *Klinefelter's syndrome*, wherein an apparent male has 47 or more chromosomes (extra X chromosome(s)). These conditions are once again due to chromosome mistakes and are genetic abnormalities rather than hereditary ones. In fact, people of the Turner and Klinefelter type are sterile and therefore cannot propagate.

There is some evidence to suggest that males with sex chromosome complement XYY (i.e. an extra Y chromosome), show a greater criminal propensity than XY males, and evidence also exists for the possibility that tall males with larger than normal Y chromosomes show a greater tendency towards personality disorder, criminality and alcohol abuse.

Sex-linkage

In the examples given earlier of modes of transmission of a dominant and a recessive disorder, namely Huntington's chorea and phenylketonuria, the abnormal genes are situated on autosomes, and males and females are equally affected. Genes are also transmitted on the one pair of sex chromosomes, and when a particular trait is so transmitted the inheritance is said to be sex-linked.

The transmission of the effects of an abnormal gene situated on a sex chromosome may lead to a higher incidence of a particular disorder in one sex.

Functional psychiatric illnesses

Turning now to what are known as the functional psychiatric illnesses in which there are as yet no clear cut anatomical or biochemical abnormalities, the following points may be made.

Heredity is widely accepted as being the most important factor in the development of manic-depressive psychosis (page 199).

Hereditary factors also play a part in the development of schizophrenia (page 180), and are also considered to play a part in psychosomatic illnesses.

As a factor in the causation of neuroses, there exists much controversy. If, according to a purely dynamic viewpoint, anxiety or unconscious conflict is the basic factor in the production of neurotic illness, hereditary factors may still be invoked to account for the variety of clinical manifestations of neurotic disorders.

To whatever extent hereditary factors (i.e. genetic make-up) are essential in the development of functional psychiatric illnesses, they cannot be regarded as sufficient cause for the development of such illnesses. It fits the available evidence better to see hereditary factors as predisposing a person to such an illness, while other stress factors inside or outside the individual precipitate the development of functional psychiatric disorders.

In other words, apart from the relatively few exceptions due entirely to hereditary factors and mentioned earlier in this chapter, hereditary defects are generally regarded as producing a tendency to develop a certain form of illness (a predisposition). Such illness may never appear clinically if environmental factors are not also adverse.

Constitution

The term constitution is used here to refer to a person's make-up in respect of physique, personality and intelligence. One's constitution is relatively fixed and is determined largely by hereditary factors and also by early environment.

German measles (rubella) in a mother in the first trimester (first three months of pregnancy), birth injury, early central nervous system disease and other environmental experiences may influence the development of physique, personality and intelligence.

These early factors affecting constitution obviously overlap with what is referred to as remote environment. Before looking at the question of remote environment however, mention will be made of the relationship between body build and temperamental traits.

Body build

The first work in this area was that of Kretschmer (1936), who divided body build into three major types, namely—pyknic, asthenic and athletic (he also decribed a fourth group, namely dysplastic, in which the body build combined features of the other three types). Kretschmer considered that individuals possessing a pyknic physique (short neck, large trunk well covered with fat and having slender limbs) were liable to manic-depressive illness and showed cyclothymic traits. The personality attributes of such a person were equated with what Jung had referred to as the personality characteristics of the extravert. The asthenic (lean or skinny) individual was seen generally to be of a quiet and shut-in disposition corresponding to Jung's introversion. Such people, according to Kretschmer, were more likely to develop schizophrenia. He considered that epileptics and people with 'epileptoid' (explosive) personalities were predominantly of athletic physique.

Sheldon, unlike Kretschmer, did not correlate physical characteristics with the liability to develop mental illness, but correlated physical dimensions with temperament. Rather than speak of types as did Kretschmer, Sheldon and his co-workers undertook large series of photographic studies and the measurement of normal individuals, and classified people as falling within the dimensions of endomorphy, mesomorphy and ectomorphy, which correspond largely with Kretschmer's pyknic, athletic and asthenic types. These physical dimensions were correlated by Sheldon with three temperamental dimensions, namely:

endomorphy—viscerotonia, evidenced in relaxation, sociability and love of comfort,

mesomorphy—somatotonia, in vigour and assertiveness; and

ectomorphy—cerebrontonia, evidenced in restraint and inhibition.

Other workers have added to the evidence of Kretschmer and Sheldon, and it may be stated definitely that body build and temperament are closely connected.

The picture is not clear as to the relationship borne by physique and temperament to the later development of mental illness as proposed by Kretschmer, but there appears to be some evidence to show that physical and temperamental make-up bear a relationship to the development of at least some neurotic reactions. It cannot be assumed however, that an individual possessing a particular physique or temperament will develop, or is even likely to develop, a particular form of illness.

The evidence that constitution is a factor in the development of some forms of psychiatric illness is another argument in favour of hereditary predisposing factors in the development of psychiatric illness; for constitution, as defined above, is known to be dependent largely on hereditary factors.

It will probably take many decades of study of generations of families before really conclusive evidence can be deduced regarding the place of hereditary and constitutional factors in the development of psychiatric illness.

Early, or remote environment

It is somewhat artificial to deal with an individual's remote past as a separate entity, unrelated to factors operating later in life, but it is perhaps worthwhile to take a brief overview of this period, bearing in mind that one's early years do not necessarily set the seal on the development of later psychiatric illness.

Both adverse physical (or organic) and psychological factors may be operating in the early environment predisposing a person to later mental illness. We have already touched upon some hereditary and physical factors in earlier sections of this chapter, and will deal with certain organic factors shortly, and also in later relevant sections on specific conditions. So, at this point, we shall merely review some psychological factors operating in infancy and childhood.

In Chapter 6 we noted that, in our culture, conflict or anxiety arises mainly out of aggression, sexuality and separation, the effect of the latter probably being related to dependency needs. In early life the child who does not find satisfaction of dependency needs in his particular world at that time (the family circle) may have inordinate dependency needs extending into adult life.

J. Bowlby (1951) showed that the absence of a mother (maternal deprivation), particularly between the ages of 6 months and 2 years, may create marked disturbances in infants and young children. There is evidence that repeated separations may later lead to serious personality disturbances.

A child may also, as a result of parental attitudes, be unable to deal in a healthy way with aggressive feelings and sexuality. We have seen that conflict arises out of the collision between demands of the id, or basic drives, and the child's developing superego, determined largely, it is thought, by the attitudes of parents and of the society in which the child lives. It would appear that the less the environment allows discharge of basic drives or healthy sublimation of same, the greater the tendency for development of mental disorders in later life. This, of course, is not a plea for complete permissiveness towards children. Failure to imbue reasonable behavioural limits in children may, at a later stage, lead to open conflict with society.

Unresolved difficulties in the areas mentioned may be factors in the habitual employment of unsatisfactory defence mechanisms, setting the pattern for later unsatisfactory reactions to stress, which reactivate the areas of conflict. Certain less pathological mechanisms may prove insufficient to cope with the internal stress or conflict set up, and may give way to more unhealthy defence mechanisms, with resultant psychiatric illness.

It would also seem true that, unless a child has some fairly strong consistent figure with whom he can identify, that part of his personality derived from the world outside him fails to develop, and he becomes as flotsam in life's varied currents.

Psychological factors

We have touched upon the importance of psychological factors in early life determining patterns of reaction and setting the stage for unhealthy reactions to stress. It has been pointed out that unsatisfactory ways of dealing with dependency needs, aggression and sexuality, may lead to psychiatric illness; that patterns set up in early life may persist into adult life; that under stress there may be a mobilisation of the earlier modes of reaction. At this point, brief comment will be made on the more specific role of dependence, aggression, and sexuality in the development of psychiatric illness. This will be followed by other possible stress situations which may precipitate psychiatric illness, namely the critical periods of normal life—marriage and parenthood, pregnancy, occupation, combat, bereavement and migration.

Dependency

Dependency needs may be inordinate, due perhaps to a failure to satisfy these in early life. Among more self-evident causes this may arise from needs within the parents (frequently the mother) to keep the child dependent on them, never giving him the opportunity to fend for himself.

An over-dependent person will be placed under considerable stress if he suddenly assumes a position of responsibility, or loses those on whom he has been dependent.

An interesting phenomenon is the denial of some adults of any dependency needs. Such an adult may have, earlier in life, been frustrated and humiliated in his attempts to be himself or exert himself, through over-solicitous care by parents fulfilling their own needs to have someone dependent on them. Some of these people find it difficult to accept help when it is offered, even if badly needed by them. Others avoid like the plague the formation of any interpersonal relationships. The history of these people may show evidence of the loss of someone on whom they were once dependent. They are now unwilling to develop further relationships which once again may disappoint them.

Aggression

Apart from ill-defined hereditary factors, aggression is seen as arising out of frustration of basic needs in early childhood. These may be the need to be loved, the need for food, the need to explore, the need for expressing one's individuality.

The realisation on the part of a child that there are others to share his mother's love may lead to frustration and anger. A situation of rivalry may develop towards brothers or sisters (sibling rivalry) and persist into adult life.

There is little point in developing further this theme of frustration of basic needs. You are well able to delineate the possibilities.

The most satisfactory or healthy way of dealing with aggressive drives is through the ego defense mechanism of sublimation, by which the drives are channelled into acceptable pursuits. Failure to utilise this mechanism may lead to the use of other less satisfactory ones. Without going into the particular mechanisms involved, we shall look briefly at some forms of behaviour produced by inordinate aggressive drives.

1. The aggressive person may be so afraid of aggressive or destructive impulses that he withdraws or becomes extremely anxious when placed in a position wherein these impulses may be discharged, for example, in military combat or other fighting situations.
2. If aggressive feelings have been held towards a peron who dies or is injured in some way, this in a sense constitutes proof of the destructive power within one, and feelings of guilt and depression may result. This may be seen in an ongoing group therapy situation where one of the members, for some unknown but innocuous reason, misses a group session. The other members may feel responsible as a result of the destructive impulses they harbour against the member, and therefore feel guilty.
3. The person who, in earlier years, has exhibited temper tantrums may become fearful of the loss of control evident in such outbursts. This may lead to self-effacement and an inordinate desire to please people, in short a flight from any action that may be felt as aggressive, because such people are afraid their aggressive drives will overflow reducing them to a chaotic and helpless state.

4. On the other hand, some people with very little superego control or 'conscience' may, without any anxiety, channel their aggression into anti-social activities.
5. A particularly difficult situation arises when anger is felt towards a person on whom one is still dependent. A display of anger may alienate the person who satisfies dependency needs, and anger is therefore suppressed.

Sexuality

In terms of sexuality, persons with persistent immature attitudes towards sexual functions appear to be predisposed to psychiatric illness.

The results of immature attitudes towards sex are seen, for example, in: the persistence of exhibitionistic tendencies in both males and females; difficulties in assuming the sex role determined by one's physical make-up (i.e. male or female), sometimes associated with a need to prove ones sexuality by numerous ephemeral 'affairs'; the maintenance of an attitude towards sex that equates it with sin or naughtiness; envy of the attributes of the opposite sex.

Critical periods of normal life

In an earlier section the point was made that conflict with, or stress from the outside world merely mobilises 'internal anxiety', which is determined by unconscious conflicts. Particular stresses are associated with certain periods of normal life; few people, if any, travel untrammelled through the experiences of adolescence, middle age and old age. Each experience requires some adjustment, and in the person predisposed to psychiatric illness, aspects of these experiences may lead to a breakdown of adequate mental functioning.

Adolescence

The adolescent has four main areas in which adjustment is necessary:

1. The first lies in the modification of his concept of parental figures. As a young child, one's security is dependent on the omnipotence invested in parents. When the child discovers, as he must, that parents are not all-knowing and all-powerful, he may feel anxious and insecure. The adolescent may then place other people outside the family in the position of supreme counsellors. These, too, are to be found wanting, as nobody can reasonably satisfy a demand to be omnipotent.

   In adolescence, there is a drive for emancipation and independence and a tendency to devaluate parents. This drive immediately sets up fears and conflicts within the child arising from a struggle between still present dependency needs and the striving for independence.
2. The adolescent assumes standards of morality, of right and wrong acceptable to the adult world. These standards are not simply a reflection of the standards of his elders, but are something that becomes part of himself and are modified or determined largely by the standards of the society in which he lives.
3. He needs to identify with the sex role for which he is biologically

determined. The person who is physically a boy is expected by society to think and behave like a boy. The girl is expected to show the attributes of feminity expected by the culture or society in which she lives. These attributes include aspects of dominance and submission and will obviously vary from culture to culture.

4. The fourth area of adjustment facing the adolescent is in the realm of his educational and vocational future. Decisions, often with far-reaching effects, may have to be made. The final choice in terms of vocation is probably determined by unconscious needs that seek expression in one's life work. Other factors include values placed on particular jobs or professions by groups with whom the adolescent is in daily contact. Such groups include the family, peer groups, the broader community and ethnic (racial) groups.

Through early relationships with people, and by the process of identifying with them, the growing child's ego and superego develop. It is as if he takes in aspects of parents and other people around him, and these become part of his personality by the process of identification.

As he achieves successes in school, work, social relations etc. the adolescent's sense of his own identity, being more than just the sum of those qualities taken in from others, begins to emerge. Struggles in the four abovementioned areas of adjustment are involved in the process of achieving a sense of identity, which, when fully developed, implies a clear picture of oneself as an individual operating within and belonging to a group, without feeling that one's individuality or identity will be swamped by the group. This struggle is referred to as the identity crisis of adolescence.

It is quite usual to observe indecision and changes in attitude from one extreme to another produced by conflicts in the areas mentioned. This cannot be regarded in any sense as abnormal. However, in susceptible young people, there is little doubt that unresolved conflicts in any of these areas can precipitate definitive psychiatric illness.

Middle age

Without stating definite age limits for this period of life, there are a number of areas where adjustment is necessary as the vigour and achievements of a full adult life decline. Numbered among these are a decline in physical capabilities, altered relationships with children, the responsibility of ageing parents, and one's occupation.

Each man and woman is faced with a fall-off in physical prowess and attractiveness. This is accepted by most with reasonable equanimity, but if great value has been placed on such attributes, adjustment to their loss may prove difficult. The menopause, to the uninformed woman in this period of life, may be misconstrued as the end of her sexual life. Most males will lose at least some of their sexual vigor, and may, in our culture at least, involve themselves in more committee, club and pub life, perhaps heightening their spouse's concern over their failing attractiveness to their marriage partner.

In middle life there may well be concern over the children's final education and vocational choices and over their establishment in worthwhile jobs. One's children, now adolescents or young adults, will have their own adjustments to make, leading often, as indicated earlier, to a virtual renouncement of their parents. For the parent whose needs are met by having someone dependent on him, this constitutes a major loss. Such parents may, of course, later satisfy this need by doting on the grandchildren. For some childless people, the future indeed looks bleak with pending old age and no family support in view, emotional or otherwise.

Old age

In the present day in most cultures, advances in the treatment of lethal physical illnesses have played their part in increasing the life span of our populations. The result of this is more old people who are potential sufferers from the psychiatric disorders that occur at this period of life.

Old age itself brings a number of pressures to bear which may lead to breakdown. Among these may be numbered decline in physical and intellectual capacities, physical illness, retirement from occupations, and loneliness. One could give many examples of such factors operating and the student should be alert to detecting them in his patients, bearing in mind that there are usually a number of factors operating simultaneously.

Seen at a hospital was a man of 65, recently compulsorily retired from work. His only complaint was a pain in the right foot, and this along with some slight defect in his visual fields first led to the possibility of some organic brain lesion. On psychiatric examination it became evident that he was depressed, though his general appearance did not suggest this. Within a few days of admission he had cut his throat in a determined attempt to shuffle off this mortal coil. Fortunately, with the appropriate treatment, namely, suturing his throat, and electroconvulsive therapy, he recovered.

The factors in this case were: firstly, retirement from a position where he was contributing something, and where he felt he was a useful member of society; secondly, there had been some fall-off in his intellectual capacity and his wife had to take over the home financial management, signing cheques etcetera which, as head of the house, he had always done; thirdly, he obviously felt acutely his loss of physical prowess, as he reiterated the fact that, 'this (the painful foot) is the foot that kicked many goals in football'. So we see that retirement and failing intellectual and physical capacity, along with the loss of his captaincy of the domestic situation, which was a severe loss in terms of his need to dominate, all played their part in the production of his depressive illness.

Among illnesses common in late age are angina pectoris, arthritic conditions, gynaecological problems in women, and prostatic hypertrophy in men. More and more long-standing friends die as one ages. One's children may become neglectful as they develop problems with their own families, or they may simply become intolerant of their aged parents' or relatives' demanding, childish, peevish and perseverative attitudes, something not uncommon in old age if interests become restricted. New ideas cannot be taken in, and the old persons' thoughts come to settle on themselves. Whatever the factors in the particular case, the aged person feels lonely and rejected by family, friends and society generally. Such a state of loss produces depression and despair, particularly in a person with weakened or no spiritual roots.

Marriage and parenthood

The state of marriage may well trigger off conflicts in the sexual sphere associated with guilt over the sexual act. It may produce difficulties where the appetite for sexual satisfaction is disproportionate in partners, leading to feelings of resentment and frustration. Marriage also involves a break from parental support in many instances. Even if parental support is not withdrawn, social attitudes may demand of the young couple that they behave independently.

On the other hand, in what is called the extended family, where grandparents and other relatives are involved with the married couple and their children, a multiplicity of different stresses may occur depending on attitudes and consequent behaviour of relatives.

A person bringing into a marriage his or her dependency needs, expecting them to be met by the marriage partner, may place crippling emotional demands on that partner. There may exist differences in attitudes with respect to having children. Such differences may exist at unconscious levels in spite of the couple, at a conscious level, being agreed on a particular line of action. Marital disharmony is frequently blamed for psychiatric disability but it must be remembered that it is often immaturity or neurotic needs in one or both partners that leads to marital disharmony. It is an interesting fact that particular psychiatric illnesses occur more frequently among single and divorced people (at least in our culture), suggesting some disorder in personality preventing such people from contracting a satisfactory marital relationship.

Pregnancy

What, to most people, is a normal and happily anticipated event as part of a marriage can raise anxiety in terms of possible relationships that may develop between parent and child. Old unconscious conflicts or unhappy associations with respect to the mother-child relationship may be triggered off in the parent-to-be.

At a conscious level the mother-to-be wonders whether she will be able to cope with parenthood, and, perhaps at a more unconscious level, anxiety, more relevant to her own feelings as a child towards her own mother, is rekindled. On the other hand, some women never feel better than when they are pregnant. Physical factors appear to have little if any part to play in the development of symptoms in pregnancy, for we have all seen cases where the husband of the pregnant woman experiences similar anxieties and even develops symptoms present in some pregnancies, for example, morning sickness (Couvade Syndrome).

Occupation

There is little doubt that certain disorders occur with more frequency in people working in particular occupations. Peptic ulceration, for example, occurs with greater frequency in bus drivers and crane drivers than in the general population. Here, conditions of stress seem to be important. Certain occupations or professions may place a person at risk in terms of abuse of drugs or alcohol, due to subcultural determinants or ready availability of these agents upon which one may become dependent.

It is socially acceptable to attribute psychiatric illness to the pressures of overwork. In actual fact, it is probably not 'overwork' or work stress that leads to breakdown, but something in the person himself. Many people strive competitively in jobs as a defence against anxiety and feelings of inferiority, thus working under continuous pressure from within. Others have difficulties with authority figures in work situations which may be an extension of childhood attitudes towards their own parents.

Promotion may involve responsibility with which the worker feels he cannot cope, or it may mean loss of the personal friendship of his previous peers. Being passed over for promotion, and more importantly, loss of a job, may produce serious sequelae in terms of gross loss of self-esteem apart from the obvious financial loss.

We have to think also of those psychiatric illnesses which may be completely unrelated to the work situation, but which will have far-reaching effects on a person's efficiency. For example, where there exists an upward swing of mood, a person may at first work extremely hard, and later quite ineffectively as deterioration continues. The depressed worker will lose interest in both his job and his colleagues. It is socially acceptable to blame work for one's indisposition or inability to cope, but it is probably more frequently the case that personal difficulties or personality weaknesses are the cause of failure in work situations, rather than that work stress leads to maladjustment.

Combat

The soldier finds himself under a multiplicity of stresses. These briefly, are related to the type of combat and the job in which he is engaged, whether he is in the front line or some supporting unit, the country in which he is serving, factors at home, loss of mates, and miscellaneous factors.

With respect to type of combat, the length of operations undertaken and the number of contacts made with the enemy have a bearing on production of psychiatric symptoms. In jungle warfare, even without contact with the enemy, one is under continuous strain resulting from the possibility of being seen without being able to see the enemy, and under tension where there is the possibility of treading on mines. To make contact with the opposing forces is often felt by the infantry soldier as a relief when he has been expectantly tense for a period of time. To sit back and receive artillery or mortar fire without being able to hit back constitutes another type of stress.

The soldier filling a position known to be associated with a high injury or mortality rate has that much more burden to bear. The officers under most stress will be those responsible for decision-making in operational units. For example, if most operations are carried out in company strength, greater stress can be expected to fall upon the company commander than upon the battalion or platoon commander.

A different type of stress occurs in troops in support areas. They may become bored, and sometimes cannot accept the fact that they are just as important in the scheme of things as those who squeeze triggers, fire artillery weapons or mortars, or drive tracked vehicles.

Good leadership will do much to prevent these support troops, as well as front line troops, from developing a low standard of morale and exhibiting behaviour disturbances.

The country in which one is serving is important from a cultural stand-point, as well as from the effects of its terrain, vegetation and climate. The soldier, whether as part of civil aid programmes or at times of leave, must of necessity come into contact with local people whose culture and customs may be quite strange to him. Romantic involvement directed towards a permanent relationship may throw up vast religious differences, or the soldier may find his bride unable to leave her country for one reason or another. If prostitution is an accepted practice in a country, the soldier, who in any case is taking a chance that he may not survive the war, has great pressures upon him to seek refuge in the arms of a prostitute or to prove his manliness while he can. If this occurs, it may later be attended by marked guilt, particularly if he has some attachment at home.

Where drugs prohibited at home are freely available in the country where one is serving, under tensions that exist in warfare, the possibility of the development of drug dependence exists, as well as the conflict associated with drug taking.

Mail from home becomes extremely important to the person serving overseas. If it does not arrive or bears unhappy or unsavoury news this may precipitate anxiety. Sickness or other domestic stress at home will concern the soldier more than usual, as he is far removed and feels impotent because he can do little to help or right the situation whatever it might be. His wife being pregnant when he leaves for overseas may constitute a problem for the soldier. He may feel he is letting his spouse down by not being with her. It may also be difficult for him to find a suitable listener to whom he can air his own conflicts both about the realistic situation and about his conflicts over fatherhood.

Loss of mates is one of the greatest demoralisers the soldier has to face. This applies to mates being wounded and returned home or killed in action. The team that trained together is no longer a team. Mutual support, trust and friendship are lost. After a time, the soldier may not wish to make an effort to integrate new members into his section. This may reach the extreme of open hostility being shown to reinforcements. Apart from this important element of loss, the death or injury of a mate brings home some of the realities of warfare and the fact that death or injury could well have been the survivor's lot. The latter, with instincts of self-preservation, may have anxieties liberated relating to death or mutilation. It is an interesting fact however, that many front line troops utilise a denial mechanism, believing they will not be killed. This may crumble however, following minor wounding or some near misses.

Among miscellaneous factors may be quoted that an exclusive male society, particularly in isolated units, may lead to the emergence of homosexual conflict. A soldier may be terrified of his aggressive drives. Here he is, a soldier, whose role is to kill or capture the enemy, and his fear of his own aggressive impulses and his habitual avoidance of showing aggression comes into conflict with his conscious role as a soldier. Yet a third factor in this miscellaneous group is poor placement of personnel. For example the man who, in civil life, has been engaged in artistic pursuits is possibly not the best choice as an infantry soldier.

No specific mention has been made of stress factors in seamen and airmen, though many of the above will apply and others will be added. For example, the navy pilot who has to land his plane on the deck of a carrier, which a matter of seconds, rather than minutes, before landing looks no bigger than a postage stamp, develops peptic ulcers much more readily than his navigator or observer. The latter is not involved in this split-second decision making and learns to sit and take what comes.

Bereavement

Following the loss of a close friend or relative, it is normal for the survivor to pass through a period of grief and mourning. Cognizance of this fact is indeed taken in certain religious persuasions where a specified time for, and form of, mourning is virtually mandatory. The person who has suffered loss usually makes adjustments through mourning, and thereafter carries on with the matter of living in a satisfactory way.

Some people however, develop psychiatric symptoms following loss. It would seem that those most at risk are people who have depended heavily on the love and protection of the deceased person. Also, they may have suffered a loss of love or a loved person early in life, or they may have felt uncertain of being loved in their childhood.

Depressive illnesses are probably the most common form of psychiatric illness occurring after bereavement. It is frequently found that the relationship between the bereaved and the lost relative has been a complicated one. Feelings of resentment or rivalry towards the deceased may have been harboured, as well as loving feelings. The former, which amount to aggressive attitudes on the part of the bereaved, may lead to strong feelings of guilt and self-blame.

Migration

Migration to a new country produces its own problems, especially if there is a language difficulty. The migrant may feel isolated, he may have to adjust to different customs and different attitudes, and one should always be sensitive to possible areas of stress in our migrant population.

A special problem is seen to exist for female migrants who may be slow to learn the language of their new country. Their husbands work and become acculturated. Their children learn the new language quickly, and readily adapt to new modes of living, growing away in interests from their relatively house-bound mothers. Lack of facility in the new language makes it difficult for such mothers to embrace outside interests, and they can be virtually left out on a limb. This is but one example of the possible stress factors that may affect a newcomer to a country.

Socioeconomic and cultural factors

A person's socioeconomic or class position in the community would appear to have a bearing on the likelihood of his developing obvious psychopathology. In small communities, there is not such a gradation in the state of affluence as exists in large industrialised areas. In most studies undertaken, the highest rate of psychopathology has been found in the lowest economic stratum of the population studied. The term 'socioeconomic' is used because in most populations a low social position goes hand in hand with a low economic position, and it is difficult to determine their individual effects. However, studies in Sweden on a particular community showed a reversal of the usual findings, namely, that in the community under study, those in the lowest socioeconomic level showed least psychiatric disorder. This would seem to indicate that particular social legislation and cultural attitudes may remove some of the difficulties present in communities of low socioeconomic standards.

Basically the problem with poverty is not lack of money, but the inability to enjoy the multiple advantages associated with affluence.

With respect to sociocultural factors, we can perhaps more readily separate out the cultural from the social. Culture may be defined somewhat narrowly as 'those aspects of a way of life of a given population that sets them apart as different from other groups'. In this fairly limited sense, anthropologists have described what would appear to be psychiatric disorders whose content and manifest behaviour is peculiar to particular cultures. People undergoing cultural change involving alteration in social roles are at far greater risk that when traditional cultural norms prevail. An example of this is the sudden urbanisation of people previously living a tribal existence. They move to the city, away from the sanctions and support of a tribal system, and are unable to adjust healthily in the new situation. It would appear that mental health is considerably better in integrated than in disintegrated communities. Integration or disintegration here refers to sociocultural dimensions. Sociocultural factors are difficult to measure, and involve appraisal of poverty-affluence dimension, the overall coherence or confusion of culture values, the viability of the religious system, the stability of families and a host of other variables. The measurements of these require the expertise of the social scientist as well as that of the psychiatrist. This is a growing field, and future investigations will no doubt add much to the understanding of human behaviour, and provide means of dealing with some of the factors responsible for the development of certain psychiatric disorders.

11

THE PSYCHIATRIC HISTORY; NURSING NOTES

In most branches of medicine, there is the opportunity to observe actual lesions or undertake physical examinations using, if necessary, a variety of simple or complex aids in order to validate the impressions given by a patient's history, and to arrive at a diagnosis. Though it is important to use a thermometer, stethoscope, sphygmomanometer and ophthalmoscope, when examining psychiatric patients, in the vast majority of cases these will provide little information. One has to rely heavily, in fact, on verbal material presented by the patient, his friends and relatives, and on a thorough examination of the patient's mental state.

A psychiatric history will be seen to embrace the complexity of factors that are implicated in the causation of psychiatric illness outlined in the previous chapter. During and after the taking of a psychiatric history one weighs up the relevance of the various factors that are brought to light.

Though it is not always possible, on the basis of an initial psychiatric interview, to develop a really sound formulation covering diagnosis, dynamic factors and prognosis, it is important to strive to do so in order that relevant management procedures can be embarked upon as early as possible.

In this chapter, the outline of a method of recording a psychiatric history, developed at the Maudsley Hospital and modified locally, will be used. I would stress that this is a formula for recording a history and psychiatric examination, and patients or relatives should not be required to state facts in the order outlined. Such rigid adherence to a set pattern of history-taking can stifle a patient's nuances of concern, leading to an imprecise formulation. One should, however, learn to record material in a standard form, remembering to cover each item in the history schema. If this is done, important areas are less likely to be overlooked, and if the patient has omitted to give information in some areas, these can be opened up to him.

Interviewing a patient

A few simple comments about interviewing or history-taking are worth making, and one should always be aware of these in the interview situation.

An interview involves an exchange of feeling and words between two people. The patient is not like a machine, to whom you put a question with the result that a fitting and consistent answer issues forth. The interviewer's attitude will very much govern what type of reply is given, or even whether a reply is given at all. Even if the interviewer says nothing, attitudes of acceptance, understanding, non-acceptance, impatience, incredulity, disagreement, intolerance, displeasure, or censure, to name just a few, will be felt by the patient, encouraging or inhibiting the patient's verbal communication, at least on particular topics. The spoken or unspoken display of attitudes, which inhibit free verbal expression by the patient are to be avoided.

Rather than attempting to stick to such rules as, 'Don't argue', 'Don't be impatient', and so forth, it is perhaps more helpful to see oneself as working with the patient, helping him to paint a clear picture. To this end, your attitude should be one of empathy, understanding and encouragement. At all costs avoid putting your preconceived ideas into the patient, lest an inaccurate sketch result.

Patients may, even in an early interview, cast the interviewer in a particular role or roles on the basis of transference. Some transferences may be helpful in the interview situation, others not. Until one has the feel of what is helpful and what is not, it is sound practice to remain relatively neutral.

Interviews may be unstructured, so allowing the patient free rein to talk, or structured in terms of questions and answers. Certain patients discourse at great length, giving what amounts to unnecessary details before reaching a relevant point. In terms of the economy of the interviewer's time and the necessity to obtain an overall picture, it may be necessary to circumvent such detail for the present, with the understanding that an opportunity will be given later to ventilate the material which one must accept as important to the patient.

If an interview is conducted on the basis of question and answer, the patient may be unable to develop themes of importance; also, in a structured interview situation, it may be impossible to elicit mild thought disorder in some patients suffering from schizophrenia.

In practice one generally tries to be non-directive, but interviewing usually involves both a free and a structured approach.

A number of clinics utilise questionnaires to be filled in by patients. This, no doubt, is a saving of staff time, but one wonders whether such a practice introduces an impersonal element, leading to the loss of potential therapeutic value in the face-to-face interview situation.

There are those who are eminently satisfied with the questionnaire procedure, but for the majority of psychiatrists who know that therapy commences at the first interview, the questionnaire method does entail a lost therapeutic opportunity.

Whether it is sound practice to take notes while a patient is speaking will not be discussed at length. But this question should be under consideration with each new patient one sees. A paranoid patient may object if the interviewer is writing. Patients may withhold information in certain areas of the history regarded by them as personal. Other patients may feel that too little importance is being placed on their words if they are not written down.

The good student will, of course, by study and practice be so conversant with the history headings that he or she, after hearing a patient's story, will be able to write it up later without missing any relevant facts. The same will apply to the documentation of the patient's mental state examination.

Information from other sources

In the assessment of a psychiatric problem, it is particularly important to obtain information from sources other than the patient, if at all possible. The patient, as a result of his illness, may not be seeing things literally and figuratively as they are seen by others. Obtaining independent evidence and meeting people who know the patient will help the interviewer to weigh the evidence given by the patient. What a relative or friend has to offer may suggest that the patient has been withholding important facts, or has for one reason or another placed an erroneous construction upon certain events. This would cause one to look more closely at the possibility that the patient is deluded, or that he at least holds over-determined or overvalued ideas.

How many of us have heard one side of a story from a patient and been convinced that the attitude of the spouse for example, has contributed much to the present picture, only to appreciate on hearing the other side, that we were indeed gullible not to have suspended our judgment before weighing another point of view?

On the other hand the 'patient' may be nearer the truth in his statements and not as emotionally disturbed as the relative. Fixed and erroneous attitudes in a relative may produce stress, precipitating breakdown in the person subsequently admitted to treatment. It could be that the relative is sicker in a psychiatric sense and more in need of help to make satisfactory adjustments in life.

Now we shall turn our attention to a format for recording the psychiatric history and examination of a patient. It will become evident that facts under most headings, but not all, can be completed at the first interview. Fig. 10 depicts areas in a patient's life that require study.

Outline of psychiatric history and examination of patient

1. Patient's name and age

2. Reason for admission or referral

   For example, wandering at night, taking an overdose of tablets, neighbours complaining to police.

3. Present complaints and their duration

4. Present illness

   A detailed chronological account of the illness from the earliest time a change was noticed. Obtain approximate dates which will

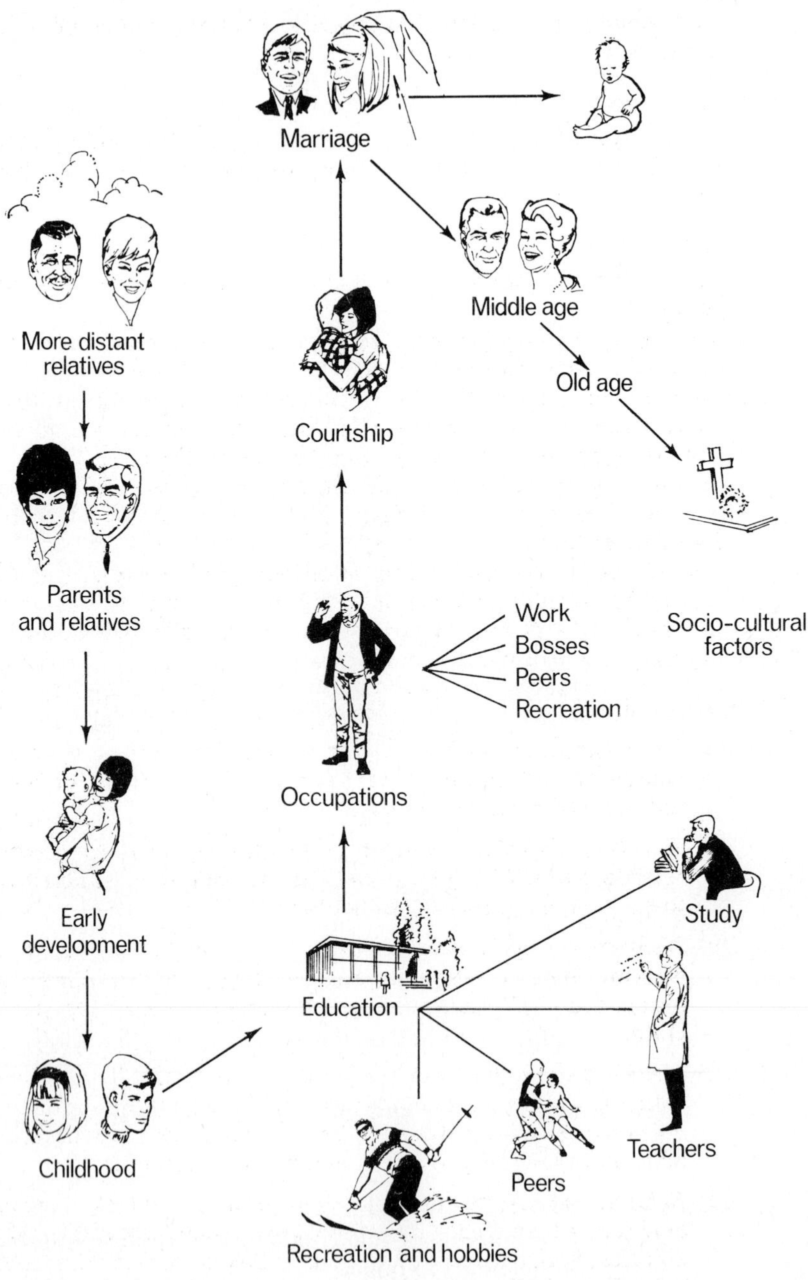

Fig. 10

permit a sequence of various symptoms. (The accounts of relatives and friends may, in many instances, be required. The informant's relationship to the patient and his reliability should be assessed and noted. Views expressed by informants should be kept separate from the main body of the history, but could follow the same outline given here.)

5. System review

A brief record of symptoms present in any of the bodily systems e.g. respiratory system, alimentary system, genito-urinary system.

6. Family history

Father: health, age or age at time of death; cause of death; personality; occupation.
Mother: health, age or age at time of death; cause of death; personality; occupation.
Siblings: enumerated in chronological order of birth (including miscarriages and stillbirths); with Christian names, ages, marital condition, personality, occupation, history of illnesses.
Social position and general efficiency of the family, including any familial diseases e.g. alcoholism, abnormal personalities, mental disorder, epilepsy.
Record home atmosphere and influence, particularly any salient happenings among parents and the rest of family during the patient's early years, the emotional relationship with parents, siblings, or with any other important figure.

7. Personal history

(a) *Date and place of birth*: mother's condition during pregnancy, whether full-term birth and normal delivery; breast or bottle fed; time of weaning; feeding difficulties.

(b) *Early development*: delicate or healthy baby; precocious or retarded; time of teething, talking and walking; cleanliness as to excreta; habit training difficulties.

(c) *Neurotic symptoms* in childhood: e.g. night terrors, sleep walking, temper tantrums, bed wetting, thumb sucking, nail biting, food fads, stammering, mannerisms, fear states, model child.

(d) *Health during childhood*: infections (especially if associated with high fever or mental symptoms); chorea; infantile convulsions; play—e.g. spontaneous games in childhood, make-believe, organised games, especially in adolescence.

(e) *School*: age of beginning and finishing; standard reached; evidence of ability or backwardness; special abilities or disabilities; hobbies and interests; relationship with schoolmates; attitude to teachers; attitude to study.

(f) *Occupations*: age of starting work; jobs held in chronological order with wages, dates and reasons for change; satisfaction in work; present economic circumstances; ambition, satisfaction or reasons for dissatisfaction; attitude to employers and workmates.

(g) *Sociocultural factors*: e.g. record any evidence of sociocultural disintegration and difficulties arising from uprooting of migrant patients.

(h) *Service or other war experience*: seen by psychiatrist or invalided out; disability pension.

(i) *Sexual and marital history*:

(i) Menstrual history: age at first period; acceptance and adjustment, regularity, duration and amount; pain; psychic changes; date of last period; climacteric symptoms.
(ii) Sexual inclinations and practice: sexual information, how was it received; masturbation, age, frequency, guilt; sexual fantasies; prudery; homosexuality and other sexual deviations; heterosexual experiences apart from marriage; venereal diseases.
(iii) Marital History: duration of acquaintance and of engagement before marriage; the husband's (or wife's) age, occupation and personality; their compatibility; mode and frequency of sexual intercourse; sexual satisfaction, disinclination or impotence; contraceptive measures; marriage forced by pregnancy; fidelity of partner.
(iv) Children: chronological list of children including miscarriages and abortions, giving ages, names, and personalities; attitude towards children; psychiatric state of children.

(j) *Medical history*: chronologically and in detail, list all illnesses, operations and accidents.
(k) *Previous mental health*: detail psychiatric conditions and treatment given. Include dates, duration, nature of treatment and hospitals concerned. Detail psychiatric symptoms for which treatment has not been received, and psychiatric disturbances or character abnormalities noted by relatives and friends, but not by the patient.

8. Personality before illness

Adequate evaluation may be difficult. Aim at a description of a person, not a type. The following areas are important to examine:

(a) *Social relationships*: particularly to the family, friends and fellow workers. Describe modes of handling interpersonal relationships (e.g. by dependency, aggressive leadership etc.); the presence of traits such as sensitivity, suspiciousness, jealousy, seductiveness, shyness, fussiness, rigidity, resentfulness, egocentricity, or lack of confidence.

(b) *Intellectual activities and interests, hobbies and recreations.*

(c) *Mood*: whether it is cheerful, despondent, anxious, worrying, optimistic, pessimistic, self-depreciating, satisfied, over-confident, stable, fluctuating (with or without provocation), controlled or demonstrative.

(d) *Standards*: moral, religious, social, economic, practical. This includes evaluation of superego function. (Remember that moral views held with extreme rigidity are often reaction formation against underlying opposing trends).

(e) *Energy, initiative.*

(f) *Fantasy life*: daydreaming—frequency, content.

(g) *Habits*: eating (fads); sleeping; excretory functions; alcohol; tobacco; drugs.

(h) *Defensive pattern*: assess whether patient has dealt with previous problems in a healthy way (e.g. appropriate direct response or sublimation) or by such mechanisms as denial, projection, repression or regression. Has he shown little capacity for postponing his impulses. Has his life-pattern been inconsistent. Such an assessment helps one in gauging the patient's ego strength.

9. Physical state

Note relevant points from referral source, or from examination carried out on admission if patient is hospitalised, plus anything noted or elicited at interview.

10. Mental state

This has been dealt with fully in Chapter 7 and the main headings only will be included at this point. The student should study once again the details included in the documentation of the psychiatric history and examination of the patient:

(a) General appearance.
(b) Behavioural patterns.
(c) Form of speech.
(d) Content of speech.
(e) Mood.
(f) Intellectual functions.
(g) Insight and judgment.

11. Reports

Special investigations—physical, psychological or social.

12. Summary and formulation

(a) A review of relevant aspects of illness; personal history, personality and findings on examination.

(b) Diagnosis and differential diagnosis are to be considered on three levels:

(i) descriptive diagnosis, e.g. schizophrenia, paranoid type.
(ii) dynamic diagnosis, by which is meant an evaluation of the patient's current stresses (physical, psychological, social and cultural), the psychological manoeuvres employed to deal with them, plus a similar evaluation, where indicated, of his previous personality dynamics.

(iii) anatomical, physiological and pathological diagnosis, in cases where this is relevant.

(c) Suggested treatment.

(d) Prognosis; for the present illness, and long term.

Further points relating to above outline

Depending on the age of the patient being interviewed, different areas of the history will require more or less detailed exploration.

Though such a history-documenting schema may at first sight appear tedious and even quite dull, its proper application can produce a living and colourful picture of the patient who has been interviewed and examined.

One point that interviewers frequently overlook is to ascertain the duration of an illness, or more precisely, at what point in time a change occurred in the patient. This will be indicated if a history is taken and documented as in the above outline and will enable the interviewer to search for appropriate stress factors.

It may be found that the illness has had either an insidious or a sudden onset, which may prove of prognostic significance.*

On the other hand, an 'illness' may be part of, or an extension of, a patient's particular mode of life as portrayed in the section of the history entitled 'Personality before illness'.

From the point of view of subsequent research of the type styled 'retrospective studies', complete histories are essential.

The worker in psychiatry must be thoroughly conversant with a reliable outline for the history and examination of a patient. A sound knowledge of such will prove a useful tool, the most frequently used and refined implement in one's diagnostic armamentarium. Also, it will provide essential background for initiating a rational management programme.

Nursing notes

There are three major practical reasons for the nurse keeping adequate nursing notes:

1. *Supplementation of patient's history*

It is extremely unlikely that the psychiatrist or social worker gleans all the relevant facts from a patient and his relatives even over a number of interviews. The nurse, who spends the most time with the patient and who has opportunity to speak with relatives and friends, may learn previously undisclosed facts. Such details may be relevant to the patient's present state or may indicate potential difficulties for the patient in returning, for example, to the home or work situation. These facts should be documented in the manner prescribed in your particular hospital or clinic. The doctor, on reading such notes, will be able to add to the total picture and will refine the management programme accordingly.

* Prognosis: prediction or forecast of future course of illness.

2. *Communication about the patient's current state*

Communication about a patient's current behaviour and thoughts expressed is of vital importance to the whole team involved in the patient's management. This applies to all treatment areas and to all types of patients. However, in an admission area where patients are frequently more floridly disturbed, adequate communication, particularly between changing shifts, assumes very great importance. Though life usually flows relatively smoothly in an admission ward, major catastrophes can and do occur if adequate communication between staff members is not maintained. Remember that you may be the only person told by the patient that he or she feels life has become unbearable and that it would be better if it were all over. You may, through your dealings with a patient, become aware that he is auditorily hallucinated, has begun to withdraw from social contact, appears more tense and agitated, or appears to be more drowsy or excited following the visit of 'friends'. The latter reaction should raise the suspicion of drug dependence.

The possibilities for such observations are legion and but a few have been mentioned. What sort of things does one look for? This question is simply answered by references to Chapter 7, Psychiatric symptoms and signs.

Built into the procedure of many wards is the healthy habit of verbal communication between shifts, the outgoing shift 'handing over' to the new. Do not leave it at the level of verbal communication. Make sure you have documented your observations precisely. Your notes can form the basis of the hand-over discussion.

In the case of P.R.N. or S.O.S. medications* particularly, provision is usually made for these to be documented on a 'special medication sheet', but it is sound practice for this information to be repeated in the nursing notes covering your shift in order that the oncoming shift will be fully aware of medications already received by the patients.

3. *Value of notes in legal proceedings*

It must be remembered that Nursing Notes may be subpoenaed, usually as part of the patient's case history notes, in legal proceedings. They may find their way into Children's Courts, Coroner's Courts, and into courts dealing for example with criminal offences, divorce and compensation.

Bearing this possibility in mind, one appreciates more the necessity for being precise in observation, and concise, simple and straightforward in written comments.

The fact that nursing notes may enter the legal arena should lead the nurse to be circumspect in what she writes. If in any doubt consult the team leader, the psychiatrist.

A 'Don't' and a 'Do' in entering up nursing notes

Don't use technical terms. Say in simple language, precisely what the patient tells you or what you observe.

---

* P.R.N.: *Pro re nata*—for a special emergency or sudden development.
S.O.S.: *Si opus sit*—if it is necessary.
Although different interpretations may be given to these shorthand directions, it is customary for 'P.R.N.' to signify 'as required', and for time intervals to be specified; and for 'S.O.S.' to signify that the medication is to be given once only.

To write, 'Mrs X is auditorily hallucinated' means something but not enough. It would be better to write, 'This morning Mrs X heard an imaginary male voice which she believed to be coming from the ceiling fan through Police transmission, telling her that she is a prostitute', or 'Mrs X while getting off to sleep, heard the voice of her deceased husband calling to her'.

In the first instance, the strong possibility is that Mrs X is suffering from a paranoid schizophrenic illness, while in the second she may be experiencing hypnagogic hallucinations of less dire clinical import. Apart from the time at which an hallucinatory experience occurs, the content of hallucinations or delusions may be of paramount importance in eliciting problem areas.

Again, to write 'Patient withdrawn' could mean that the patient concerned was avoiding social contact generally or with a particular group, that he appeared to be preoccupied with his own thoughts, or that he refused to talk. It is far better to describe the circumstances and the patient's behaviour, than to affix an imprecise and maybe incorrect shorthand description.

Do write the date of, and add your signature to, your entry in the Nursing Notes.

12

ORGANIC PSYCHOTIC CONDITIONS

INTRODUCTION

Organic psychotic conditions are syndromes in which the essential features are impairment of:

1. Orientation
2. Memory
3. Comprehension
4. Calculation
5. Learning capacity
6. Judgment

Added to these essential features there may occur shallowness or lability of affect, or a more persistent disturbance of mood, lowering of ethical standards and exaggeration or emergence of personality traits, and diminished capacity for independent decision.

Usually a number of these abnormalities are found to exist together in the one patient.

Some patients with organic psychotic conditions recover completely while others are left with residual symptoms and signs depending on the nature and severity of brain damage which may or may not be reversible. The terms 'acute brain syndrome' and 'chronic brain syndrome' used to be applied to these respective conditions. These terms have been replaced by 'delirium' and 'dementia'. The term *delirium* includes organic psychoses with a short course in which the essential and accompanying features mentioned above are overshadowed by clouded consciousness, confusion, disorientation, delusions, illusions, and often vivid hallucinations usually of a visual nature.

The term *dementia* is applied to organic psychoses of a chronic or progressive nature which if untreated are usually irreversible and terminal.

Before turning our attention to the diagnostic entities falling within the rubric of organic psychotic conditions the following is submitted as a useful way to group the most common causal factors leading to the development of these conditions, excluding those present at birth which are described later in the section on mental retardation (Chapter 24). The table shown does not indicate a complete differential diagnosis, and workers in tropical areas for example would need to add endemic medical conditions to their check list. These conditions would include cerebral malaria, typhoid fever, scrub-typhus, trypanosomiasis etc:

Primary brain degeneration
—senile dementia
—presenile dementia—Alzheimer's disease
Pick's disease
—Huntington's chorea

Space-occupying lesions
—benign tumours, subdural haematoma
—malignant tumours—primary
secondary

Infection
—syphilis, encephalitis, meningitis
—brain abscess, systemic infections

Drug or poison intoxication
—amphetamines, barbiturates, bromides, alcohol, carbon monoxide, lead, arsenic, mercury, petrol

Cardiovascular disorders
—cerebral arteriosclerosis, cerebral embolism, cerebral haemorrhage, arterial hypertension, heart disease

Anoxia
—from any cause

Metabolic, endocrine or nutritional disorders
—hypoglycaemia, complications of thyroid, pituitary and adrenal disorders, avitaminosis

Other physical causes
—uraemia, liver failure, anaemias

Trauma to brain

Epilepsy

The organic psychotic conditions resulting from the above causal factors will not be described in the order given here but will follow that of the I.C.D.

SENILE AND PRESENILE ORGANIC PSYCHOTIC CONDITIONS

Senile dementia, simple type

A gradual impairment of bodily and mental functions is natural in man's progress to the grave. In some individuals however, the mental deterioration outruns the bodily, and the term senile dementia is applied to such a condition. To be more specific, the diagnosis of senile dementia is applied to 'dementia occuring usually after the age of 65 years in which any cerebral pathology other than that of senile atrophic change (atrophy = wasting), can be reasonably excluded.'

Senile dementia may occur with relatively slight pathological changes in the brain, while in other cases, well-marked changes may be observed post mortem in an individual who showed few or no symptoms during life. Macroscopically, the demented brain shows generalised shrinkage of the cerebral cortex, particularly in the frontal lobe, and consequent widening of the sulci.

Aetiology

The social and medical advances which have been largely responsible for bringing about an increased expectation of life, give rise to a greater population at risk.

There is some evidence for a genetic factor in the development of the condition.

Senile dementia occurs more commonly in women, the ratio of females to males being approximately 2:1.

Social, environmental, and personality factors appear to play a large part in the development of clinical deterioration.

Clinical picture

Approximately 50% of sufferers are said to follow a pattern of simple intellectual deterioration, wherein the six basic mental state abnormalities become more and more obvious.

Failure of memory first becomes apparent in the inability to remember proper names. Loss of memory may lead to daily or even hourly repetition of the same story, the patient being unaware of having previously recounted it. When the sufferer from senile dementia is asked what he did earlier in the day he may confabulate, giving details of activities which could not possibly have been carried out. Loss of interest in the present and the failure to receive new impressions leads to a retreat into the past, and childhood scenes are remembered as if they happened yesterday. There is poverty of ideation often leading to the repetition of platitudes. An inability to sympathise with others and a reluctance to recognise their deficiencies lead the old man or woman to become peevish and unreasonable.

Management

Psychotherapy is of little or no use in the deteriorated patient when memory may not even extend from one session to the next. No specific physical or drug treatment prevents or reduces the pathological changes underlying senile dementia.

The principal management of dementing aged people in a hospital situation involves social and milieu therapy. A balance has to be struck between structuring rigid routines in the day's activities and providing fresh activities which will stimulate mind and body. The aged person perhaps feels more secure in routine repetitive situations, but if these are all that is provided, institutionalisation will result and the pleasure and satisfaction of achievement in activities relevant to his declining abilities is lost. Group meetings, television, newspaper clubs, occupational therapy groups and excursions may all contribute to the well-being of these patients.

The simple procedures of maintaining reasonable daytime activity plus regular toilet habits can do much to ensure that these aged patients sleep well without sedation, and what is more, have dry nights.

One's aims in rehabilitation are limited by the fact that we are dealing with a person whose brain manifests an impairment of function which will most certainly deteriorate further.

Much can be done in the community to prevent unnecessary hospitalisation of people suffering from senile dementia. Removal from the well-known local geography of the home into a new environment may lead to confusion and even disturbed behaviour. Against this, has to be balanced the stresses experienced by the family of which the old person is a member. Regular visits by community nurses to assist in actual nursing procedures required, can ease the family's anxiety arising largely out of a lack of expertise.

If hospitals are prepared to admit the dementing patient for a time, once or twice a year, this gives the younger members of the family some respite from what can be a formidable task, that of caring for the aged.

Presenile dementia

This is a 'dementia occurring usually before the age of 65 years in patients with relatively rare forms of diffuse or lobar cerebral atrophy. Such dementia occurs in Alzheimer's disease and Pick's disease of the brain.'

Alzheimer's disease

This is said to be the most common of the dementias occurring before the age of 60.

Aetiology. The aetiology of the condition is unknown, though families in which a hereditary disposition exists have been reported. The pathological changes in the brain are widespread, involving the frontal, temporal and parietal lobes, and basal ganglia.

Clinical Picture. The clinical picture is frequently described in three stages:

1. The first symptom to attract attention is loss of memory. Severe spatial disorientation also occurs at an early stage, and patients may become lost even in their own homes.

2. Focal symptoms, due to damage to specific functional areas of the brain, are: aphasia, apraxia (the inabiiity to carry out deliberate voluntary movements), and agnosia (the inability to recognise the nature or use of objects, including parts of the body). Extrapyramidal symptoms, rigidity, and alteration in gait occur so that it resembles that of a puppet. Echolalia and logoclonia (the incomprehensible repetition of syllables) may be present, Epileptiform convulsions occur in 25-30% of cases.

3. Marked dementia, flexion contractures, restlessness, emaciation and a decline to a vegetative existence constitute the terminal picture. Patients with confirmed Alzheimer's disease usually live for 2-5 years, depending to some extent on the management of intercurrent illness. Some cases are reported to have survived for over 15 years.

Treatment. There is no specific treatment, and we are limited to drug therapy for agitation, the maintenance of nutrition, the prevention of bedsores and the application of general management principles, outlined under the section on treatment of senile dementia.

Pick's disease

This rare condition is said to affect females and males in the ratio of 2:1.

The atrophic changes in the brain are more selective than in Alzheimer's disease, affecting mainly the frontal and temporal cortical areas.

The condition is due to the effects of an abnormal single dominant autosomal gene.

Clinical picture. This is a slowly progressing dementia, first evidenced by intellectual impairment, characterised by difficulty in concentration and attention, and easy fatiguability. Memory becomes impaired to a gross degree. The patient's affect is flat, and he becomes inert, apathetic and lacking in spontaneity. Symptoms arising from focal cortical lesions are primarily aphasias, apraxias, and agnosias. Restlessness may develop, and speech deteriorates to meaningless and incoherent jargon.

Moral and ethical control of behaviour is lost early, leading, not infrequently, to activities which may come under police attention.

The presence of depression, delusions or hallucinations is rare in Pick's disease. Epileptic seizures, though uncommon, may occur.

The final picture is similar to that seen in Alzheimer's disease. Death occurs within 2 to 11 years. The average duration of life following its onset is stated to be 5 years.

Management. There is no known treatment, and management revolves around the care of the patient's general health, as well as environmental measures applicable to any illness in which dementia is a feature.

Senile dementia, depressed or paranoid type

This condition is described as 'a type of senile dementia characterised by development in advanced old age, progressive in nature, in which a variety of delusions and hallucinations of a persecutory, depressive and somatic content are also present. Disturbances of the sleep/waking cycle and preoccupation with dead people are often particularly prominent.'

The additional symptoms to those of the simple type of senile dementia are probably attributable to the person's premorbid personality and previous modes of adjustment to life. Oncoming deafness also appears to precipitate paranoid symptoms.

The question of testamentary capacity comes into the picture when the sufferer from senile dementia, probably with unmasked paranoid personality traits, becomes suspicious of the family and alters his will.

The management of these patients is as for simple senile dementia with the early addition of a suitable medication such as a phenothiazine or butyrophenone derivative. Depression may be helped by giving ECT—widely spaced to avoid further memory defect and confusion.

Senile dementia with acute confusional state

This is the term used to describe 'senile dementia with a superimposed episode of acute confusional state'.

If the underlying precipitating factor leading to the confusional state can be identified it should be appropriately managed. Precipitating factors include intra- or extracerebral toxic, infectious, metabolic or other systemic disturbance.

Arteriosclerotic dementia

The I.C.D. defines this as

> dementia attributable, because of physical signs (on examination of the central nervous system) to degenerative arterial disease of the brain. Symptoms suggesting a focal lesion in the brain are common. There may be a fluctuating or patchy intellectual defect with insight, and an intermittent course is common. Clinical differentation from senile or presenile dementia, which may coexist with it, may be very difficult or impossible.

The disorder usually manifests itself in the sixth decade, but may be present as early as the middle forties, with men more commonly affected than women. There may occur one or more cerebrovascular accidents or strokes prior to the onset of symptoms. Hypertension is present in about half of these patients.

Clinical picture

The patient usually comes under notice as a result of the sudden onset of a confused or delirious state in which he may be incoherent and restless, and may experience hallucinations. A careful history will frequently indicate that for some months the patient has had an increase in headaches, has experienced dizziness, faintness or increased fatiguability, and may have suffered from transient 'blackouts' or short-lived focal neurological symptoms. The nature of these focal symptoms will depend on the site or sites of the impaired blood flow to the brain. Insomnia, usually difficulty in getting off to sleep, is common early in this disease.

Of the six basic symptoms occurring in organic psychotic conditions memory is usually the first mental function affected, and this consists in amnesia for recent events.

Personality is preserved and insight is maintained at least in the early stages of the disease. The retention of insight into his state of deterioration may be most distressing to the patient.

The mood generally shows marked fluctuation, the patient being easily moved to tears or laughter. This emotional lability, together with a marked fluctuation in the course of the illness, helps in distinguishing the condition from senile dementia in those cases occurring later in life. For hours, or even days, the sufferer from arteriosclerotic dementia may appear quite lucid, only to return to a state of confusion and disorientation. Those who have nursed these patients will be only too aware of the great restlessness and confusion that may be present after nightfall.

A 'catastrophic reaction', wherein a patient may withdraw, become depressed, or show signs of anxiety and distress leading to aggressive behaviour, is not infrequent in these patients when faced with a task they are unable to carry out. Short-lived paranoid delusions, along with hallucinatory experiences are not uncommonly seen, and depressive symptoms, also usually short-lived, may be a feature.

A progressive or episodic decline in intellectual functions occurs. It is stated that the average life expectancy from date of onset of the illness is something over four years, though figures quoted differ considerably.

With improved physical care and modern medications, some patients may survive is a demented state for 15 years or more, death usually resulting from infection, cerebral haemorrhage or thrombosis, or from myocardial infarction.

Management

General management in the later stages is as for senile dementia; night sedation however, will probably be more necessary in sufferers from arteriosclerotic dementia.

ALCOHOLIC PSYCHOSES

Alcoholic psychoses are described in the I.C.D. as organic psychotic states due mainly to excessive consumption of alcohol. Defects of nutrition are thought to play an important role. In some of these states withdrawal of alcohol can be of aetiological significance as it is in the first condition to be described, namely, delirium tremens.

Delirium tremens

Delirium tremens (DTs) is an acute or subacute organic psychotic state due to the lowering of the blood alcohol level following diminution in alcohol intake after a heavy prolonged bout of drinking. It rarely occurs in people who have not suffered serious dependence on alcohol for at least a few years.

Clinical picture

The sufferer, for some considerable time, may have experienced episodes of the so-called tremulous state manifested by psychomotor agitation without evidence of auditory or visual hallucinations. The fully-developed withdrawal syndrome known as delirium tremens is characterised by clouded consciousness, disorientation, fear, illusions, delusions, hallucinations of any kind, notably visual and tactile, and restlessness, tremor and sometimes fever.

Generalised epileptic seizures may further complicate the picture and, in fact, delirium tremens is not infrequently ushered in by a grand mal epileptic seizure. Other symptoms and signs associated with the condition at some stage include: an internal abdominal quivering, epigastric in site and referred to as 'butterflies in the stomach'; muscular cramps affecting principally the muscles concerned with locomotion; nausea and vomiting; insomnia; tachycardia and a rise in blood pressure. Hyperacusis may also be complained of. The hallucinations which occur are usually of a frightening or even terrifying nature.

The death rate in delirium tremens ranges from 10%-20%, and illnesses complicating the condition account for much of this mortality, the most common of these being pneumonia and liver disease. A group of people die following a state of hyperthermia (40° C or higher), frequently manifesting convulsions, and finally dying in a state of coma and vascular collapse. Dehydration may be an important factor in this group.

Management of delirum tremens

TREATMENT FACILITIES

Delirium tremens requires hospitalisation. Treatment should preferably be carried out in a special unit that can handle the physical complications which may exist, rather than in a situation where there are multiple pressures on staff, arising from patients with a variety of psychiatric conditions and the presence of a large admission rate.

Long-term treatment of alcohol addiction should be initiated along with medical management of the acute toxic state. This is a rational preventive approach as 25%-50% of patients with multiple episodes of delirium tremens may be expected to die within five years. (See page 255).

COMPLICATIONS

Complicating conditions should be sought diligently, and treated appropriately at the first possible moment. An argument for handling patients on a special unit is that staff there could be expected to develop a subtlety of judgement in detecting and handling complications. Whether prophylactic antibiotics are used would depend to a large extent on the staff and attending doctor's ability to frequently assess the patient's physical state.

Any patient in a state of acute withdrawal, who has a history of prior seizures, or who has marked tremor and clonic jerks suggesting impending seizures, should be given prophylactic anti-convulsants on admission.

PATIENT'S IMMEDIATE ENVIRONMENT

As the majority of patients start to misinterpret external stimuli and enter delirium tremens at darkness, particularly when they are on their own, it is sound practice to leave a night light burning. This enables the patient to utilize external orientating cues. Members of staff should be present with patients in their waking periods, talking to them by name, identifying themselves, and explaining possible visual misinterpretations (illusions). Such actions strengthen the patient's link with reality, and the tendency for him to disorganise is lessened. Such a role is an ego-supporting one, and is made possible through the development of a relationship between staff and patients wherein they can temporarily rely on staff members for the assessment of reality.

FOOD AND VITAMINS

Upper gastrointestinal symptoms are treated with aluminium hydroxide, and a bland diet is given when the patient is able to accommodate same. Though vitamin deficiency has no necessary part to play in the development of delirium tremens, thiamine deficiency is implicated in the development of Wernicke's disease and Korsakov's psychosis, and in alcoholic polyneuropathy. However, as the nutritional state of patients in delirium tremens is usually very poor, vitamins, particularly the B group, must be considered mandatory, at least in the initial stages of treatment. For example, it is a reasonable practice to mix and give intravenous Parentrovite (B group and Vitamin C) for 3-5 days.

HYDRATION

Adequate hydration of patients in acute alcoholic withdrawal states is of paramount importance, and with the use of suitable drug medication, the oral route is usually quite feasible. Intravenous fluids and electrolytes should rarely be required, but if dehydration is marked and difficulty exists in using the oral route, intravenous fluids must be given.

DRUGS

One is faced with a bewildering array of drugs and regimes used in the management of delirium tremens. Before dealing with a number of these, two important principles in the use of drugs for the treatment of acute alcoholic withdrawal states should be stressed:

(i) Drugs should be given as near as possible on a round-the-clock basis and not 'P.R.N.' or 'as required'.

(ii) As there is some evidence that drugs given in standard doses may worsen rather than improve the clinical manifestations in alcohol withdrawal states, one must not give too little of the medication decided upon.

TIME-HONOURED REMEDIES

Barbiturates, paraldehyde and chloral hydrate have their place in treatment if given at regular intervals. For example, paraldehyde up to 10cc. I.M. may be given at 4-hourly intervals, with chloral hydrate added at 6-hourly intervals if agitation is present.

MORE RECENT REGIMES

(i) Haloperidol (Serenace) 10-20 mg I.V. or I.M. with amylobarbitone sodium 250 mg or 500 mg I.V. on admission. Then 5-10 mg haloperidol I.M. 6th hourly for the next few days depending on the patient's condition. A medium acting barbiturate, for example amylobarbitone sodium, may be added at night if necessary. Paraldehyde 10cc orally or I.M. may be given as well, though this is rarely necessary. Extrapyramidal side-effects of haloperidol are controlled by benztropine mesylate (Cogentin) 2 mg daily which may be given I.V. or orally, or by procyclidine hydrochloride (Kemadrin) 5 mg B.D. orally.

(ii) In patients with no history of peptic ulceration and no vomiting, the following regime may be followed: Chlormethiazole (Hemineurin) 0.5 G, 4 capsules statim then 3 at night depending on time of commencement of treatment. Dosage is then reduced: 2nd day—2 capsules mane, 3 capsules midday, 3 capsules at night; 3rd day—1 capsule mane, 1 capsule midday, 2 capsules at night; 4th day—1 capsule mane, 1 capsule midday, 1 capsule at night; 5th day—one capsule at night only.

(iii) In patients with a history of peptic ulceration, or if they are vomiting or extremely restless or agitated, Chlorprothixene (Taractan) 30 mg ampoule I.M. is given statim. This is repeated in 4-6 hours if the patient is still restless. On the second day in the early morning, a second injection of chlorprothixene 15-30 mg is given I.M., and chlordiazepoxide (Librium) 20 mg T.D.S. orally is commenced after reassessment of the patient. If night sedation if required, diazepam (Valium) 5-10 mg orally is usually sufficient.

These are but three proven regimes that are in use. There are doubtless other therapists with particular personal regimes. In our present state of knowledge, one should not be dogmatic about which regime is best. Whatever drugs are used, of utmost importance is the provision of adequate treatment facilities, dealing with complications early, the patient's immediate environment, vitamins, adequate hydration, and the giving of medication in adequate amounts on a round-the-clock basis.

An attempt to deal with the problem of Alcohol dependence syndrome has led to the development of the withdrawal and motivational unit wherein many clients are managed in states of withdrawal, including delirium tremens (page 257).

Korsakov's psychosis, alcoholic

Korsakov's (also spelt Korsakoff's) psychosis, alcoholic is

> a syndrome of prominent and lasting reduction of memory span, including striking loss of recent memory, disordered time appreciation and confabulation, occurring in alcoholics as the sequel to an acute alcoholic psychosis (especially delirium tremens) or, more rarely, in the course of chronic alcoholism. It is usually accompanied by peripheral neuritis and may be associated with Wernicke's encephalopathy.

Other basic features of organic psychotic conditions are also present. The syndrome was first described in 1887 by Korsakov, who labelled it polyneuritic psychosis. It was subsequently called Korsakov's psychosis or the amnestic confabulatory syndrome. The pathological findings in the brain include lesions consisting of haemorrhages, proliferation of capillary endothelial cells and destruction of nerve cells and fibres, situated mainly in the grey matter surrounding the third ventricle and aqueduct, the mammillary bodies, the brainstem and the dorsomedial nuclei of the thalamus.

Korsakov's psychosis or syndrome may be due to factors other than alcoholism resulting in thiamine (Vitamin B_1) deficiency. These factors include: persistent vomiting associated with toxaemia of pregnancy, chronic arsenical gastritis, chronic poisoning with lead or other heavy metals, nutritional deficiences associated with starvation, beriberi and pellagra, vascular disease and brain trauma. When due to factors other than alcohol the condition is classified as Korsakov's psychosis or syndrome (nonalcoholic).

Wernicke's encephalopathy

Although Wernicke's encephalopathy is not classified under 'mental disorders' but under another rubric in the I.C.D., brief mention will be made of this disorder first described in states of malnutrition by Wernicke in 1881. The condition is of acute onset and potentially fatal, manifest by confusion, memory loss, apathy and confabulation. Of physical signs and symptoms, disturbance of gait, diplopia (double vision) and impaired lateral gaze due to paralysis of the third and sixth cranial nerves are the most pronounced. Somnolence, stupor and coma may supervene. If the patient survives the acute phase he is left with a residual Korsakov's psychosis. The common factor in both Wernicke's encephalopathy and

Korsakov's psychosis appears to be thiamine deficiency, and some writers speak of the Wernicke-Korsakov syndrome to describe the association of both conditions. Wernicke's encephalopathy is a medical emergency and 100 mg of intramuscular thiamine should be given immediately the diagnosis is made.

Alcoholic dementia

Classified as 'other alcoholic dementia' this consists of a 'nonhallucinatory dementia . . . in association with alcoholism but not characterised by the features of either delirium tremens or Korsakov's psychosis'.

Treatment of the alcoholic dementias

Already mentioned as an emergency measure in the management of Wernicke's encephalopathy is the giving of intramuscular thiamine.

In the late stages of alcoholic dementia and in Korsakov's psychosis cerebral changes may not be completely reversible. However, one must persevere with a strict management programme which involves prolonged hospitalisation, for with cessation of drinking, intensive treatment with vitamins, particularly the B group, and adequate nutrition, improvement may occur over many months. It is said that in six months to two years, 25 per cent of cases presenting with Korsakov's psychosis can fully recover with adequate management, and an additional 50 per cent will improve significantly. One has certainly seen patients who were apparently hopeless prospects with grossly disorganised intellectual functions able to once again cope with work, even of a semi-technical nature. Regular follow-up is mandatory, and programmes such as are mentioned later under the management of the alcohol dependence syndrome should be seriously considered (page 255).

It must be remembered that alcoholic psychoses are very frequently accompanied by physical pathology apart from the neurological changes in the central and peripheral nervous systems already mentioned. Cirrhosis of the liver, with the possibility of ultimate liver failure and hepatic coma, is not uncommon. Portal hypertension with increased pressure in the veins that pass to the liver may develop, and this can result in bleeding, manifesting itself as haematemesis (vomiting of blood) and malaena (black stools due to altered blood). With respect to the peripheral nervous system pathology mentioned above, the condition arising due to thiamine deficiency is peripheral neuritis. This presents with paraesthesia such as tingling, pins-and-needles and numbness in the periphery of all limbs, frequently accompanied by severe pain. Motor weakness may follow, leading for example to foot drop, and the patient may become ataxic or unsteady in his gait.

Chronic gastritis occurs, giving rise to morning vomiting and gross interference with appetite and digestion. This should be differentiated from the anorexia associated with psychotic depressive illnesses. Lack of thiamine may occasionally lead to cardiac failure.

The good psychiatrist or nurse is aware of the possible physical complications in his patients, and will never fail to see the patient as a whole, and not simply as somebody existing only above the bridge of the nose.

It is obvious that early consultation with experts in internal medicine is in the best interests of the patient when physical complications are present.

Alcoholic hallucinosis

Classified as 'other alcoholic hallucinosis' this condition is

> a psychosis of less than six months duration, with slight or no clouding of consciousness and much anxious restlessness in which auditory hallucinations, mostly of voices uttering insults and threats, predominate.

The state may occur during continued drinking by the patient, but is more in evidence from one to a few days after ceasing alcohol intake. Some patients who have suffered from alcoholic hallucinosis are said to become schizophrenic, but whether the condition is related to schizophrenia is unclear.

Clinical picture

Usually the sole manifestation of the disorder is the occurrence of auditory hallucinations, which may be threatening, accusatory, and fear-producing. A patient may attack his believed persecutors. Delusions may be present in many cases, but auditory hallucinations are the prominent feature of this disorder. Visual hallucinations rarely form part of the clinical picture. Intellectual resources remain unaffected, and the sensorium is clear. Depressive symptoms may occur, and suicidal attempts are not uncommon. The usual course of the condition runs a few days to a month, but recurrences are common if further alcohol is taken. Cases have been recorded lasting 3-4 months after the cessation of alcohol. The treatment is to hospitalise the patient, withdraw alcohol, and give medication to calm him. The phenothiazines and antidepressant drugs are frequently indicated, and adequate nutrition and vitamin supplements are necessary.

Pathological drunkenness

This term is applied to

> acute psychotic episodes induced by relatively small amounts of alcohol. They are regarded as individual idiosyncratic reactions to alcohol, not due to excessive consumption and without conspicious neurological signs of intoxication.

Alcoholic jealousy

Also known as alcoholic paranoia the term is used to describe

> a chronic paranoid psychosis characterised by delusional jealousy and associated with alcoholism.

There occur poorly systematised delusions of persecution, delusions of marital infidelity, morbid jealousy, and aggressive violent behaviour.

Alcohol *per se* cannot be regarded as the cause of alcoholic paranoia. It is a complicating factor, inasmuch as intake of alcohol may be symptomatic of inner tensions related to a poorly developed personality which does not permit the formation of satisfactory heterosexual relationships; again it is considered that the use of alcohol weakens repression, and forbidden homosexual impulses rise to the surface to be defended against by the development of a paranoid delusional system. Alcohol, taken in quantity, can and does reduce potency. This, in itself, may cause panic if further doubt as to the sufferer's masculinity is engendered. The combination of jealousy and lessened potency, increased sexual desire due to intoxication, and decreased consideration and affection, may cause aversion in any wife. The slightest sign of reluctance on her part leads to anger, resentment and further suspicion and jealousy. The alcoholic cannot tolerate the fact that he is a failure in married life, and he projects his failure on to his wife.

Treatment

Hospitalisation, reduction or elimination of alcohol intake if this can be achieved, and giving one or more of the phenothiazine drugs constitute the main areas in management of such patients. Prognosis on return to the original environment is only fair.

DRUG PSYCHOSES

The I.C.D. describes drug psychoses as

> syndromes that do not fit the descriptions of the nonorganic psychoses and which are due to consumption of drugs (notably amphetamines, barbiturates and the opiate and LSD groups) and solvents. Some of the syndromes in this group are not as severe as most conditions labelled "psychotic" but they are included for practical reasons.

Three major groupings are described:

1. The *drug withdrawal syndrome* which includes states associated with drug withdrawal ranging from severe (*cf.* delirium tremens in alcohol withdrawal) to less severe states characterised by one or more symptoms such as convulsions, tremor, anxiety, restlessness, gastrointestinal and muscular complaints, and mild disorientation and memory disturbance.
2. *Paranoid and/or hallucinatory states* induced by drugs which are states of more than a few days but not usually of more than a few months duration, associated with large or prolonged intake of drugs, notably of the amphetamine and LSD groups. Auditory hallucinations usually predominate, and there may be anxiety and restlessness.
3. *Pathological drug intoxication* involves individual idiosyncratic reactions to comparatively small quantities of a drug, which take the form of acute, brief psychotic states of any type.

Following this introduction from the I.C.D. we shall turn our attention to the effects of a number of individual drugs. At this stage a brief description will be given of amphetamines, barbiturates and bromides. The effects of the opiates, LSD and other hallucinogens are described in a later chapter entitled 'Alcoholism and drug dependence' (page 251ff.) and they should be studied along with the following descriptions.

Amphetamines

It might be expected that the consumption of large quantities of amphetamines would lead to clouding of consciousness with delirium and excitement. This does occur, but in the majority of people, the clinical picture after long continued excessive consumption of amphetamines resembles that of paranoid schizophrenia, with ideas of reference, paranoid delusions, and hallucinatory experiences with no demonstrable clouding of consciousness.

One patient seen in an admission centre was a truck driver who took up to one hundred 5 mg tablets of amphetamine sulphate on a five hundred mile journey. He was admitted to hospital after seeing Lilliputian figures on the dashboard of his truck and a sailing boat in the middle of the road.

Treatment

Therapy is symptomatic. A protective, quiet, constant environment plus the giving of tranquillising drugs if necessary, is usually all that is indicated. The psychotic symptoms usually disappear within a few days of stopping the drug, but may persist for several weeks.

Barbiturates

These are cortical depressants, and act in much the same way as alcohol or a general anaesthetic agent. The clinical picture may vary from a state of drunkenness to one of drowsiness and stupor. Excessive dosage can lead to coma and death. Some patients, as in a drunken state from alcohol, are confused, disoriented, and have slurred speech and ataxia. Others develop a persistent hypomanic state interrupted by periods of restlessness and irritability, while some may remain for a time in a subdelirious state. Apart from the above effects of the barbiturates themselves, the effects of sudden withdrawal of these drugs may lead to convulsions and delirium tremens. Status epilepticus may occur following the sudden cessation of a large and prolonged intake of barbiturates. It has been stated by one authority that in addicts who have taken 0.8 G or more of a medium-acting barbiturate daily for some 3 to 6 weeks, sudden withdrawal will produce convulsions in 3 out of 4 cases, and delirium in 4 out of 5 cases.

Treatment

In view of the possibility of delirium or convulsions developing during the withdrawal state, it is sound practice to administer a barbiturate, for example, sodium amylobarbitone, in doses reducing by 100 mg per day. Other general aspects of management are similar to those for delirium tremens to be mentioned later. In fact, the principles applied in the management of DTs will be suitable for the management of patients suffering from acute brain syndromes, arising from a variety of causes.

Bromide and bromureides

Following excessive or continued use of these drugs, which accumulate in the body, a frequent clinical picture is one of confusion, slurred speech, and ataxia. The most common symptom which can lead to misdiagnosis is depression, and probably many patients admitted to hospital and diagnosed as suffering from a depressive illness are really only showing the effects of bromide intoxication. Treatment consists in giving copious fluids, for example, one gallon per day if there are no physical contra-indications to this amount. Some therapists give large amounts of sodium chloride to hasten the excretion of bromide. In practice, however, it suffices to give a large quantity of fluid along with a normal salt-containing diet. Other aspects of management will depend on the patient's mental state.

Other drugs

Apart from the drugs mentioned above and in Chapter 17 it is well to remember that certain other substances commonly used in medical practice may also lead to drug psychosis. Included among these are digitalis, the belladonna alkaloids, cortisone and its derivatives, adrenocortecotrophic hormone (ACTH), thiocyanates used in hypertension, penicillin, disulfiram (Antabuse), and many more.

TRANSIENT ORGANIC PSYCHOTIC CONDITIONS

These are

> states characterised by clouded consciousness, confusion, disorientation, illusions and often vivid hallucinations. They are usually due to some intra- or extracerebral toxic, infectious, metabolic or other systemic disturbance and are generally reversible. Depressive and paranoid symptoms may also be present but are not the main feature.

In making diagnoses under this heading the associated physical or neurological conditions must also be stated.

Two main diagnostic categories are included. The first is the *acute confusional states*, which is short-lived, lasting hours or days, and covers the following acute states: delirium; infective psychosis; psycho-organic syndrome; psychosis associated with endocrine, metabolic or cerebrovascular disorder; as well as the epileptic confusion and twilight states.

The second category is the *subacute confusional state* in which the symptoms are usually less florid than in the acute states. They last for several weeks or longer, during which they may show marked fluctuations in intensity. The following subacute states are included: delirium, infective psychosis, organic reaction, post traumatic organic psychosis, psycho-organic syndrome, and psychosis associated with endocrine or metabolic disorder.

The management of these acute and subacute states is principally that of the underlying physical or neurological condition plus symptomatic management of mental state abnormalities, depending on their severity.

OTHER ORGANIC PSYCHOTIC CONDITIONS (CHRONIC)

Three categories of disorders are listed here. The first is *Korsakov's psychosis or syndrome (nonalcoholic)* which has received mention on page 152.

The second covers dementia in: cerebral lipoidoses, epilepsy, general paralysis of the insane, hepatolenticular degeneration, Huntington's chorea, multiple sclerosis, and polyarteritis nodosa.

The third classified as 'other' covers states that fulfil the criteria of an organic psychosis but do not take the form of a confusional state, a nonalcoholic Korsakov's psychosis, or a dementia. Included in this third category are mixed paranoid and affective organic psychotic states and epileptic psychosis NOS. Instead of attempting to cover all diseases associated with transient and chronic organic psychotic conditions a selection of some will be made. It must be remembered that these conditions may, or may not, depending on their severity and stage of devopment, lead to symptoms classifiable as transient or chronic organic psychotic conditions.

Huntington's Chorea

This hereditary condition results from the transmission of single abnormal dominant gene, and so theoretically may affect 50% of each generation.

Pathological changes are degenerative and progressive in nature, involving mainly the cerebral cortex and basal ganglia.

Clinical Picture

Symptoms appear most frequently between the ages of 30 and 40 years, though onset may be much earlier or much later in life.

Initially, there occurs restlessness, clumsiness and purposeless involuntary movements which may be converted by the sufferer into something that appears purposeful. The involuntary movements are choreo-athetoid in nature. Choreic movements are quick and jerky, while athetoid movements have a sinuous quality. This combination of movements comes to involve the fingers, face, and muscles concerned with speech including the diaphragm. The latter produces great difficulty in speech, resulting in explosive articulation. Gait becomes ataxic, and in fact, all voluntary muscles are affected, and all develop some degree of hypertonicity, sometimes producing peculiar postures.

Mental symptoms occur in all cases and take the form of a progressive dementia with apathy, impairment of comprehension, and loss of memory.

Emotional instability, manifest by outbursts of irritability and destructiveness, is common. Depression often colours the picture and there is a not unexpected tendency for patients to suicide. The mood of some patients may fluctuate between depression and euphoria. Paranoid ideation may develop in some, such a development being dependent on a patient's premorbid personality and other psychosocial factors.

The disease is progressive and incurable, death usually occurring in 10-20 years, but in some families the condition may be protracted in the sufferer over several decades.

Management

Management is as for any dementing process. In addition, phenothiazines, chlordiazepoxide or diazepam may give some relief from the musclar hyperactivity.

SPACE-OCCUPYING LESIONS

Cerebral tumours

Mental symptoms suggestive of a cerebral organic state may develop before there is neurological evidence of a cerebral tumour. Personality changes may well occur if the frontal lobes are involved. Tumours may give rise to, or precipitate symptoms of, a variety of psychiatric disorders.

Increased intracranial pressure, the rapidity of development of which depends on a number of factors including the rate of growth of the tumour and its site, may produce headache and vomiting.

A persistent or recurrent headache, aggravated by exertion, for example stooping to tie up one's shoe laces, warrants examination of the fundi to exclude the pressence of papilloedema, which is swelling of the optic disc (nerve head) caused by increased intracranial pressure.

Chronic subdural haematoma

A subdural haematoma is a collection of blood between the outer and middle coverings of the brain, that is, between the dura mater and the arachnoid mater. It may follow a severe head injury in which case it becomes immediately apparent that it constitutes a neurosurgical problem. However even relatively trivial head injury such as a fall on the forehead or occiput may lead to rupturing of cortical veins as they cross the subdural space and a slow leak of blood into the subdural space occurs. If there are recurrent small leaks of blood, the haematoma which becomes covered by a fibrous membrane, may develop in size and produce the clinical picture of an expanding space-occupying intracranial lesion, and it is difficult to differentiate clinically from a growing cerebral tumour. This slowly developing haematoma is referred to as a chronic subdural haematoma.

Clinically there is a latent period before symptoms appear that may range from days to months. Headaches develop and become more frequent and intense. Drowsiness, forgetfulness and confusion become apparent, and stupor and coma may supervene. A marked and common feature is the fluctuation in symptomatology from day to day and even from hour to hour.

Thorough neurological examinations, charting of pupil sizes, and ophthalmoscopic examinations to detect developing papilloedema are mandatory.

The treatment is surgical and consists in the evacuation of the haematoma.

INFECTIONS

Central nervous system syphilis

Neurosyphilis was formerly a common condition in general and psychiatric hospitals, but more effective treatment in the primary and secondary stages has made neurological involvement much less frequent. A rise in the admission rate of people suffering from tertiary syphilis was noted in certain English hospitals, and documented in 1960. This may have been due to the curing of one venereal disease, gonorrhoea, by treatment inadequate to cure an unnoticed and concomitant syphilitic infection. Adequate surveillance of cases should obviate this eventuality. Syphilis is due to infection by a spirochaete, Treponema pallidum. Two types of central nervous system syphilis will be described.

Meningoencephalic syphilis (dementia paralytica, general paralysis, G.P.I.)

Meningoencephalic syphilis or general paralysis of the insane (G.P.I) is a manifestation of the tertiary stage of syphilis, and, as the name implies, the brunt of the attack by the spirochaete is borne by the meninges and the substance of the brain. Gross pathological changes include cloudy and thickened meninges, atrophy of the cerebral convolutions, particularly over the anterior two-thirds of the brain, dilation of the ventricles, and a compensatory hydrocephalus. The latter consists of an increase in the amount of cerebrospinal fluid in the ventricles and around the brain, compensating for the loss of cerebral tissue in the confines of the skull.

CLINICAL PICTURE

The first symptoms of general paralysis occur 5-25 years after the primary infection, the usual interval being 10-15 years. Both physical and mental symptoms and signs are present.

PHYSICAL SIGNS

Physical signs which may or may not be apparent before mental symptoms have developed include, pupils which are small, unequal and irregular in outline, and which do not react to light but react to accommodation (Argyll Robertson pupils); irregular coarse tremor of face, lips and tongue, leading to gross dysarthria; tremor of hands, and incoordination of all movements. Epileptic attacks may occur, as may a transient hemiplegia, aphasia or hemianopia (loss of half of visual field). Upper motor neurone lesion signs, incontinence of urine, and optic atrophy leading to blindness, may also occur.

MENTAL SYMPTOMS

The most outstanding feature is the progressive destruction of all mental functions. The history given by the patient may be unreliable, and relatives may have noticed him misplacing articles, or repeating the same story several times, due to loss of recent memory. There may be disorientation in time, and affective changes may be apparent early. Euphoria or a feeling of well-being is most characteristic. On the other hand, the patient may become apathetic and dull, or anxious with emotional instability.

Sudden acts of violence or bizarre unpredictable behaviour may occur as a result of the gross loss of judgment characteristic of the disease. The grandiose delusions which are sometimes present are usually transitory in nature. As the disease progresses, dementia becomes marked, perhaps more than in any other psychiatric illness.

The condition may mimic a variety of psychiatric illnesses. Symptoms which may be present, and which may suggest other psychiatric disorders apart from those in which simple dementia occurs, include hypomania, depression, delirium or confusion, and schizophreniform symptoms. From this list, it can be seen how important it is to have a Wasserman Reaction or other tests for syphilis performed on the blood and cerebrospinal fluid of any patient over the age of 40 years who shows any signs of dementia, whether or not he manifests other psychiatric symptomatology. If a test on the CSF of any patient showing signs of dementia is not carried out, syphilis may be missed.

Meningovascular neurosyphilis

In this form of the illness, the spirochaete attacks the meninges and blood vessels of the brain. The important pathological change is cerebral softening resulting from occlusion of arteries by the syphilitic process.

CLINICAL PICTURE

The common clinical manifestation is apoplexy or stroke resulting in hemiplegia, sometimes associated with aphasia. Mental symptoms are those of a chronic brain syndrome, and may be indistinguishable from those of a meningoencephalic syphilis, depending on the extent of the vascular damage and cerebral softening. The early stages of the disease however, show a marked fluctuation in severity. It develops more acutely than meningoencephalitic syphilis, the patient generally has more insight, tremor is uncommon, and focal symptoms due to cerebral softening are more prominent. The prognosis is far better than in G.P.I. if the condition is diagnosed early and appropriate treatment given.

Treatment of central nervous system syphilis

This consists in giving penicillin in adequate dosage, and it is claimed that 15-25 million units in divided doses will effect a cure. Post-treatment surveillance at regular intervals is essential and follow-up may be necessary for a number of years. This consists of taking cerebrospinal fluid by lumbar puncture and submitting it to cell counts and other tests, including a W.R. or equivalent test. Response to therapy depends on the extent of brain damage prior to the commencement of treatment.

Encephalitis

The term 'encephalitis', meaning an infection or inflammatory process of the brain, is, by common usage, restricted to viral infections of the brain, and many different types of virus have now been isolated. The clinical picture is one of an acute brain syndrome with a variety of neurological signs, depending on the sites of insult to the brain.

Some of the encephalitides may lead to severe irreversible impairment of intellectual function with marked symptomatology. On the other hand, some may be so mild as to be undiagnosed at the time of illness, the development of Parkinsonism* later in life (post encephalitic Parkinsonism) suggesting that a previous mild pyrexial illness was indeed encephalitis.

The child's brain reacts to encephalitis in a different way from that of the adult. Following the acute attack, a child frequently shows gross

* The term Parkinsonism is derived from Parkinson's disease (paralysis agitans) which is a primary degenerative disease of the brain of unknown cause, occurring usually between the ages of 50 and 60 years. The main features are rigidity and tremor of voluntary muscles, and salivation. Another cause of Parkinsonism is atheroma of cerebral vessels supplying the basal ganglia.

Parkinsonism also occurs as a side-effect of large dosage of some of the drugs used in psychiatry today, notably phenothiazine derivatives and the butyrophenones.

personality changes. He may be untruthful, overactive, aggressive, and may impulsively carry out acts of cruelty or destructiveness. Following encephalitis, intellectual functions in children may or may not be impaired.

METABOLIC, ENDOCRINE OR NUTRITIONAL DISORDERS

Hypoglycaemia

The condition of hypoglycaemia, meaning lowered blood sugar or glucose, may arise from a number of causes apart from the rarely occurring cryptogenic or idiopathic hypoglycaemia wherein no cause is demonstrable. Hypoglycaemia may arise from a functional disorder of the beta cells of the Islets of Langerhans in the pancreas, with the glucose level in the blood being lowered by over-production of insulin. It may also be due to a tumour of the islet cells of the pancreas, be associated with chronic liver disease, and of course, occur when overdoses of insulin are given to patients suffering from diabetes mellitus.

A man in his late twenties was presented some years ago to a group of doctors in a London hospital. This young man, previously a brilliant student with a doctorate, showed marked signs of dementia. He had an insulin-producing islet-cell tumour of the pancreas which was not diagnosed before repeated and persistent hypoglycaemia had led to severe brain damage.

Clinical picture

Apart from the severe state of dementia that may occur, the early symptoms are similar to those of an anxiety neurosis, with flushing of the skin, sweating, tachycardia, tremors, headache, dizziness, nausea, weakness and syncope or fainting. At least some of these symptoms are due to a homeostatic reaction on the part of the body wherein adrenalin is released in an effort to convert liver glycogen to glucose, and so restore the glucose level in the blood. Numbness and tingling of the extremities, tongue and lips, may develop and there may be muscular twitching and even convulsions. Other mental symptoms may include confusion, drowsiness, auditory and visual hallucinations, or illusory phenomena. Hypoglycaemic coma may supervene.

An example of the effects of low blood sugar was seen in a man of middle age found directing traffic at a street intersection. He was brought to a London observation ward by police, and was found to be a sufferer from diabetes mellitus whose blood sugar had dropped very low due to injudicious use of insulin.

Thyroid disorders

Hypothyroidism

Hypothyroidism is due to deficiency of thyroid hormone. This deficiency, if occurring from birth, gives rise to cretinism, which will be described in the section on mental retardation. Thyroid deficiency commencing in adulthood leads to the development of myxoedema in which psychiatric symptoms may be apparent before physical signs and symptoms are obvious.

CLINICAL PICTURE

There occurs a progressive slowing down and falling off in all mental functions. Sufferers become apathetic, dull and drowsy and display memory defects. Anxiety and irritability may occur, but a more common picture is one of complete sluggishness with little evidence of emotion.

Depression and paranoid symptoms may be of psychotic intensity. The term 'myxoedematous madness' is applied to such a state, which may also feature hallucinations and phases of excitement. Such symptoms probably depend on the previous personality of the patient, the psychotic symptoms being a reaction of the personality to the mental and physical state produced by thyroid lack, or may be the result of the organic insult of thyroid lack itself.

TREATMENT

Treatment consists in giving Thyroid extract 60 mg or *l*-thyroxine sodium B.P. 0.1 mg daily, increasing the dose no more frequently than every 10-14 days, owing to the delay in eliciting a response. Adjustment of dosage level will depend on such factors as the patient's symptoms, the resting pulse rate, and body weight. Mental state abnormalities usually clear along with the myxoedema.

Hyperthyroidism (Grave's Disease)

Hyperthyroidism or thyrotoxicosis results from excessive production of thyroid hormone. Mental changes are essential features of this illness, and they often give the appearance of being an exaggeration of the patient's previous personality. The sufferer is persistently on the move, suffers from insomnia, is distractible, lacks concentration, and is impatient and irritable. Noise intolerance may be a marked feature. Mood may be either one of hypomania or depression. The latter is not accompanied by the retardation of thought or action seen in some depressive illnesses. Underlying the prevailing mood there is always a feeling of anxiety or fear.

Associated with severe thyrotoxicosis, a psychotic state may supervene, features varying from manic excitement with delusions and hallucinations to psychotic depressive symptoms or delirium.

TREATMENT

This is primarily medical or surgical, but psychotherapy has its place as an adjunct in management.

Pernicious anaemia (Addisonian pernicious anaemia)

Pernicious anaemia is a megaloblastic anaemia caused by failure of absorption of Vitamin B_{12} (cyanocobalamin) from the alimentary tract. The primary cause is the lack of Castle's intrinsic factor from the gastric secretions, this factor being necessary for the absorption of Vitamin B_{12}. Untreated, this illness may be accompanied by mental symptoms. Somnolence and apathy may be present. Manic states and depression are reported, but the most common mental accompaniments of the condition are a paranoid psychosis and tactile hallucinations, these latter probably not being truly hallucinatory in nature, but the result of nerve damage. Disorientation, drowsiness and delirium may also occur.

When a psychotic state accompanies pernicious anaemia, it is sometimes referred to as 'megaloblastic madness'.

Treatment

Psychotic symptoms settle as the blood picture is stabilised. Treatment is essentially that of pernicious anaemia, namely a regime of Vitamin B_{12} injections which it is necessary to continue indefinitely.

CEREBRAL TRAUMA

Fractures of the skull tend to be associated with brain damage, but the brain may escape injury even with a severe skull fracture. Conversely, brain damage may occur without fracture of the skull. Contrecoup lesions are areas of contusion or laceration to areas of the brain opposite the point of trauma.

Trauma to the brain may produce symptoms which are reversible or irreversible. Two reversible clinical conditions described are concussion and traumatic coma.

Concussion

A state of concussion is one in which there is immediate but usually transient loss of consciousness due to a head injury, for example, the usual knockout in boxing. A complete transient flaccid paralysis occurs. The brain probably shows contusion (bruising) with little or no laceration. There is frequently amnesia for events occurring just prior to the injury (retrograde amnesia). If unconsciousness is prolonged, there may be a sudden waking, or a period of confusion with disorientation following an injury, though the injured person shows no evidence of abnormality. Where the amnesia occurs following head injury, the term anterograde or post-traumatic amnesia is applied. A young doctor complete with crash helmet, following a fall from a motor scooter, remembered details occurring up to within a second of the accident. The next recollection was that of thanking a truck driver who had given an eye-witness account to the police and who was climbing back into the cabin of his truck. A kindly old lady living nearby had apparently invited the police and victim in for a cup of tea, and the next recollection was for the few seconds it took to walk off the road. After mounting the footpath there was an amnesic gap sufficient for the party to have settled in the front room of the house, and tea to have been made and poured. The doctor 'awoke' in strange surroundings to be told he had expressed concern about his motor scooter. He had no recollection of expressing consternation. Light dawned. Of course, he was on his way from home to work at his hospital. The police phoned the hospital, and apparently no sooner was the receiver replaced that a Senior House Officer materialised. The time required to travel from the hospital to the house in question was at least 15 minutes, indicating that a third amnesic episode had occurred. This anecdote is an example of the occurrence of short periods of anterograde amnesia with some islands of memory, during which time the injured party behaved in a normal fashion, having no recollection of the amnesic periods.

The symptoms frequently following concussion are headache, dizziness, apathy, dullness, inability to concentrate, difficulty in recall, irritability, easy fatiguability, decreased tolerance to light, heat and alcohol, exhaustion and insomnia. These symptoms usually subside in less than six weeks without signs of residual damage.

Should unconsciousness last more than two hours, it is highly probable that laceration of the brain, as well as contusion, has occurred.

Management

Rest in bed with full nursing care, close observation, including charting of temperature, pulse, respiration, and size of pupils, is essential. A constant watch is kept for signs of delayed bleeding which may give rise to mental confusion, headache, an increase in pupil size and other neurological signs. Relapse after a 'lucid interval' is usually due to a subdural haematoma. A subdural haematoma caused in this way may not show itself until weeks, months or even years after injury.

Traumatic coma

Coma is usually diagnosed if the patient is unconscious for several hours. It may persist for days or weeks. Extensive contusions and lacerations of the brain are usually present. The recovery phase is characterised by fluctuating stupor of variable depth, restlessness and disorientation. There may be transient periods of clarity followed by more stupor before recovery finally takes place.

Late effects of cerebral trauma

Both organic and functional factors play a part in the late effects of brain trauma.

Organic defects consist of dementia and irreversible personality changes both of which are fortunately rare, post traumatic epilepsy, chronic subdural haematomata, and focal neurological symptoms. Repeated small injuries to the brain appear more prone to produce dementia and personality change. This is seen in punch-drunk boxers.

Among personality changes that may last are those arising from severe injuries to the frontal areas of the brain, including the standard prefrontal leucotomy operation (page 320). Resultant symptoms and signs comprise the frontal lobe syndrome, features of which include:

1. Reduction in drive, inertia, apathy, somnolence.
2. Affective deficit, the exhibition of less concern for others, less sympathy, and more selfishness.
3. Lack of restraint evidenced principally in speech and temper which usually subsides rapidly, tactlessness.
4. Intellectual impairment—patchy amnesias and defective retention and recall.

It is now known that the 'frontal lobe syndrome' may occur with extensive lesions in other parts of the brain as well as the frontal lobes.

Head injury to the young infant or child may give rise to a developmental defect in intelligence.

Some defects seem to have a combined functional and organic basis. The name 'post-concussional' or 'post-contusional' syndrome is given to these. The injury is frequently trivial, and common complaints are headache, giddiness, difficulty in concentration, and anxiety. If compensation is at stake for the injury sustained, it is quite possible that some of the complaints form part of the picture of so-called 'compensation neurosis'. Such complaints may clear when payment of compensation has been made.

Functional psychiatric disorders in people so predisposed, may occur following even trivial head injury. Perhaps the injured person may have developed for example, a schizophrenic illness, a depressive psychosis, or a neurotic illness without the occurrence of the accident. There are instances however, where a trivial incident may be perceived by the patient as a threat to life, in which case an illness of psychotic intensity may be precipitated.

A male storeman in his early thirties was struck on the head by a box of lard. This did not injure his scalp nor his skull, neither was he concussed. He presented with symptoms as described above under 'post-concussional syndrome', and quickly developed a psychotic depressive illness which eventually required electroconvulsive therapy for its amelioration. This was a compensation case, but it is stretching the imagination somewhat to see his terminal psychotic state as part of a 'compensation neurosis' or a self-willed state. Such cases can provide figurative headaches for those responsible for the process of law.

EPILEPSY

It is becoming common practice to refer to 'the epilepsies' rather than to 'epilepsy', as many clinical variants of epilepsy exist, and already in this section on organic brain syndromes we have noted that epileptic seizures or convulsions occur as symptoms of a number of disorders.

An epileptic seizure is a state produced by an abnormal excessive neuronal discharge within the central nervous system. Two aetiological groups are described:

1. Primary (idiopathic or cryptogenic) epilepsy.
2. Secondary (symptomatic) epilepsy.

The most likely causes of epilepsy presenting at different ages (after Penfield and Jaspers) are as follows:

	Age	Lesions
Infancy	0-2 years	Birth injury, degeneration, congenital abnormality.
Childhood	2-10 years	Birth injury, fever, thrombosis, trauma, idiopathic.
Adolescence	10-20 years	Idiopathic, trauma, birth injury.
Youth	20-35 years	Trauma, neoplasm.
Middle Age	35-55 years	Neoplasm, trauma, arteriosclerosis.
Senescence	55-70+ years	Arteriosclerosis, neoplasm.

Primary epilepsy

Many years ago, the greater proportion of recurrent seizures were considered to be primary or cryptogenic, meaning that the cause was hidden or unknown. Hereditary or constitutional factors leading to a low fit threshold were considered to be causal. With more refined techniques of investigation however, for example electroencephalography and its modifications, and other ancillary investigations, the relative number of primary cases is now smaller, as it has become possible to demonstrate pathology, previously undetected.

Secondary epilepsy

Secondary epilepsy may be due to either intracranial (local) or extra-cranial (general) causes which are listed below.

1. *Intracranial Causes*
   - (a) Space-occupying lesions, e.g. cerebral tumours, abscesses.
   - (b) Vascular lesions, e.g. cerebrovascular disease both acute and chronic, hypertensive encephalopathy, cerebral thrombophlebitis.
   - (c) Brain injury, including birth injuries, that give rise to cerebral scarring, atrophy.
   - (d) Inflammatory diseases, e.g. meningo-vascular syphilis, G.P.I., cerebral cysticercosis, meningitis and encephalitis.
   - (e) Degenerative diseases, e.g. presenile dementia.
2. *Extracranial Causes*
   - (a) Cerebral anoxia from heart block, asphyxia or carbon monoxide poisoning.
   - (b) Metabolic disturbances e.g. uraemia, hypoglycaemia, alkalosis, hepatic failure.
   - (c) Poisons such as alcohol, cocaine, lead, ether, cardiazol.
   - (d) Undetermined causes e.g. seizures associated with teething and febrile illnesses in childhood.
   - (e) Eclampsia.

Precipitating factors in epilepsy

Epileptic attacks may be precipitated by such factors as fatigue, excitement, boredom (especially in petit mal), inadequate food intake, excessive consumption of alcohol, sensory stimuli, e.g. flickering light including TV, reading, sexual intercourse.

A young boy was able to produce seizures by passing his hand quickly back and forth across his face in sunlight. Seizures have been reported where the sufferer has been driving along a tree lined road with sunlight flickering through the branches. A male patient usually had his seizures on the way home from work. It was unlikely that a hypoglycaemic factor was involved, so perhaps emotional factors centred around the domestic situation may have been the precipitating ones. A male patient who had not told his wife-to-be of previous unfortunate episodes, and who was apparently not well stabilised on drugs, featured in a divorce court following a grand mal seizure that occurred while attempting sexual intercourse on the first night of marriage.

As well as an aetiological classification, epilepsy is classified clinically in terms of the type of seizure and related electroencephalographic findings.

Two types of seizure are described, generalised (centrencephalic), and local (or focal).

Generalised seizures

Generalised (centrencephalic) seizures are the result of abnormal neuronal discharges occurring in the grey matter at the base of the brain and in the upper brain stem, involving the reticular activating system.

Consciousness is dependent on the proper functioning of the reticular activating system, and there is always a loss or diminution of consciousness when a generalised seizure occurs.

There are four types of generalised seizures:

1. Major seizures (grand mal).
2. Minor seizures (petit mal).
3. Myoclonic seizures (myoclonic jerks).
4. Akinetic seizures (drop attacks).

Major seizures may be primary or may result from the spread of an abnormal neuronal discharge from a focal cortical area to the centrencephalic region.

The term minor seizure or petit mal should be restricted to a particular form of primary epilepsy to be described below. Myoclonic and akinetic seizures may occur as primary epilepsy, but similar seizures may occur as a manifestation of secondary or symptomatic epilepsy in some cases where diffuse brain damage exists, and in a familial type of epilepsy.

Minor seizures, also referred to as absences, and myoclonic and akinetic seizures, when these latter are primary in nature, all show similar generalised 3 per second spike and wave complexes in the electroencephalographic tracing. These three clinical conditions, when primary in nature, are referred to as the 'petit mal triad'.

Major Seizures (grand mal, generalised convulsions)

Some patients have warning of an impending attack, which may consist of tension, irritability or some other change of mood, lasting hours or days. An aura probably does not occur in primary grand mal epilepsy originating in the centrencephalic region.

There are three phases described:

1. *Tonic Phase.* Usually without warning, the sufferer suddenly loses consciousness and falls to the ground in a state of rigid extension. There may be a cry due to spasm of respiratory and glottal muscles. Cessation of respiration leads to cyanosis. Urination may occur. This tonic phase may last from 5-40 seconds during which time the patient displays intense tonic spasms of face, trunk and limbs.

2. *Clonic Phase.* The tonic spasm gives way to a series of jerky movements involving the musculature of the face, trunk, arms and legs. In this

stage the tongue may be bitten, the patient frequently froths at the mouth, and incontinence of urine or faeces or seminal emission may occur. The clonic phase may last 40-60 seconds.

3. *Flaccid Coma.* This stage supervenes upon the clonic stage. The patient's clonic movements having gradually subsided and ceased, he relaxes and breathes deeply and stertorously while in a comatose state. Muscles have no tone and are in fact quite flaccid. This state may last for half an hour with consciousness gradually returning and leaving post ictal (post fit) symptoms of headache, confusion and drowsiness, or the patient may pass directly into a state of natural sleep.

A condition known as Todd's paralysis is described, in which, following a grand mal attack exhaustion of the cerebral neurones may lead to a paresis lasting up to 24 hours.

MANAGEMENT OF THE SEIZURE

Rarely does a patient come to any harm during a seizure. He should be gently restrained if there is a possibility of his injuring himself against hard objects. A clear airway is maintained by turning him on his side and holding the lower jaw forward, a procedure which is impossible before the flaccid stage is reached. Forcible attempts should not be made to open the mouth as teeth may be unnecessarily damaged. During the clonic phase, a rolled up cloth held in the angle of the mouth may help to prevent biting the tongue or cheeks.

The patient usually recovers spontaneously with no complications. Should a second seizure follow without consciousness being regained, this could be the start of status epilepticus, and medical attention should be obtained.

SOCIAL IMPLICATIONS

Epilepsy is not yet a disease that society accepts, and among other things, this can lead to the sufferer being made to feel 'different', experiencing difficulties in employment, and to parental rejection, often compensated for by over-solicitude. The questions of type of occupation, motor vehicle driving, marriage, pregnancy and travel must be considered in the light of the nature of the epileptic seizures whether they have a genetic basis or not, and the effectiveness of drug therapy. In general, one would encourage the sufferer to lead as normal a life as possible. Obviously dangerous situations such as working at heights, swimming unattended, and perhaps in the majority of instances, driving motor vehicles should be avoided.

DRUG THERAPY

As a general rule, a person who has suffered epileptic seizures should continue to take his medication for at least two years after cessation of seizures. Also, in changing from one drug to another, the dosage of the drug in use must be gradually reduced while its successor is being introduced and gradually increased. Maintenance dosage of anticonvulsant drugs, as with any other medication, should be the lowest dosage consistent with control of the condition.

Mention will be made of a number of drugs in common use, and adult dosage only will be stated.

Phenobarbitone

This is an effective, safe, and cheap anticonvulsant, having an effect both on the cortex and on the reticular formation. It may be used on its own, but it is frequently used in supplementing the effect of other drugs such as phenytoin, and to confer protection from seizures during sleep by giving one dose at night, and using a less sedative drug by day. Dosage: 60-100 mg once or twice daily.

Primidone (Mysoline)

This drug is preferably used in combination with phenobarbitone.
Dosage: 100-250 mg B.D. or Q.I.D. It is usual to start with 250 mg at bedtime and gradually increase the daily amount.
Toxic and side effects: The principal side effect is a sedative one. Vertigo, ataxia, diplopia and skin rashes may occur. Among more serious side effects are megaloblastic anaemia and possibly leucopenia.

Phenytoin Sodium (Dilantin)

This is the drug of choice in the treatment of grand mal epilepsy.
Dosage: 60-200 mg B.D. or T.D.S.
Toxic and side effects: Gastric upset which is alleviated by taking the drug with meals or with milk; dermatitis which may be accompanied by fever and eosinophilia; hyperplasia or hypertrophy of the gums; hirsutism (hairiness) particularly of the limbs; nystagmus and ataxia; megaloblastic anaemia, leucopenia, agranulocytosis, thrombocytopenia (reduction in platelet count). Symptoms of depression, intellectual deterioration, a schizophrenic-like psychosis and peripheral neuropathy appear in rare instances after many years of taking this drug.

A most uncommon complication is enlargement of lymph glands, liver and spleen. This settles on withdrawal of the drug.

Methoin (Mephenytoin, Mesontoin, Mesantoin)

This drug is probably a more powerful anticonvulsant than phenytoin, but its marked toxicity on the bone marrow and the liver cause its use to be restricted to those cases unresponsive to less toxic drugs.
Dosage: 50-100 mg T.D.S. or Q.I.D.

Carbamazepine (Tegretol)

This drug is chemically related to imipramine. It is not given as a drug of first choice in grand mal epilepsy but has its main use in supplementing the longer established drugs when these prove inadequate.
Dosage: 100-200 mg B.D.-Q.I.D.
Toxic and side effects: Skin reactions, drowsiness, dry mouth and gastro intestinal disturbances. Jaundice and aplastic anaemia are reported to have resulted from its use.

Post-ictal automatism

On occasions, a grand mal attack is followed by a twilight state (post-ictal automatism) in which occurs a state of disturbed consciousness lasting from a few minutes to several days. In this state, the patient may move around without apparent impairment of functions, and even undertake a journey without being aware of having done so (fugue). Anxiety, paranoid ideas, hallucinations or aggressive behaviour may be present.

Grand mal status (status epilepticus)

Generalised convulsions, or grand mal attacks, may occur in a series, separated by minutes or hours, the patient not fully recovering but remaining confused between attacks. This is a serious state requiring urgent management. If untreated, the patient may become comatose and attain a body temperature as high as 41° C. The term status epilepticus also embraces unilateral convulsive status and minor epileptic status. We shall now deal with the management of generalised convulsive status or grand mal status which, as inferred above, constitutes a medical emergency.

MANAGEMENT

Suppression of seizures is accomplished by giving Diazepam (Valium) 1-2 mg per year of life to a maximum of 10 mg I.V. or I.M., repeated if seizures recur. It is also common practice to give phenytoin sodium (Dilantin) 20-30 mg per year of life up to a maximum of 250 mg I.V. The adult dosage of other drugs which may be used are as follows:

Sodium phenobarbitone 200 mg I.M.; Sodium amylobarbitone as a 5% solution given at a rate of 1 cc per minute I.V. until seizures cease or until 10 cc (500 mg) have been given; Paraldehyde 10 cc I.M.; thiopentone I.V. in a 2½% solution until convulsions cease.

Maintenance therapy may be commenced by giving sodium phenytoin (Dilantin) 250 mg I.M. at the same time as the drug is given I.V. for the suppression of seizures. Sodium phenobarbitone may be given I.M. as well. Once control of convulsions is achieved and the patient is conscious, oral anticonvulsant therapy is instituted.

During status epilepticus, the nurse must ensure that a clear airway is maintained by positioning the patient, using a simple airway and aspirating saliva. Oxygen will reduce cerebral anoxia and may help in controlling seizures. In rare instances, tracheotomy and assisted respiration may be required. The importance of maintaining a satisfactory fluid balance in patients in status epilepticus for any length of time cannot be overemphasised.

Petit mal (*minor epilepsy, absence or lapse attacks*)

Attacks of petit mal consist of short lapses in consciousness lasting up to a few seconds. The condition mainly occurs in children. In an attack, the sufferer quite abruptly ceases what he is doing, may stare and roll his eyes upwards, and is unresponsive. Twitching of eyelids and fingers at the rate of 3 per second may occur. Immediately after an attack, he may continue with what he was doing and may not be aware of the episode. Sometimes as many as 100 attacks a day occur, in which case the term pyknolepsy is applied. It is evident that, if a school age child has many attacks a day, his educational attainments will be grossly hampered.

The condition may disappear in adolescence or be replaced by grand mal seizures, and though rare, it may be seen in adults. The EEG picture is one of 3 per second spike-and-wave complexes seen in all leads.

DRUG TREATMENT

Troxidone (Tridione) and Paramethadione (Paradione)

These two drugs are chemically related and are given in similar dosage of 300-600 mg T.D.S. or Q.I.D. Toxic and side effects: Sedation, photophobia (inability to tolerate glare or bright light), skin rashes, neutropenia (diminution in neutrophils in blood), agranulocytosis, aplastic anaemia and kidney damage. In addition, these drugs have a tendency to provoke grand mal seizures. To counteract this, phenytoin is prescribed along with troxidone or paramethadione. A night time dose of phenytoin may be all that is necessary. Alternatively, phenobarbitone or primidone may be given in place of phenytoin.

Ethosuximide (Zarontin)

This preparation is available in capsules or as syrup. As with troxidone, ethosuximide has a tendency to precipitate grand mal seizures, and the use of a drug suitable for control of grand mal epilepsy may be indicated concurrently.

Dosage: One capsule (250 mg) daily for one week; two capsules daily for second week. The dose can be increased by one capsule per week until side effects occur, or up to a maximum of 6-8 capsules per day, the usual dose being 4-6 capsules daily.

Toxic and side effects: The evoking of grand mal seizures, anorexia, nausea and vomiting, skin rashes, leucopenia or pancytopenia (a diminution of all cellular elements in the blood).

Phensuximide (Milontin), methsuximide (Celontin)

These are two drugs chemically related to ethosuximide. They have similar toxic and side effects to ethosuximide except that there is less tendency for phensuximide to evoke major seizures, and methsuximide does not appear to have this effect at all. Methsuximide, apart from its use in petit mal, is sometimes useful in the treatment of focal (cortical) seizures.

Acetazoleamide (Diamox)

A sulphonamide derivative, this drug is used as an adjuvant to troxidone, paramethadione, ethosuximide, phensuximide, or methsuximide therapy when these drugs are not sufficiently effective alone.

Dosage: 250 mg once daily to T.D.S.

Side effects: Included are paraesthesias, some anorexia and mild gastrointestinal upsets. Drowsiness and confusion have been reported, as well as headache. Acetazoleamide has a diuretic action also, and there is a slight risk of renal calculus formation.

Myoclonic Seizures and Akinetic Seizures

Myoclonus is regarded as resulting from a hyperexcitable neuronal system. Attacks consist of sudden jumps or jerks of various parts of the body, particularly the limbs. It may be associated with akinetic or atonic seizures, in which there is sudden loss of muscle tone with alteration of consciousness. The patient, if standing, may drop to the ground. Major seizures may also be present in the same patient.

Primidone (Mysoline) is of value in myoclonic epilepsy.

Local (or focal) seizures

In contradistinction to generalised seizures, in which the abnormal neuronal discharge originates in the grey matter at the base of the brain and in the upper brain stem (centrencephalic region) and in which alteration in consciousness occurs, in local seizures the abnormal neuronal discharge usually commences in part of the cortex as a result of underlying pathology, and consciousness is not lost. Focal cortical seizures must be regarded as secondary or symptomatic in nature, and efforts should be made to elicit the underlying pathology.

The symptoms present in local epilepsy will depend entirely on the area of cortex which is experiencing the abnormal neuronal discharge. Thus, seizures arising in the motor cortex may result in movements of a limb or part of a limb, usually clonic in nature; seizures arising in the somatosensory area may produce paraesthesias; lesions in the occipital cortex may produce impairment of vision or flashing lights, and, if the adjacent temporal lobe is also affected, distinct visual hallucinations may occur; seizures in the frontal cortex may produce 'forced thought' and turning of head and eyes. Abnormal electrical discharges affecting the temporal lobe or its related structures are common, and special comment will be made below on this type of local or focal epilepsy, known as temporal lobe epilepsy.

Spread of local discharge

An abnormal electrical neuronal discharge may remain localised. It may spread to adjacent areas of cortex giving rise to what is termed a Jacksonian march or Jacksonian seizure in which, for example, the hand may first show clonic movements, spreading in progression to the wrist, forearm and upper arm.

If the local discharge spreads to the upper brain stem or centrencephalic area, a grand mal or generalised seizure will result. This state of affairs, wherein symptoms of local epilepsy precede a grand mal seizure, gave rise to the concept of an aura (or warning) preceding generalised convulsions. The aura is really a local epileptic discharge already in progress. Some people when experiencing such local epilepsy seem able, almost by an act of will, to prevent its spread to the centrencephalic area, so forestalling a grand mal seizure.

Figure 11 shows some of the cortical areas that may be affected, and the approximate position of the centrencephalic area.

Temporal lobe epilepsy

Temporal lobe seizures constitute about one third of all epilepsies. The reason for this frequency is related to the vulnerability of the temporal lobes to damage, thus readily producing epileptogenic foci, that is, areas where abnormal neuronal discharges are initiated. Damage to the temporal lobe is caused by anoxic changes during the birth process, acceleration-deceleration head injuries occurring in later life, involvement of the temporal lobe in infective processes spreading from the middle ear and mastoid, and other vascular and neoplastic lesions that can affect any part of the brain.

CLINICAL PICTURE

The symptoms of temporal lobe epilepsy vary widely depending on the area of abnormal electrical discharge. One or more of the following may occur:

1. Epigastric sensation: This used to be regarded as an aura of grand mal epilepsy but it is a local seizure wherein an unpleasant sensation commences in the pit of the stomach (epigastrium) and rises to the chest and throat. It may be accompanied by paraesthesia of the mouth and lips.

2. Changes in perception: Objects may seem smaller (micropsia) or larger (macropsia), dimmer or brighter. Sounds may seem louder or distant.

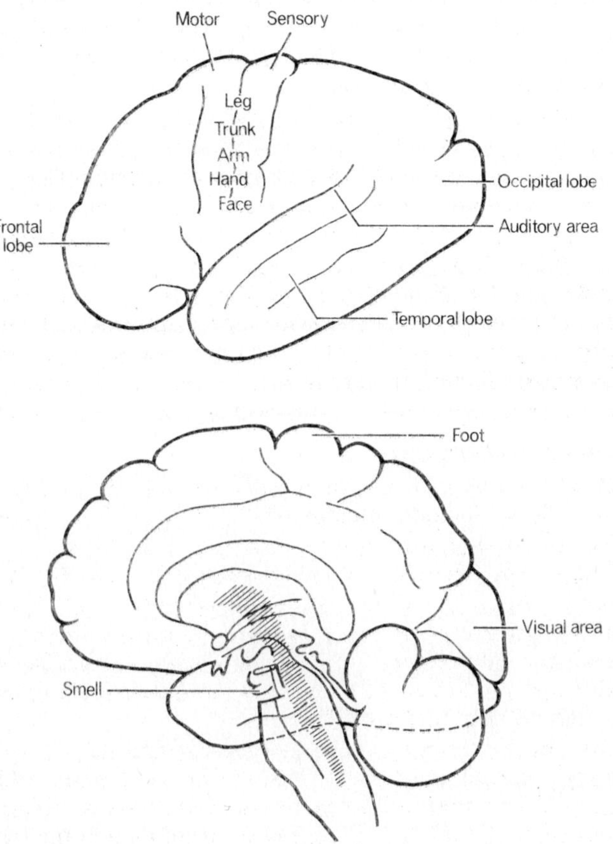

Fig. 11. Cortical areas and centrencephalic area (shaded)

3. Hallucinations: These may be olfactory, gustatory, visual or auditory. Abnormal electrical discharge in the temporal lobe may also produce vertigo.

4. Changes in the quality of familiarity: This is really a disturbance of memory. Patients may have a sense of familiarity with an unknown environment (déjà vu) or may feel their present situation has been previously experienced (déjà vecu). Changes in the quality of familiarity may lead to a feeling that the patient can predict what will happen in the immediate or more distant future. Patients may also feel unfamiliar in an environment or situation they know well (jamais vu).

5. Changes in thought: Patients may experience the phenomenon of forced thinking in which a thought, word, sentence or piece of music may obtrude itself into consciousness. The thought may be a whole complex memory or sequence of memories accompanied by a sensation of time rushing by or standing still (panoramic memories).

6. Dreamy states: These are feelings of unreality (derealisation or depersonalisation).

7. Primary automatism: The patient may go through a stereotyped set of actions such as making a bed or dressing. This automatism is to be distinguished from the automatism that follows a grand mal seizure and which receives mention on page 170.

8. Affective disorders: Paroxysmal disturbances in mood are not uncommon. These may range from anxiety or terror, to pleasure and ecstasy. Depression and paranoid feelings may also occur. There may be a mixture of these feelings which rarely last for more than a few minutes at most. Some states are described in which depression is present for up to two weeks. Patients with repeated depressive or schizophrenia-like episodes should not be diagnosed as suffering from these functional illnesses without having previous electroencephalographic studies.

As with other cortical areas affected in local epilepsy, the abnormal discharge may remain localised, spread to adjacent cortical areas, or may spread to the centrencephalic area giving rise to a grand mal seizure.

Drug treatment of local epilepsy

Drugs used in the treatment of grand mal seizures are used to control local seizures. These include phenobarbitone, primidone, phenytoin, carbamazepine. In addition, methsuximide (Celontin) which is used in the treatment of petit mal seizures is sometimes effective in the control of cortical seizures. Apart from the above-mentioned drugs, sulthiame (Ospolot) has its main role in the treatment of local epilepsy. Where phenytoin produces side-effects without adequately controlling cortical seizures, its dosage is reduced, and sulthiame is concurrently introduced.
Adult dosage: 100-200 mg B.D. or T.D.S.
Toxic and side effects: These include gastrointestinal upset, headache, hyperventilation, paraesthesia, drowsiness and confusion. Sulthiame does not seem to have a toxic effect on the bone marrow or kidneys. It is stated that sulthiame should not be used with primidone in the treatment of temporal lobe epilepsy, as the combination may produce psychiatric symptoms.

ethosuximide
sodium valproate.

Surgical treatment

Surgery is mainly directed towards the removal of intracranial pathology leading to epilepsy, for example meningiomata, and to the removal of cortical epileptogenic foci. Such treatment is only carried out in specially equipped units and when the more conservative measures have failed.

Twilight States

These are states characterised by a disturbance in consciousness during which the patient is not prostrate but is able to act more or less automatically. They may have forensic implications if acts of violence are carried out in this abnormal mental state. Three conditions are included:

1. A post-ictal twilight state or automatism may follow a grand mal seizure (page 170).

2. Ictal twilight states, sometimes called psychomotor seizures, may begin with alteration in consciousness with no other warning, or they may follow a temporal lobe discharge with features mentioned above, the discharge having spread from the temporal lobe to the centrencephalic area. This state often starts with searching movements of head and eyes, lip smacking, masticatory movements and swallowing. The patient becomes disoriented and only vaguely aware of his surroundings, wanders around aimlessly and responds inappropriately to external stimuli. He may display complex automatisms. The state may last 5-10 minutes, or longer. Agitation and fear may become marked, and aggressive acts may occur, particularly if restraint is applied. Other patients may behave in an apparently purposeful and well coordinated manner, with complete or partial amnesia for a period of time lasting hours or even days. Fugue states, lasting minutes or days, may occur in which the patient undertakes a journey, regains consciousness in a diffèrent location, and has no recollection of events occurring in the intervening time. Such ictal twilight states may be difficult to differentiate from an hysterical fugue or from malingering.

3. Petit mal status is an uncommon condition in which the clinical picture may include confusion, confused behaviour, or mental dullness lasting up to several days and characterised by difficulty in concentration and slowing of thought processes. The electroencephalograph in these cases is characterised by continuous or nearly continuous generalised spike and wave patterns.

Late effects of epilepsy

Epileptic personality

There is no convincing evidence that sufferers from epilepsy show a characteristic pre-morbid personality. Once fits have occurred however, many patients, though by no means all, show definite personality changes. These consist of slowness and rigidity in thinking and reaction, self-centredness, hypochondriasis in some instances, and the maintenance of fixed attitudes or opinions. Some sufferers show a profound deterioration in intellectual functions, become cirsumstantial, quarrelsome, irritable and aggressive. This train of characteristics has a multiple aetiology, including social rejection, the depressant effect of some anticonvulsants, institutionalisation in some cases, the underlying pathology associated with epilepsy, and the anoxic effects on the brain sustained during seizures.

Schizophrenia-like psychoses of epilepsy

These states were described by Slater and Beard in the British Journal of Psychiatry, January, 1963. Symptoms of schizophrenia may appear years after the onset of epilepsy, mainly temporal lobe epilepsy, the average time lapse being 14 years. The states are indistinguishable clinically from schizophrenia. On statistical grounds, there is little doubt that epilepsy, and more specifically the duration of epilepsy, is a causative factor in the development of these psychoses. The development of a psychotic picture is independent of the severity of seizures, aetiology of the epilepsy, amount of medication taken or the effective control or otherwise of the seizures.

Recent developments

New drugs have been introduced to the treatment armamentarium during recent years. Clonazepam (Rivotril) is a new benzodiazepine derivative and clinical trials suggest that is has a wide spectrum of activity. Another drug is sodium valproate (Epilim) which also on the basis of controlled trials seems assured of a useful place in the management of a variety of seizures. The interested student is referred to larger texts on these new medications.

Methods of long-term intensive monitoring of epileptic patients are being refined. The process requires frequent, and accurate recording of the clinical seizures, the electrical manifestation of these seizures, and the serum concentration of the antiepileptic drugs circulating in the blood to combat these seizures. Simultaneous monitoring of these three factors is essential. Apart from the estimation of serum antiepileptic drug concentrations, techniques used are videotape recording, the telemetered E.E.G., and the E.E.G. digital cassette recording system. Patients who have suffered recurring seizures for many years and have failed to respond adequately to antiepileptic drugs using conventional approaches are candidates for intensive monitoring. Intensive monitoring is sufficiently expensive to preclude its use when conventional management techniques will suffice. It is estimated that less than five per cent of all epileptic patients should require intensive monitoring.

Carbon monoxide poisoning

While dealing with the organic psychotic conditions, some brief mention will be made of the effects of carbon monoxide poisoning, for although it falls under another rubric in the I.C.D. it may have marked effects on cerebral function.

A detailed description of carbon monoxide poisoning will not be given, as this will be found in standard text books of forensic science.

Since carbon monoxide reduces the oxygen-carrying capacity of the blood due to the formation of carboxyhaemoglobin, the signs and symptoms of carbon monoxide intoxication are those characteristic of oxygen lack in the tissues, and particularly those in the central nervous system. Psychiatric and neurological sequelae will depend on the length of exposure and the concentration of carbon monoxide inhaled. It is stated that a patient poisoned with carbon monoxide is not likely to have serious sequelae if he regains consciousness within one hour of removal from a toxic atmosphere.

A person exposed to carbon monoxide will be seen to exhibit a cherry red colour of the mucous membranes, finger nails, and skin generally. The major psychiatric sequela of carbon monoxide poisoning, often due to the inhalation of coal gas, is gross memory deficit, and a patient may not remember incidents or statements from one minute to the next. Unfortunately, this condition may be permanent.

Treatment

Treatment of the unconscious patient consists in intubation and giving 100% oxygen. An intravenous drip is set up, and at this stage the help of an expert in the use of a hyperbaric chamber should be sought. If cardiac arrest supervenes, 100 ml of 8.4% sodium bicarbonate solution is given intravenously and external cardiac massage instituted. Hypoxia damages brain tissue much more readily than cardiac muscle, and if the cardiac arrest is due to hypoxia and not to some other cause, the brain will already be extensively and irreparably damaged.

Patients with residual mental symptoms of dementia are managed on the lines outlined in the treatment of senile dementia.

SPECIFIC NON-PSYCHOTIC MENTAL DISORDERS FOLLOWING ORGANIC BRAIN DAMAGE

This category of disorders has no place in a section dealing with Organic Psychotic Conditions but as the disorders do not warrant a separate chapter they will be dealt with here. The frontal lobe syndrome and the post concussional syndrome have been described elsewhere, but in keeping with the policy in the rest of this text to quote freely from the I.C.D. glossary they will be mentioned again along with 'Cognitive or personality change of other type' and that recurring category called 'other'.

Frontal lobe syndrome

This category includes the lobotomy syndrome and the post leucotomy syndrome or state. It entails

> changes in behaviour following damage to the frontal areas of the brain or following interference with the connections of those areas. There is a general diminution of self-control, foresight, creativity and spontaneity, which may be manifest as increased irritability, selfishness, restlessness and lack of concern for others. Conscientiousness and powers of concentration are often diminished, but measurable deterioration of intellect or memory is not necessarily present. The overall picture is often one of emotional dullness, lack of drive and slowness; but particularly in persons previously with energetic, restless or aggressive characteristics, there may be a change towards impulsiveness, boastfulness, temper outbursts, silly fatuous humour, and the development of

unrealistic ambitions; the direction of change usually depends upon the previous personality. A considerable degree of recovery is possible and may continue over the course of several years.

Cognitive or personality change of other type

This term embraces

chronic, mild states of memory disturbances and intellectual deterioration, often accompanied by increased irritability, querulousness, lassitude and complaints of physical weakness. These states are often associated with old age, and may precede more severe states due to brain damage classifiable under dementia of any type or any condition or aetiological factor in the transient organic psychotic conditions.

The terms 'mild memory disturbance' and 'organic psychosyndrome of nonpsychotic severity' are subsumed under this heading.

Postconcussional syndrome

This term refers to

states occurring after generalised contusion of the brain, in which the symptom picture may resemble that of the frontal lobe syndrome or that of any of the neurotic disorders, but in which in addition, headache, giddiness, fatigue, insomnia and a subjective feeling of impaired intellectual ability are usually prominent. Mood may fluctuate, and quite ordinary stress may produce exaggerated fear and apprehension. There may be marked intolerance of mental and physical exertion, undue sensitivity to noise, and hypochondriacal preoccupation. The symptoms are more common in persons who have previously suffered from neurotic or personality disorders, or when there is a possibility of compensation. This syndrome is particularly associated with the closed type of head injury when signs of localised brain damage are slight or absent, but it may also occur in other conditions.

There are numbers of synonyms for this syndrome mentioned in Appendix I.

Other

Disorders resembling the postconcussional or postcontusional syndrome, associated with infective or other disease of the brain or surrounding tissues are included in this category.

13

OTHER PSYCHOSES

In this section, which deals with psychoses other than organic psychotic conditions, we shall look at schizophrenic psychoses, paranoid states, affective psychoses, and other non-organic psychoses. Psychoses with origin specific to childhood, although under this category of disorders, will be dealt with later, in the chapter on child psychiatry.

SCHIZOPHRENIC PSYCHOSES

The general picture of schizophrenia was known in the early 1800s, and numerous names were given to the condition as it appeared in different patients. In France, Morel, in 1856, applied the name demence precoce to an adolescent boy who became gloomy, silent and withdrawn. Emil Kraepelin, in 1896, made the distinction between dementia praecox and manic-depressive psychosis, deterioration commonly occurring in the former and not in the latter. Kraepelin came to recognise three types of dementia praecox, namely, hebephrenic, paranoid and catatonic. Eugene Bleuler, in 1911, saw the syndrome described by Kraepelin, not as a condition necessarily progressing to dementia or deterioration, but as a disorder characterised mainly by an alteration in the faculty of association, and by a splitting of the basic functions of the personality. He named the condition 'schizophrenia', which means literally 'split mindedness', and added a fourth type, namely simple schizophrenia, to the three types described by Kraepelin. A number of other sub-types have since been added to these four generally-accepted basic schizophrenic syndromes, all of which will be described below. In addition, Langfeldt, in 1939, proposed two separate groups of schizophrenic illnesses, namely process schizophrenia with a propensity for deterioration in the sufferer, and the schizophreniform psychoses, or reactive schizophrenias, which have a good prognosis. There appears to be no conclusive proof as to whether two such qualitative types of schizophrenia exist or whether the clinical pictures are dependent solely on the severity of the same type of schizophrenic process.

Although the description of the schizophrenic psychoses included in the I.C.D. glossary is lengthy and may overlap with other material presented in this chapter it will be quoted in full:

> A group of psychoses in which there is a fundamental disturbance of personality, a characteristic distortion of thinking, often a sense of being controlled by alien forces, delusions which may be bizarre, disturbed perception, abnormal affect out of keeping with the real situation, and autism.

Nevertheless, clear consciousness and intellectual capacity are usually maintained. The disturbance of personality involves its most basic functions which give the normal person his feelings of individuality, uniqueness and self-direction. The most intimate thoughts, feelings and acts are often felt to be known to or shared by others and explanatory delusions may develop, to the effect that natural or supernatural forces are at work to influence the schizophrenic person's thoughts and actions in ways that are often bizarre. He may see himself as the pivot of all that happens. Hallucinations, especially of hearing, are common and may comment on the patient or address him. Perception is frequently disturbed in other ways; there may be perplexity, irrelevant features may become all-important and, accompanied by passivity feelings, may lead the patient to believe that everyday objects and situations possess a special, usually sinister, meaning intended for him. In the characteristic schizophrenic disturbance of thinking, peripheral and irrelevant features of a total concept, which are inhibited in normal directed mental activity, are brought to the forefront and utilized in place of the elements relevant and appropriate to the situation. Thus thinking becomes vague, elliptical and obscure, and its expression in speech sometimes incomprehensible. Breaks and interpolations in the flow of consecutive thought are frequent, and the patient may be convinced that his thoughts are being withdrawn by some outside agency. Mood may be shallow, capricious or incongruous. Ambivalence and disturbance of volition may appear as inertia, negativism or stupor. Catatonia may be present. The diagnosis 'schizophrenia' should not be made unless there is, or has been evident during the same illness, characteristic disturbance of thought, perception, mood, conduct, or personality—preferably in at least two of these areas. The diagnosis should not be restricted to conditions running a protracted, deteriorating, or chronic course. In addition to making the diagnosis on the criteria just given, effort should be made to specify one of the following subdivisions of schizophrenia, according to the predominant symptoms.

'One of the following subdivisions' refers to the clinical types of schizophrenia described later.

Incidence and prevalence*

The incidence of an illness refers to the number of new cases in a given population, occurring within a specified period, for example one year. In a six-month survey conducted by the author in 1965 on admissions to the then sole government psychiatric facility serving the north-east quarter of the Sydney metropolitan area, with a population of approximately 500,000 there were seventy-four new cases of schizophrenia admitted and these comprised 19% of new admissions.

If one knew the numbers of all new cases from the area detected and/or treated by all the private and general hospital facilities in the same period of time studied, one would be in a position to work out the incidence of schizophrenia in this particular population.

As well as new admissions suffering from schizophrenia, there are also those who are readmitted with this diagnosis (eighty-four in the above survey), and those who are maintained in the community following discharge from treatment facilities. If one adds all these together, an idea of the prevalence of this illness can be arrived at.

The prevalence of an illness refers to the number of cases, either new

* Some general remarks on incidence and prevalence are made as students will find these terms used in many texts.

or old, occurring in a given population at any specified period of time. This is usually expressed as a percentage or as a number per so-many thousand population. Prevalence rates for schizophrenia vary enormously from study to study and from country to country, partly due to different diagnostic criteria and partly due to target populations studied. One type of target population could be hospital populations, which reflect prevalence rates rather than incidence in communities. Omitting sociological factors for the moment, hospital populations vary enormously in the percentages of different diagnostic categories admitted, depending for example, on admission policies and on other available treatment facilities. In the small survey mentioned above, it was found that of all admissions in a six-month period, 24% were diagnosed as suffering from schizophrenia.

On a visit to a large hospital in the Peoples' Republic of China in 1973, the author was informed that 70% of the patients admitted were suffering from schizophrenia. This does not necessarily mean that the incidence or prevalence of schizophrenia is higher in the population served by this particular Chinese facility than in the population of the north-east quarter of Sydney. One found, in fact, that many other diagnostic categories found their way into the so-called traditional hospitals, and so the special psychiatric facility's clientele consisting of patients with more serious disturbances over-represented the prevalence of schizophrenia in its catchment area.

With these sorts of difficulties in estimating prevalence rates it is not surprising that published figures vary between 0.3 and 3%, with a median of 0.8 to 1%. This means that, overall, 0.8 to 1% of the assessed world population can be expected to be suffering from schizophrenia.

Aetiology

The aetiology or causation of schizophrenia still remains one of psychiatry's great challenges.

No one specific cause of schizophrenia has been found, and it is indeed possible that a number of factors may be implicated in its development. We shall look at some of these.

Heredity

The weight of evidence which is supported by 'twin studies' strongly suggests that genetic factors have a part to play in the aetiology of schizophrenia. The mode of inheritance, however, is far from being clearly defined. Theories relating to this include the monogenetic theories, a two-gene theory, and polygenic theories.

Currently it would appear that a polygenic theory is considered most likely. The future sufferer inherits a predisposition to the illness and it requires stressful life events to elicit schizophrenia.

It would seem quite possible for there to be a number of differing genetic defects leading to the various clinical manifestations of this disorder, but such a statement is purely hypothetical at this stage of knowledge of the aetiology of schizophrenia.

Constitution

PHYSIQUE

Kretschmer showed there to be a greater incidence of people of asthenic body build among sufferers of schizophrenia.

PERSONALITY

The most common pre-psychotic personalities are:

(a) the schizoid personality who is aloof, detached, less emotional than the average person, and less involved. He is very sensitive, and because of his over-sensitivity, defends himself by this type of withdrawal.

(b) the 'stormy personality' (Arieti). People with a stormy personality did not, in earlier life, find a defence in emotional detachment. They probably tried many manoeuvres to cope with life's pressures, for example, submissiveness, aggression and even schizoid detachment. The variety of responses to other people is probably influenced by inconsistencies in parents. Such stormy personalities are very vulnerable to stress, and life is a series of crises. They sometimes resort to excessive use of drugs and alcohol to abate the storms. There is no relationship between level of intelligence and the tendency to develop schizophrenia.

PHYSICAL FACTORS

1. No convincing evidence relating endocrine disorders to schizophrenia is forthcoming.
2. There are no definitive neuropathological changes in the brain in schizophrenia.
3. Some writers claim that a greater proportion of abnormal electroencephalographic changes occur in the sufferer from schizophrenia, but this is both doubtful and not definitive.
4. Biochemical findings are inconsistent and the significance of any abnormal findings is hard to interpret. An abnormal retention of nitrogen was found by R. Gjessing (1939) in certain recurrent catatonic states, the condition being called periodic catatonia. This is treated successfully with a low protein diet and thyroxine. Such patients are said also to respond to neuroleptic drugs. Some more recent work points to a possibility that faulty metabolism of adrenalin may give rise to adrenochrome which, like lysergic acid and mescaline, can produce disturbances resembling schizophrenia. The so-called 'model phychoses' produced by these drugs however, probably bear little relationship to schizophrenia.
5. Physical illness may precipitate a schizophrenic reaction in a person so predisposed. However, an interesting observation is that patients with long-standing schizophrenia may become more rational in the course of an intercurrent physical illness.

Psychological factors

General psychological stress factors which may precipitate a schizophrenic illness in a person so predisposed are dealt with in Chapter 10. There are no specific psychological factors to which the development of schizophrenia can be attributed. A great deal of work has been carried out in an attempt to clarify the role of psychological factors in the genesis of schizophrenia, but none of the work is conclusive. We shall look briefly at some areas of study:

1. Adolf Meyer who stressed the unity of the individual's psychological and biological functioning, preferred to study his patients longitudinally in a temporal sense, and saw psychotic illnesses as 'reactions', and in 1906 suggested that schizophrenia could be a 'habit deterioration'.

2. Theodore Lidz and others at Yale undertook pioneering investigations into the intrafamilial environment in which schizophrenic patients grow up. The Yale group commenced their intensive investigation of schizophrenic families in 1952, though Lidz himself had begun studying the topic in 1940. It is stated that families of schizophrenic patients are, in general, not happy ones, displaying conflict, tension and anxiety in the formative years of the patient. Lidz refers to marital schizm and marital skew as two types of pathology, existing in parents of the families studied. To quote from his book *Schizophrenia and the Family:*

> In those families that we have designated as 'schismatic', the parents were in open conflict, trying to coerce each other, each encountering from the other either defiance, or, at best, a temporary hostile and resentful submission. Each undercut the worth and self-esteem of the other and divided the family, the mother wooing the children to side with her, and the father wooing them to side with him in the conflict, each parent fostering distrust and devaluation of the other. The widely discrepant attitudes and directives of the parents cannot be integrated within the single child—irreconcilable parents become irreconcilable introjects . . . Not all of the parents (in skewed families) were in overt conflict. In the families that we have termed 'skewed' . . . the serious personality problems and devious ways of the dominant parent were not countered by the spouse. The patient, in contrast to his siblings, is the object of a particular intrusiveness by the dominant parent, usually the mother, which blurs the ego boundaries between parent and child and ties the patient to satisfying the parent's needs and to continue a primary relatedness with her. The boy's differentiation from the initial symbiotic bond to his mother and the development of identification with his passive father are impeded. The symbiotic attachment leads to confusion of sexual identity, incestuous concerns, and a greater assimilation of the disturbed parent's devious and paralogical ways.

3. G. Bateson *et al.*, in 1956, published a paper on the double-bind hypothesis of schizophrenia. They proposed the double-bind as an aetiological mechanism for the development of thought disorder in schizophrenia. Briefly, it would seem that the basic ingredient in a double-bind situation in a family is a parent who gives two contradictory communications simultaneously to a child. A double-bind situation may be said to occur also when the content of what is said conflicts with the affective component of the communication. It must be stated that there is little agreement among workers in this field about what elements are necessary to produce a double-bind situation. There is no evidence that double-bind communication is necessarily pathological, nor does there

appear to be any evidence that it is related to the production of thought disorder in schizophrenia.

4. The concept of the 'schizophrenogenic mother' enjoyed a vogue. Such a mother was said to be overambitious, extremely rejecting or obsessively anxious in the future sufferer's formative years. It is also stated that mothers of schizophrenics completely dominate the lives of their passive husbands and children. They may be mothers with nebulous ego boundaries who treat their child as an extension of themselves, intruding into the child's world while oblivious of the child's needs and wishes. It can be inferred from Lidz's writings that there is no one specific personality pattern that fits the so-called schizophrenogenic mother.

These are but a few of the unsuccessful attempts to determine a specific psychological factor in the genesis of schizophrenia.

Social and cultural factors

Schizophrenia occurs in every country and in every culture. It is more frequent in urban than rural areas and in industrial rather than non-industrial areas. Its greater frequency among migrants probably has nothing to do with the process of migration nor with difficulties in adaptation to a new culture, unless the sufferer is so predisposed. One study on migrants to the United Kingdom showed that a significant number of those who developed schizophrenic illness in the United Kingdom were unsettled wanderers in their own country before migration, having moved from rural or provincial areas to the capital city in their own country. There is a higher incidence of schizophrenia in the centre of a city with its social disorganisation, than at the periphery. There is no evidence to suggest that life in city centres is a factor in the causation of schizophrenia. It could well be that people so predisposed, or with some forms of the developed illness, drift to city centres.

The problems surrounding research into the aetiology of schizophrenia are enormous. To date no simple answer has been found to account for this baffling psychiatric disorder. Probably many factors play their part. As a general statement, it would seem that to develop the disorder, an hereditary predisposition is a prerequisite. Schizophrenia as a clinical entity may never develop unless one or more of the other suggested aetiological factors also operate.

Basic symptoms and signs

In a condition about whose nature there are varying authoritative opinions, it is to be expected that text books will differ in their delineation of basic symptoms and signs. Some symptoms are regarded as primary, arising directly out of the schizophrenic 'process', and others as secondary, being in the nature of the person's response to the changes wrought in him by the primary symptoms. There is no general agreement as to which symptoms and signs are primary or basic and which are secondary. There are, however, symptoms and signs of high diagnostic value whether one regards them as primary (basic) or not. These will now be described:

1. *Thought disorder*

This is a disturbance in the process of thinking, and shows in the patient's speech. Manifestations of what is essentially a failure in normal associations or linkages of ideas include thought blocking, pressure of thoughts, incoherence, neologisms. These symptoms are described on pages 68 and 88, and reference should be made to these sections. The ability to think in the abstract is commonly lost, and thinking becomes concrete. Concrete thinking is not pathognomonic of schizophrenia however, as it occurs also in organic psychotic disorders and in mental retardation.

2. *Loss of ego boundaries*

A characteristic of most schizophrenic illnesses is a disturbance of ego function or loss of ego boundaries, discussed earlier in Chapter 8. The following may be seen as the result of such disturbance or loss of 'ego-feeling' or 'self-experience':

(a) Outbursts of impulsive and often unpredictable behaviour, in some instances thought to be due to failure of ego control over id drives, were common before the advent of the major tranquillising drugs.

Many people working with schizophrenic patients have been surprised at unexpected acts of aggression directed towards them by patients. This is less likely to occur if one has developed some degree of rapport with a patient. A nurse should exercise extreme tact, and may be well advised to stay out of striking distance on initial confrontation with some sufferers from schizophrenia.

(b) Some people launch into disclosures of intimate details of their sexual lives, their misdemeanours and their obscene or anti-social wishes, to virtual strangers. When such lack of restraint dictated by society's norms is evidenced, one is likely to be witnessing the result of disturbed ego functioning.

(c) Loss of ego boundaries may give rise to delusions of influence or passivity feelings in which the patient feels influenced or driven by outside events or people, or he may feel that his thoughts are read and controlled by someone or something in the external environment. On the other hand he may believe that his thoughts and actions have far-reaching effects on people and situations in the outside world.

(d) The fusion of the patient's identity with objects or people in the outside world may cause him to react to stimuli applied to another person or object. The author has observed a patient wince with a pain in the leg and comment on this, when another patient's leg knocked against a low table.

(e) The individual's perception of his own body may be so grossly distorted that he may see himself as ugly or misshapen, and he may even be perplexed as to whether he is male or female.

(f) Depersonalization or derealization, also experienced in less serious psychiatric conditions, may result from loss of personal identity.

3. *Withdrawal from reality*

Bleuler stressed what may be termed the dereastic attitude present in schizophrenia. The schizophrenic patient progressively loses interest in people around him. It is not unknown for a schizophrenic patient to initially transfer his interest from people to an animal, for example, a dog or a horse. He may develop an inordinate interest in politics, philosophy or religion, perhaps in an effort to stop the process that is enveloping him. Such pursuits, however, lead to little or no action. His thinking becomes more and more governed by his inner wishes and fantasies than by external realities, a type of thinking known as autistic thinking. Wishes, day dreams and fantasies assume greater importance than people or events in the outside world.

4. *Alterations in affect*

A disturbance of affect may be the first indication of a developing schizophrenic illness, evidenced by an increasing failure to respond in a normal fashion to people or events. There may occur emotional blunting or flattening, progressing to gross apathy, or incongruous or inappropriate affect.

5. *Disturbances of volition*

The most common disturbance is blunting of the will power. This can occur early in some clinical types of schizophrenia when the patient may be unable to make decisions or to act on them. He may in fact simply not go to work, but spend the days lying around inactive. Inactivity may also be seen in so-called 'burnt out' or residual schizophrenia. A housewife, a patient previously obsessional in her household chores, and recovered from more florid psychotic symptoms, found that she simply could not activate herself to tidy her home, and this non-volitional state pervaded other areas of previous activity.

Apart from indecision due to weakening of will power, there is often a stubborn persistent negative attitude to any requests. This is known as negativism. Ambivalence in schizophrenic patients is probably due to the weakening of volition.

Passivity phenomena, mentioned above and resulting from a disturbance of ego boundaries, may be regarded as a disturbance of volition. Many catatonic symptoms are probably the outward expression of a disturbance of volition.

6. *Delusions and hallucinations*

When taken in conjunction with other symptoms and signs, delusions and hallucinations are of high diagnostic value.

Clinical types of schizophrenia

There are nine main diagnostic categories described. It must be remembered that the clinical pictures presenting in patients do not always fit the classical text book decriptions, and one patient may present with features of more than one clinical type. Occasionally a patient may present with the main symptoms of one clinical variety of schizophrenia at one time, and at another, show features associated with a different clinical type.

1. *Simple type*

Of the simple type or schizophrenia simplex the I.C.D. glossary states:

> A psychosis in which there is insidious development of the oddities of conduct, inability to meet the demands of society, and decline in total performance. Delusions and hallucinations are not in evidence and the condition is less obviously psychotic than are the hebephrenic, catatonic and paranoid types of schizophrenia. With increasing social impoverishment vagrancy may ensue and the patient becomes self-absorbed, idle and aimless. Because the schizophrenic symptoms are not clear-cut, diagnosis of this form should be made sparingly, if at all.

The principal symptoms and signs elicited on mental state examination are shallowness of emotional response and absence of will and drive. It is very likely that a number of these patients go unrecognised. For example, a person who does not keep a job, develops dissolute habits, displays criminal propensities, and for no evident reason sinks lower in the social scale, may be suffering from simple schizophrenia.

2. *Hebephrenic type* (*Hebe*: Goddess of Youth)

This is

> a form of schizophrenia in which affective changes are prominent, delusions and hallucinations fleeting and fragmentary, behaviour irresponsible and unpredictable and mannerisms common. The mood is shallow and inappropriate, accompanied by giggling or self-satisfied, self-absorbed smiling, or by a lofty manner, grimaces, mannerisms, pranks, hypochondriacal complaints and reiterated phrases. Thought is disorganized. There is a tendency to remain solitary, and behaviour seems empty of purpose and feeling. This form of schizophrenia usually starts between the ages of 15 and 25 years.

Little can be added to this description save to say that some authorities rate thought disorder as the leading symptom in hebephrenic schizophrenia.

The patient may first complain of malaise and headache. He becomes depressed, irritable, dull and apathetic and tends to avoid the company of others. Work and study fall off. Depersonalization and derealization may be experienced. Distortion of body image and passivity phenomena wherein thoughts may be put into or taken out of a patient's head are not uncommon. Suicidal attempts are not infrequent. Later, the patient becomes childish with inconsequential behaviour, showing the fully-developed picture described above.

3. *Catatonic type*

This—

> includes as an essential feature prominent psychomotor disturbances often alternating between extremes such as hyperkinesis and stupor, or automatic obedience and negativism. Constrained attitudes may be maintained for long periods: if the patient's limbs are put in some unnatural position they may be held there for some time after the external force has been removed. Severe excitement may be a striking feature of the condition. Depressive or hypomanic concomitants may be present.

The I.C.D. description concentrates on the psychomotor disturbances as the essential feature of catatonic schizophrenia. At the risk of some repetition a fuller picture will now be painted.

Catatonic schizophrenia usually occurs before the age of 25 years. The outstanding feature is abnormality in motor behaviour which may take two extreme forms, generalised inhibition or excessive motor activity, referred to as catatonic stupor and catatonic excitement respectively. Intermediate states occur. In catatonic stupor there may have been a prodromal period of indefinite ill health. The patient may develop insomnia, depression, limitation of activity and a gradual withdrawal from contact with reality. Delusions of a persecutory or self-accusatory nature and hallucinations are common. A peculiar muscular rigidity which is uniform in distribution develops. Grimacing and tremors, or spasms of the facial muscles, especially a pursing or protrusion of the lips (Schnauzkramf), occur. Negativism in the form of resistance to attention, mutism and refusal of food is not uncommon. Verbigeration may occur.

In the advanced state of catatonic stupor, the patient may sit, stand, or lie in various attitudes (posturing). He is generally mute, but may verbigerate or display echolalia. Echopraxia, stereotypy and flexibilitas cerea are other common signs. Many patients appear to pass into the full-blown stuporose state relatively quickly. In these days, the earlier recognition of schizophrenia and the application of active therapies modify the clinical picture to the extent that stuporose catatonic features are now seen less often. The presence of generalised motor inhibition occurring in catatonic stupor should not lead one to conclude erroneously that the patient is oblivious of what is going on about him. A male nurse working in the bad old days 'encouraged' a male patient in a state of catatonic stupor to move along into the day room. The patient responded to treatment and was discharged home. Twelve months later, having relaxed his medication, he was re-admitted to the same hospital, this time in a more active state than on his previous admission. His first action was to kick the aforementioned male nurse in the seat of the pants, thus squaring the account.

Catatonic excitement may follow a state of catatonic stupor, or may arise *de novo*. Patients are extremely overactive, displaying purposeless and sometimes stereotyped behaviour, unpredictable to the observer because it is governed by the patient's delusions and hallucinatory experiences. Such patients may be extremely violent and resistive, and constitute a considerable nursing problem before being settled by medication or other means of treatment to be discussed below. It is impossible to establish sound rapport with such a patient while he is in this state. Before modern therapies, such patients could remain in a state of excessive movement day and night, proving impossible to feed, and in spite of other adequate nursing care, the condition not infrequently ended fatally. Speech is frequently incoherent, degenerating to the status of a word salad.

4. *Paranoid type*

The onset of this clinical type of schizophrenia usually occurs somewhat later in life than the three already mentioned, the condition evidencing itself in the late 20s and the early 30s as a rule, though it may occur at puberty, and is relatively common in the fourth and fifth decades. The condition is characterised by delusions generally of a persecutory or grandiose nature. Persecutory delusions may become systematised. Erotic, hypochondriacal and religious delusions are not infrequent. Hallucinations are common, if not always present, and are most frequently of an auditory nature. The patient may hear voices which threaten or accuse, or which to him are direct communications from God. Tactile hallucinations, interpreted by the patient for example as electricity or rays directed to part of the body are not uncommon, and hallucinations related to any of the other senses may also be present. The behaviour of these patients may be largely governed by their delusional and hallucinatory experiences and, in consequence, may be unpredicable. A patient harbouring persecutory delusional ideas will show a fairly constant attitude of hostility, aggression and suspicion. Excessive religiosity may be present.

Ideas of reference and passivity feelings may be prominent features. Other mental state abnormalities, at least in the early stages, may not feature prominently. Thought disorder is not obvious, and the affective response to delusions is appropriate. At a later stage of the illness, flattening of the affect is usually noticeable and there occur gross inconsistencies between a person's delusional belief and his actual behaviour. For example, the woman who believes herself to be of royal blood may express no objection when asked by a nurse to undertake some menial activity.

The I.C.D. glossary description of schizophrenia, paranoid type, also termed paraphrenic schizophrenia, appears to place more emphasis than is usual on disorder of thought processes, which at least in the early stages of this disorder are generally found to be intact. The following is the glossary statement:

> The form of schizophrenia in which relatively stable delusions, which may be accompanied by hallucinations, dominate the clinical picture. The delusions are frequently of persecution but may take other forms (for example of jealousy, exalted birth, Messianic mission, or bodily change). Hallucinations and erratic behaviour may occur; in some cases conduct is seriously disturbed from the outset, thought disorder may be gross, and affective flattening with fragmentary delusions and hallucinations may develop.

5. *Acute schizophrenic episode*

This term is used to cover

> schizophrenic disorders, other than those listed above, in which there is a dream-like state with slight clouding of consciousness and perplexity. External things, people and events may become charged with personal significance for the patient. There may be ideas of reference and emotional turmoil. In many such cases remission occurs within a few weeks or months, even without treatment.

This category includes: oneirophrenia (Gk. oneiros = dream), schizophreniform attach, or schizophreniform psychosis, confusional type.

6. *Schizoaffective type*

This term is applied to

> a psychosis in which pronounced manic or depressive features are intermingled with schizophrenic features and which tends towards remission without permanent defect, but which is prone to recur. The diagnosis should be made only when both the affective and schizophrenic symptoms are pronounced.

7. *Residual schizophrenia*

> A chronic form of schizophrenia in which the symptoms that persist from the acute phase have mostly lost their sharpness. Emotional response is blunted and thought disorder, even when gross, does not prevent the accomplishment of routine work.

The somewhat dehumanising term 'burnt out schizophrenic' has been applied to persons falling within this category.

8. *Latent schizophrenia*

The I.C.D. glossary states:

> It has not been possible to produce a generally acceptable description for this condition. It is not recommended for general use, but a description is provided for those who believe it to be useful: a condition of eccentric or inconsequent behaviour and anomalies of affect which give the impression of schizophrenia though no definite and characteristic schizophrenic anomalies, present or past, have been manifest. The inclusion terms indicate that this is the best place to classify some other poorly defined varieties of schizophrenia.

9. *Other*

Schizophrenia not classifiable under any of the eight above-mentioned categories is included. The terms acute (undifferentiated) schizophrenia or atypical schizophrenia are used in this category.

Prognosis in schizophrenia

The outcome is not always unfavourable, but overall, there is a general tendency in schizophrenia towards deterioration of the personality. Factors which tend towards a good prognosis are an acute onset, the presence of precipitating factors of a psychological or physical nature, a well-integrated and adapted pre-morbid personality of high intelligence, a manic-depressive heredity or the occurrence of benign psychoses in the family, the presence of catatonic or affective symptoms (depressive or hypomanic) in the illness, and the retention of a satisfactory emotional response on the part of the patient during the course of the illness. Pointers towards a poor prognosis are an insidious onset, the absence of adequate precipitating factors, onset at an early age, limited intelligence, marked schizoid features in the pre-morbid personality, the existence of schizophrenic relatives whose illness has taken a deteriorating course, and early signs of emotional flattening.

Management of schizophrenia

The question of hospitalisation will have to be considered for each individual sufferer. It is obvious that, in most instances where florid psychotic symptoms exist, destroying meaningful realistic relationships with other people, hospitalisation is indicated. There are, however, some patients who can be treated on an ambulatory or outpatient basis. If a patient requires hospitalisation and settles down on a treatment regime, it would seem important that he is not discharged prematurely before improvement is consolidated, and before sufficient rapport is established to give the incentive to continue follow-up treatment.

Psychotherapy

Formal psychotherapy has little to recommend it in the fully-developed case. In the early stages, a patient may be helped to make better social adjustment, and at least given the opportunity to maintain a personal contact whilst his world is literally falling apart.

Some workers claim to cure schizophrenia by psychotherapy alone without the use of drugs or physical treatments. One wonders at the severity of such illnesses. However, there is no doubt that, by working with the healthy part of the sufferer's ego, a helpful relationship can be formed and the patient is enabled to make better adjustments to life.

In the hospital setting, psychotherapy, which may simply mean a helping or understanding relationship on the part of team members, is an important aspect of treatment of this condition when the patient's ego boundaries are blurred and he tends to withdraw from outside contact.

Psychotherapy in a hospital setting is usually on a group basis. In terms of the patient's own future well-being, and in terms of the family's adjustment to the total situation, it is in many instances, worthwhile for the family to be involved in the treatment process.

There is also evidence that the attitudes of family members may have precipitated the breakdown, and not infrequently another family member, though able to cope in some way (possibly at the expense of the patient), is found to be more disturbed than the patient.

Drug therapy

Today, drugs play a major role in the management of schizophrenia. The major tranquillisers, for example phenothiazine derivatives and the butyrophenones, are the drugs of choice. These and other drugs are dealt with more fully in Chapter 20, and the student should refer to that chapter to learn something of dosages used, side effects, and other aspects of psychopharmacology.

Among the tranquillisers in more common use are trifluoperazine (Stelazine), chlorpromazine (Largactil), thioridazine (Melleril), fluphenazine (Anatensol), pericyazine (Neulactil), thiothixene (Navane), chlorprothixene (Truxal) and haloperidol (Serenace), the last mentioned being particularly valuable in states of catatonic excitement.

Any author who writes in a limited way about drugs must of necessity omit many that are valuable therapeutic agents, and some readers might take offence that their favourite is not mentioned. It is far better to get to know thoroughly the action of a limited number of well-tried drugs, than to use a wide spectrum of preparations, never becoming familiar with any. It is probably not so much the particular drug in a group of similarly acting drugs that counts, but the way the drug is used.

The administration of major tranquillisers must not cease too early.

Patients may be feeling and coping well, and it might be felt that medication is no longer indicated, and, as cessation of therapy may produce no apparent deterioration for some weeks (2-8 weeks), the enthusiast, either patient or doctor, who stops drugs might be lulled into a false sense of security, only to find that after some weeks, there occurs a recrudescence of symptoms. This is particularly noticeable in the sufferer from paranoid schizophrenia. A young adult male patient who felt in some way part of a spring inside a clock on the mantle shelf, lost his symptoms on treatment with trifluoperazine and was discharged from hospital. Follow-up in this instance was not possible, and feeling well, he ceased his medication only to be readmitted six weeks later, once again part of a spring inside a clock. If, as believed by many psychiatrists, each succeeding frank psychotic episode leaves a further adverse mark on the personality of the patient, then long continued treatment becomes of paramount importance. In practice, one may continue medication for up to 12 months before very gradual reduction is attempted. It is, perhaps, not a bad generality to adopt the following aphorism: 'as insulin is to the diabetic, so major tranquillisers are to the schizophrenic'. When depressive symptoms are associated with a schizophrenic illness, it is sound practice to administer one of the tricyclic antidepressants (Chapter 20) concurrently.

It is not an uncommon phenomenon for a person suffering from paranoid schizophrenia to settle on phenothiazines, only to develop features of the depressive syndrome a few weeks later (page 203). These people usually respond satisfactorily when one of the tricyclic antidepressants is added to their phenothiazine medication.

For maintenance medication of sufferers from schizophrenia who, for one reason or another, find difficulty in continuing oral medication, the depot fluphenazines may be of particular value (see page 304).

Physical treatments

(a) Insulin coma therapy was first used by Sakel in 1935. It had a vogue for two decades or more but is now little, if at all, used by British and Australian psychiatrists. It is mentioned merely for historical interest.

(b) Electroconvulsive therapy (ECT) has its place when affective symptoms colour the clinical picture. One, two or three treatments given daily may shorten the period of catatonic excitement. ECT is of value in lifting patients out of a state of catatonic stupor, and usually not more than 2-4 treatments are required. Apart from these indications, ECT is not of much value in schizophrenia when compared with the drugs now available. Some cases however, inexplicably improve with ECT when drug therapy appears to have failed. The use of 'regressive ECT' had its adherents in the past. Patients were given an intensive course of up to 20 treatments which caused gross confusion and even incontinence of bladder and bowels. They sometimes improved once they had come out of the state of profound confusion, but the long-term beneficial effects are doubtful.

(c) Leucotomy should not be considered until all other methods of treatment have been given a fair trial. Its use is limited, and paranoid schizophrenic illness where there is 'inner tension' is its main indication in schizophrenia.

Social and milieu therapy

An atmosphere is produced in the treatment situation, giving the most favourable opportunities for the patient to re-establish or maintain contact with other persons in a setting of security and trust. Staff and other patients in such a therapeutic atmosphere are accepting of the patient's behaviour and communications, which may indeed be bizarre. This sort of acceptance will help the patient to develop confidence, and in minimising anxiety, will help him to drop unhealthy defences. The student should read again Chapter 2 describing the therapeutic community which produces the kind of milieu that one is aiming for.

The nursing approach

The approach of the nurse to the patient suffering from schizophrenia cannot be formalised in any simple fashion, as a perusal of the variety of ways in which sufferers present should indicate. Certain areas require careful thought by the nurse, namely: the need to maintain or build the patient's self-esteem; the fact that the nurse is a representative of healthy reality to a patient who requires help to emerge from his own unreal world; the need to accept the patient as a person in spite of his sometimes untoward and bizarre behaviour; the need to allow a patient to use his own initiative and judgement as much as possible; the patient's needs in terms of warmth, friendliness and human contact; the necessity to encourage a patient into activity without pressurising him too much, thus causing further withdrawal; the patient's need to develop and maintain a sense of personal identity, involving such things as his own clothes, and having and caring for some personal possessions.

It is obvious that the nurse, serving as a model to the patient, demonstrating an approach to the problems of living, may be sorely tried in patience and forbearance; but such is psychiatric nursing.

Rehabilitation

Rehabilitation should be commenced the moment a schizophrenic patient enters hospital, and aspects mentioned under social and milieu therapy and the nursing approach will do much to prepare the patient for his return to life outside hospital.

The bulk of long-stay hospital patients fall into the diagnostic category of schizophrenia, and the process of institutionalisation will have left its mark on many occupying our older hospitals under a previous custodial regime. The section on rehabilitation techniques (page 328) applies to these patients.

With the development of psychiatric units attached to general hospitals, and when existing psychiatric clinics develop therapeutic community programmes for inpatients and expertise in community measures, the future may hold fewer problems in this particular area.

Community measures

Community psychiatry is described in Chapter 20. With an illness such as schizophrenia and its general tendency towards deterioration, it is not surprising that schizophrenic patients form a large proportion of people falling within the orbit of this aspect of management.

PARANOID STATES

Paranoid states are 'disorders of psychotic depth without a demonstrable physical aetiology . . . characterised by delusions, generally persecutory or grandiose, with or without hallucinations (ordinarily without). Intellectual functions may be well preserved and emotional responses and behaviour are usually consistent with the ideas held'.

Incidence

The incidence is believed to be high in the general population, but it is difficult to arrive at definite figures. Mild paranoid characteristics are found in many otherwise normal persons, and in neurotic persons who will probably never develop a paranoid psychotic illness.

Aetiology

It is stated that little evidence has been accrued to suggest that genetic factors play an important part in the development of paranoid states. A higher incidence is reported among migration and minority groups than in the general population. Isolation from other people through deafness or physical illness appears to be a precipitating factor.

Paranoid states usually develop after the age of 40, and probably never under the age of 30 years.

The psychotic picture generally arises from a background of a paranoid personality. The individual with such a personality is tense and insecure, operating at a high level of anxiety. He readily becomes suspicious and distrustful, finds it difficult to confide, and if he does place his trust in someone, expects to be betrayed. He tends to be secretive, and is basically hostile. Such a personality is also immature, and makes excessive use of denial and projection which favours delusion formation at times of stress. The transition from a paranoid personality disorder to frank psychosis with manifest delusions may be extremely difficult to date. On the other hand, adults who later develop a paranoid reaction may never have been regarded as having a paranoid personality. It is assumed however, that, arising essentially out of a distortion of early childhood development, such a person has a predisposition to mistrust others.

This factor of basic mistrust may indeed be the reason why a large proportion of sufferers from paranoid states have never married.

Freud developed the thesis that paranoid states become manifest when homosexual trends escape repression, and for years it has been considered that a person developing a paranoid state is basically homosexual. There is little clinical evidence however, to support this thesis.

Clinical picture

Four clinical types are described.

Paranoid state, simple

This is

> a psychosis, acute or chronic, not classifiable as schizophrenia or affective psychosis, in which delusions, especially of being influenced, persecuted or treated in some special way, are the main symptoms. The delusions are of a fairly fixed, elaborate and systematised kind.

Paranoia

The description given for paranoia is that of

> a rare chronic psychosis in which logically constructed systematised delusions have developed gradually without concomitant hallucinations or the schizophrenic type of disordered thinking. The delusions are mostly of grandeur (the paranoiac prophet or inventor), persecution or somatic abnormality.

Paraphrenia

Paraphrenia is the name applied to

> paranoid psychosis in which there are conspicuous hallucinations, often in several modalities. Affective symptoms and disordered thinking, if present do not dominate the clinical picture and the personality is well preserved.

The condition, as its other appellations of 'involutional paranoid state' and 'late paraphrenia' suggest, occurs later in life generally between the ages of 45 and 65 years. It is characterised by persecutory and/or grandiose delusions which lack the logical nature of the systematisation seen in the paranoid state and paranoia.

Some authorities regard paraphrenia as schizophrenia, paranoid type occurring late in life, after the personality has become stable and less likely to disintegrate.

Patients with paranoid symptoms appear to have particularly good memories, if only for detail of alleged slights, injustices or persecution. They tell their story in intimate detail, and, as their personality is generally well preserved, it may take a long time to come to the conclusion that the patient is indeed mentally ill. Again, very long examination may be necessary before the paranoid patient touches upon his delusional system, and the examiner may indeed require the attributes of a ferret to uncover the delusional material, even after abnormal behaviour of a patient has led to his referral. This may, in some cases, be the result of the patient having insight into the fact that his false beliefs will probably not be generally acceptable, so they are not brought to the fore. On one occasion, a woman was admitted to hospital for observation after lighting a fire on the fence between her home and her neighbour's house. This seemed the proper remedial thing to do, since she believed the neighbour was gassing her through the fence. It took a long time however, for this patient to admit to her persecutory delusion.

It may be extremely difficult to differentiate between schizophrenia, paranoid type and the paranoid states.

Differential points favouring a paranoid state include the following: Onset of illness is gradual and occurs at an older age; thought disorder of a schizophrenic kind is less marked or not in evidence; affect and behaviour is congruous with, and appropriate to the delusions entertained; there is little external evidence of psychiatric illness, the personality is well preserved, and the course of the illness is only gradually progressive, with the patient's mental state remaining essentially the same over one or two decades.

Induced psychosis

The I.C.D. has the following to say:

> Mainly delusional psychosis, usually chronic and often without florid features, which appears to have developed as a result of a close, if not dependent, relationship with another person who already has an established similar psychosis. The delusions are at least partly shared . . .

The condition is also known as *folie à deux* or induced paranoid disorder. Rare cases in which several persons are affected are also classified as suffering from induced psychosis (for example, folie à cinq).

FOLIE À DEUX

For the development of folie à deux (or folie imposee) special conditions are required. Firstly, one person is dominant and usually more intelligent than the other, and he or she, usually suffering from paranoid schizophrenia or a paranoid state, imposes his or her delusions on to the more passive and originally healthy partner. Secondly, there must be a close physical association in the same relatively isolated environment for a long period of time, and an intimate emotional bond between the two affected people.

The condition occurs more frequently in women than in men.

Management involves separating the recipient partner from the source of the delusion(s). The dominant initially ill partner is treated like any other patient suffering from a nonorganic psychosis. The passive partner may or may not lose his or her delusions after a period of separation. If not, neuroleptic drugs (page 297) may be of value.

Management may prove quite difficult however, as needs or deficiencies within the passive partner contribute towards the development of the state—delusions are not able to be transmitted to a mentally healthy individual. The dominant partner complete with delusions has become the key person in the life of the passive partner, and the loss on separation assumes gigantic proportions. Consequently time, psychotherapy, social therapy and interaction are often essential for a successful management outcome.

Management of paranoid states

Many patients are able to continue with their normal occupations, as they have the capacity for divorcing their delusional system from the normal stream of consciousness. Under conditions of stress, the patient may act under pressure of his delusional beliefs, and socially unacceptable behaviour may require hospitalisation. An occasional paranoid patient is highly dangerous, and under the influence of delusions, may attack his believed persecutors. Such a patient will require hospitalisation for the safety of members of the community.

Electroconvulsive therapy has little or no value in treatment. The major tranquillisers may reduce the tension arising out of delusional beliefs, and their use is advocated.

Perhaps more important than anything else, is the development of a long term relationship with a well trained psychotherapist, within which, the patient who has never really trusted anybody in his life, is given the opportunity of learning to trust somebody without being 'sold down the river'. If such a patient can learn 'basic trust', not developed in infancy and childhood, he will feel less threatened and more comfortable. In such a treatment situation and in a hospital milieu, certain general principles should be borne in mind:

1. As much freedom as possible should be given to the patient. This will be governed by the patient's potential for hostile behaviour. The person who already feels people are against him will object strongly to petty restrictions. Such restrictions merely give proof that people really are opposed to him.
2. One must always be honest in dealings with the paranoid patient. He expects to be misused or misled, and is acutely sensitive to other people's motives. If those nursing or treating him serve as consistently honest models, he may have a chance to develop some degree of trust.
3. One must listen with courtesy and understanding without condescension to the paranoid patient's delusional beliefs, neither saying one believes them—as one doesn't—nor arguing against them. If forced to make a statement about a patient's delusional beliefs, it is best to indicate that one understands the experience to be very real to the patient but that one does not see things in the same light.
4. Forcing a patient, mistrustful of his fellow men, into activities or group situations in a ward can lead only to resentment on his part. In time, he may develop enough assurance and trust to enter into group activities.
5. In general, one should avoid prying into these patients' backgrounds and activities.
6. A therapist must expect a paranoid patient to be distrustful of him, at least initially, and should not respond belligerently to a patient's accusations. The patient may even be testing the therapist to see if he can be trusted, if he is consistent, and if he can tolerate the patient's attitudes.
7. A therapist or nurse must avoid the overt show of too much friendliness or kindness, as this may be construed by the patient as an attempt to cultivate him so that his expected later rejection will be all the more painful to him. An attitude of friendly but distant neutrality is probably as much as a paranoid patient can tolerate, at least early in treatment.
8. It must be borne in mind that delusional beliefs involving other people, including staff, may lead to violence.

In many instances, the most that can be expected is that the paranoid patient will learn to trust the therapist. This state is indeed reached, much to the joy of the therapist, when the patient can accept the therapist saying, 'That's complete rubbish, so there's no point in talking about it outside this office. You can come and talk to me about it when you feel like it'. This happy state of affairs may never be achieved.

THE AFFECTIVE PSYCHOSES

The affective psychoses are

> mental disorders, usually recurrent, in which there is a severe disturbance of mood (mostly compounded of depression and anxiety but also manifested as elation and excitement) which is accompanied by one or more of the following: delusions, perplexity, disturbed attitude to self, disorder of perception and behaviour; these are all in keeping with the patient's prevailing mood (as are hallucinations when they occur). There is a strong tendency to suicide. For practical reasons, mild disorders of mood may also be included . . . if the symptoms match closely the descriptions given; this applies particularly to mild hypomania.

They may be described as non organic psychoses characterised by excessive states of depression or elation with resultant disturbances of thought and behaviour. These changes of mood are often apparently unprovoked. Affective psychoses have a strong tendency to recur, and are self-limiting.

The resultant disturbances of thought and behaviour are consistent or congruous with the prevailing mood which, as we have learned, is not the general rule in schizophrenic illnesses. It is normal for us to show some fluctuations in mood, but the elation and depression are regarded as morbid when their intensity and duration are out of all proportion to the prevailing circumstances.

Manic-depressive psychosis

Confusion frequently exists in the student's mind as to what is meant by 'manic-depressive psychosis'. The term simply refers to a group of differing syndromes which appear to have the same aetiology, and which may occur at different times in the same individual. It does not necessarily mean that a patient swings suddenly from depression to mania or vice versa. Such a condition would be classified as manic-depressive psychosis, circular type. A patient may indeed be labelled manic-depressive, even if he has suffered only one depressive episode and never a manic episode.

Incidence and aetiology

The average frequency of manic-depressive psychosis in the general population is quoted as 3-4 per thousand. There appear to be some racial differences, the condition occurring more frequently in southern European countries than in northern. Also, the presenting features of the illness may differ from culture to culture. It is stated that in Java, excitement is far more common than depression, though the overall incidence is similar to that in European countries.

The condition occurs more frequently in women than in men. In New South Wales, for example, the proportion of female to male sufferers is 2 or 3:1, and this trend is found to be world-wide.

Doubt has been cast on a previously-held view that manic depressive psychosis has a higher incidence among people in higher socio-economic groups. There is an insignificant relationship between this disorder and marital status.

Heredity appears to play an important role in the occurrence of manic-depressive psychosis. In at least 10% of cases one or other parent has suffered from the illness. An eighth to a quarter of the children with one manic-depressive parent are affected, and figures of over 20% have been recorded for the occurrence of the condition in siblings of sufferers.

There would appear to be a number of possible ways for genetic transmission relating to the development of manic depressive illness to take place. A long-held view is that it results from the effect of a single dominant gene with incomplete penetrance.

More recent studies have shown that, within some families, a dominant X-linked gene appears responsible for transmission of some factor(s) leading to manic depressive illness, and the illness has been found in some families to be associated with colour blindness, itself a sex-linked condition. The sex-linked nature of the gene could account for the higher incidence of manic depressive illness found in females. However, not all manic depressive illness arises from X-linked genes, as the condition can be transmitted from father to son; suggesting that there is more than one way for a predisposition to manic depressive psychosis to be transmitted.

It is often found that the patient's temperament has previously been depressed, elated, irritable, anankastic, or cyclothymic. First attacks are most common between the ages of 20 and 35 years, and there is a significant relationship with the pyknic body build. Attacks may arise apparently out of the blue, or be precipitated by some physical or emotional stress with a psychological basis of real or imagined loss. The author has known at least one patient who could recall the step he took on the footpath when a depression of suicidal intensity enveloped him. Knowledge of the psycho-dynamic mechanisms occurring in the development of depression is fragmentary, but the student should revise the outline given in Chapter 8.

The important precipitating factor is that of loss of a valued object. It would appear that, owing to a strong hereditary predisposition, some patients develop this illness on the basis of little or no precipitating stresses, while others, still with an hereditary predisposition of less import, require an obvious situation of loss for the development of the illness.

With respect to the symptom of elation in manic-depressive psychosis, as suggested in Chapter 8, it is very likely that a patient with this symptom has the same hereditary factors and problems as the depressed patient, but he reacts by denial of these problems and goes to the opposite extreme.

CLINICAL TYPES

The I.C.D. lists five major clinical variants of manic-depressive psychosis and provides four other labels for the purpose of classification. These are shown in Appendix I. The I.C.D. glossary descriptions state:

Manic-depressive psychosis, depressed type

An affective psychosis in which there is a widespread depressed mood of gloom and wretchedness with some degree of anxiety. There is often reduced activity but there may be restlessness and agitation. There is a marked tendency to recurrence. In a few cases this may be at regular intervals.

Manic-depressive psychosis, manic type

Mental disorders characterized by states of elation or excitement out of keeping with the patient's circumstances and varying from enhanced liveliness (hypomania) to violent, almost uncontrollable excitement. Agression and anger, flight of ideas, distractibility, impaired judgment, and grandiose ideas are common.

Manic-depressive psychosis, circular type but currently depressed

Circular type (see next definition below) in which the depressive form is currently present.

Manic-depressive psychosis, circular type but currently manic.

An affective psychosis which has appeared in both the depressive and the manic form, either alternating or separated by an interval of normality, but in which the manic form is currently present. (The manic phase is far less frequent than the depressive.)

Manic-depressive psychosis, circular type, mixed

An affective psychosis in which both manic and depressive symptoms are present at the same time.

With this brief overview we shall now look in more detail at the main clinical types.

Manic-depressive psychosis, depressed type

Clinical picture

Depression in mood occurs along with mental and motor retardation and inhibition. In some cases anxiety may be a prominent symptom. In others, perplexity, agitation or stupor may be prominent. In the latter two instances, 'agitated depression' or 'stuporose depression' are terms sometimes used to describe the clinical states. Agitation is probably more common in association with depression occurring in middle and later life. Some patients, particularly middle-aged women, are frequently wrongly diagnosed as being hysterical, or suffering from an anxiety state, when they are in fact suffering from psychotic depression. The presence of hysterical or anxiety symptoms occurring for the first time in middle life should always alert the worker in psychiatry to the strong possibility that the patient is suffering from a psychotic depression. The term 'endogenous depression' is synonymous with manic-depressive psychosis, depressed type.

The typical patient looks as he feels. Stance is bowed, movements and speech are slow, and speech lacks expression. In severe states, secretions are reduced and the patient may display an inability to cry. The mouth may be dry. A reduction in libido occurs in both sexes, and amenorrhoea may be present. There may be hypochondriacal complaints and even delusions of guilt, sin, unworthiness, or nihilistic delusions where the patient may believe his brain or bowels, or he himself does not exist. Such delusions are more common in depressions occurring in the involutional period of life. One of the early symptoms is loss of interest in work and activities which may previously have been most satisfying. Intolerance to noise and withdrawal from social contact may occur early. Patients become engrossed in their own personal world and are frequently unable to concentrate on what is going on around them.

The most prominent and important symptoms in manic-depressive psychosis, depressed type, and ones which must always be looked for if not volunteered by the patient are as follows: anorexia, which in the early stages is frequently worse in the mornings, and which may be associated with a churning or heavy feeling in the pit of the stomach; insomnia, typically late insomnia, i.e. early morning waking, but initial and middle insomnia may be present as well; diurnal variation in depression, meaning that depression is worse at a particular time of day and in the case of psychotic depressions this is in the mornings, frequently lifting for no obvious reason in the afternoon or evening. Constipation may be marked but is is by no means always present.

The sufferer tends to blame himself for his state, feels worthless, and is often unduly full of guilt and self reproach over past minor sins of commission or omission. He may temporarily lose any faith he has held, and the future usually looks black. It is no wonder that suicide is such a major hazard in sufferers from psychotic depressive illnesses.

Cultural differences influence the degree to which guilt and feelings of worthlessness are found. In Asian and African cultures feelings of shame, complaints of bodily disfunction, and loss of energy may be prominent symptoms.

Every patient suspected of suffering from manic-depressive psychosis, depressed type, should be given the opportunity of talking about, and indeed should be asked about suicidal thoughts. These may consist simply in the feeling that it would be good to be able to go to sleep and not wake up, or the patient may have contemplated suicide by one means or another, or may have made an actual attempt at self-destruction. Though in the main ready to share such thoughts, some patients do not, and one has to depend on the content of the patient's communication. A male patient when asked directly was he suicidal, denied the possibility, saying he was so unworthy he had not yet made his peace with God. The inference from this being he would not commit suicide before making such peace. Within two days, having apparently made peace with his Maker, or having decided that this was impossible to achieve, he absconded from hospital and made a suicidal attempt by drowning, fortunately unsuccessful. It is indeed a tragedy for a life to be lost through a self-limiting illness, recovery from which leaves the personality unimpaired and the sufferer once again able to enjoy life and contribute to it to the full.

One cannot overstress the importance of diligently seeking for the symptoms of anorexia, epigastric discomfort, diurnal variation in depression (worse in mornings), early morning waking, and loss of interest, in patients whose history and clinical state suggest the possibility of a depressive illness. The symptoms form part of the constellation sometimes referred to as the 'depressive syndrome'.

Variations in presentation

It is not at all uncommon for patients to present simply with a physical symptom. The male patient described in Chapter 10 with a pain in the foot was one. Among other single presenting symptoms previously investigated, and in some instances treated medically or surgically before psychiatric referral, may be included from the author's experience: dizziness; pain in the left arm in a young to middle-aged childless woman who would have nursed her offspring in that arm had she borne an infant; abdominal pain, treated unsuccessfully by appendectomy, and which cleared by the end of one week after the commencement of suitable antidepressant medication. This number could be added to, but it serves as a reminder that one should be on the alert for the not-so-obvious depression, and once again, without putting symptoms into the patient's mind, one should explore the possibility of the presence of the 'depressive syndrome'.

Some extremely depressed and even suicidal patients do not appear depressed and may even smile fairly consistently when engaged in conversation. There is something about the quality of this smile which makes one feel it is not the outward manifestation of inner calm and happiness, but the uninitiated may well be fooled by it. The depressed patient who lingers at the consulting room door disinclined to see the end of what might be termed a reasonably long and supportive interview bears watching as a potentially serious suicidal risk. A term applied to these variations in clinical presentation is 'masked depression'.

Management

Many patients suffering from manic-depressive psychosis, depressed type may be treated on an outpatient basis or from the doctor's consulting room providing the risk of suicide has been assessed as negligible, and providing relatives are supportive and understanding. The stuporose or severely agitated depressive patient will require hospitalisation. It is wise to admit to inpatient care the patient retarded in mental and physical function, for the simple reason that the retardation frequently diminishes more quickly under treatment than do the feelings of unworthiness and guilt. Early in treatment in such cases the patient may be rendered active enough to attempt suicide under the pressure of as yet unchanged or minimally changed feelings of gross unworthiness or guilt. It behoves the nurse and doctor in the inpatient situation to observe such a patient at all times in the early stages of treatment until it is certain that the mood has also lifted, thus making a suicide attempt unlikely. Formal psychotherapy is of little value in the more severe stages of a psychotic depressive illness. In terms of the sense of loss experienced by such patients however, the presence of someone with them in the early stages of treatment, even if no verbal communication is possible, is of extreme importance.

Drug therapy has assumed a major role in the management of these patients whether on an inpatient or outpatient basis. Two major groups of drugs, the tricyclids, for example amitriptyline, nortriptyline, imipramine, trimipramine, protriptyline, doxepin, and the monoamine oxidase inhibitors, for example phenelzine and tranylcypromine, are used. In general, it may be stated that the tricyclids overall are much more effective in the treatment of psychotic depressive illnesses than are the M.A.O. inhibitors which require certain rigid precautions to be exercised by the patient who is taking them. Details of these drugs are given in Chapter 20. Some general points however, will be made here. There is little difference between the antidepressant effects of any of the tricyclids mentioned, and it is a sound policy to become familiar with the therapeutic dosage and use of one or two of them. Some improvement is usually noticed in the first week of treatment, though it may not be complete for 5 or 6 weeks. If there is no indication of improvement after one week, particularly in appetite, sleep, work and general interest, then electroconvulsive therapy is usually indicated. Following recovery from a depressive episode, antidepressant medication must be continued at therapeutic levels for several months before gradual reduction is undertaken. One cannot always be sure how long a particular depressive episode will last or take to burn itself out, and sudden cessation of medication may result in a recrudescence of symptoms. This is described in Chapter 20 (page 309 and Figure 14). A female middle-aged patient, taking maintenance imipramine fifteen months after being symptom free, became severely depressed once again within a week of having her medication reduced from 100 mg per day to 75 mg per day. Depressive symptoms lifted again on resumption of the previous dosage. A return of symptoms after such a long period of maintenance therapy is not common, but the case emphasises the point made that medication should be continued for several months at least before attempting gradual reduction in dosage.

Where florid psychotic symptoms such as delusions, and more rarely hallucinations, are present, one of the phenothiazine drugs is given along with whatever specific measures are taken to treat the depression.

One of the minor tranquillisers, such as the benzodiazepine, chlordiazepoxide 10 mg T.D.S., may be given along with antidepressant medication if agitation or anxiety is marked. Alternatively, a small dose of one of the major tranquillisers, for example thioridazine 25 mg T.D.S. or chlorpromazine 25 mg T.D.S., may be given along with the tricyclic antidepressants.*

Lithium salts were shown by J. F. J. Cade, in 1949, to be of value in the treatment of 'psychotic excitement'. Lithium carbonate, the salt most frequently used, is indeed efficacious in the management of manic-depressive psychosis, manic type, and some evidence is accruing that it may be of value in the treatment of some psychotic depressive episodes (see page 314).

The giving of maintenance lithium however, lessens the number of depressive as well as manic episodes in sufferers from the cyclical type of

* The symptom of agitation appears to respond better to phenothiazines and other neuroleptic drugs than to the benzodiazepines (page 306).

manic-depressive psychosis, and has some prophylactic value in some patients who suffer from recurrent depressive episodes.

Electroconvulsive Therapy (ECT) is still the most effective form of treatment for an attack of manic-depressive psychosis, depressed type. There is, however, a greater tendency for a recurrence of depression, than in those patients who respond to antidepressant medication and continue maintenance therapy. If, along with ECT, one of the tricyclic drugs such as amitriptyline is given and continued as maintenance therapy, the relapse rate is much less marked.

Following a course of ECT given on its own, one must be particularly careful to ensure that the patient is seen 11-14 days after the last treatment, as this appears to be a critical time for relapse and possible suicide.

The number of treatments required is approximately 8. A sound rule is to give two further treatments once clinical improvement is complete, as this reduces the relapse rate.

Patients with first attacks of depression over the age of 50 years usually do very well with ECT, and it is indicated as a first line of treatment in patients who are grossly retarded or stuporose. Some advocate the use of ECT in deluded patients without first trying drugs. This will depend to some extent on the patient's suicidal propensity, which is naturally a clear indication for lifting a patient's depression as quickly as possible. Where other treatment methods have failed, leucotomy may have a place in the treatment of persistent depressive states in older patients, especially those with obsessional personalities.

When a patient is in the depths of a psychotic depressive illness, as indicated earlier, all that may be possible is to keep him company. Such patients should not be forced into group activities. As the condition improves, encouragement is given to participate in graded activities such as are provided in the unit or ward programme, so helping to restore lost confidence. Games, cooking, painting, for example may be included. As depression continues to lift, it is fascinating, in units where art therapy is available, to see colour and life come back into a patient's paintings.

In the community, preventive measures may be utilised in an attempt to minimise stress factors that may precipitate a psychotic depressive illness. After clinical recovery, follow-up of patients is of extreme importance if only to keep a check on maintenance medication. On recovery, most patients get on with the business of living, and many do not wish to be reminded of their illness or of hospitalisation.

Prognosis

The prognosis, or expected outcome, following a single attack of depression is good. With respect to the chances of having a further depressive episode, one must be guarded. If the patient has had a number of previous episodes, it is likely that more will follow. On the other hand, a patient may live for years with no recurrence. An upswing of mood, leading to the clinical picture of manic-depressive psychosis, manic type, may appear amid a series of depressive episodes. It is an impression that the patient who has not responded well to adequate dosage of a suitable antidepressant drug, frequently appears to do less well on ECT, and may indeed become a long-term visitor to the psychiatrist or treatment unit.

Manic-depressive psychosis, manic type

'Elation or irritability with overtalkativeness, flight of ideas and increased motor activity, chatacterise this type. Transitory episodes of depression may occur', but if the general picture is one of mania or hypomania, the condition is still classified under the manic type.

Incidence and aetiology

Manic-depressive psychosis, manic type, occurs much less frequently than does the depressed type. In a survey of 6 months admissions of patients to one ward of The Psychiatric Centre, North Ryde, in 1964-65, there were 114 psychotically depressed patients admitted, as opposed to 4 in the manic phase of manic-depressive psychosis. Aetiological factors are those of manic-depressive psychosis generally, and are dealt with earlier in this chapter and in Chapter 8.

Clinical picture

At home before hospitalisation, or in hospital, these patients may be trying in the extreme. They do everything to excess, talk loudly, sing loudly, put into action numerous schemes which they may never carry through. If, however, they accomplish objectives by dint of the tremendous drive possessed in the manic phase, they may indeed cause great embarrassment to families or employers. In 6 weeks before admission to hospital, a railway clerk bought and sold three cars and entered into negotiations which would have involved his Department in deals worth approximately one million pounds sterling. This arose out of his heightened self-esteem, grandiosity and complete lack of judgment. In terms of insight into their state, these patients frequently have no idea they are ill. When asked how they feel, they will say 'On top of the world', 'Never better', and if in hospital, they will query why they are there.

Such patients may be witty and penetrating in their observations, and their jovial mood is often infectious. However, some lability of mood is frequently present, transitory episodes of depression may occur, and if thwarted in their aims, these patients may become extremely irritable.

Problems are created on the ward by their tendency to interfere with ward activities. Behaviour may become destructive or degraded and may degenerate to the indecent e.g. sexual assaults and exposure. Modern methods of management do much to obviate this type of behaviour. The overactivity of the manic patient may interfere greatly with his sleep, nutrition and hydration.

Initially it may be difficult to determine whether an overactive patient is suffering from schizophrenic catatonic excitement or manic-depressive psychosis, manic type. The main differential points are as follows:

	Acute mania	*Catatonic excitement*
Behaviour	Pressure of activity, mostly purposive	Purposeless, absurd, stereotyped, often impulsive and violent
Negativism	Absent	Present
Speech	Flight of ideas	Flight of ideas, but more likely to be incoherent; may degenerate to word salad

Mood	Infectiously expansive	No rapport
Hallucinations	Absent or insignificant	Present

Management

Whether in an individual or a group setting, psychotherapy is impossible in the florid stage of the illness. In fact, there is nothing more disrupting to group therapy or to a ward meeting than to have such a patient moving restlessly about, entering into conversation with this patient and that, in fact, literally holding the floor and diverting others from any theme that may develop. These patients should not attend ward or group therapy meetings until there is reasonable reduction in their pressure of activity.

Drugs which are of value in the treatment of mania or hypomania include chlorpromazine, thioridazine, haloperidol, lithium carbonate. (See Chapter 20.)

Before the advent of suitable drug therapy, the treatment of choice was to give ECT daily, or even two or three times daily, until the condition settled. Such a procedure can still be lifesaving if the patient is poorly nourished and becomes dedydrated due to excessive activity and failure to eat or drink. In the days before major tranquillisers suitable for intramuscular or intravenous injection were available, it was not an uncommon practice to pass an intranasal or intragastric tube and give the patient fluid and nourishment by this route while he was still in a post anaesthetic or post ECT confusional state following modified ECT. This procedure was not without its risks, but these had to be weighed against the risk of a patient dying from dehydration or starvation. In some instances, the same type of feeding applied to patients in schizophrenic catatonic excitement.

In nursing manic or hypomanic patients, efforts should be made to direct activities into useful channels, not always an easy task. The very distractibility that enables one to divert a patient into some accoptable activity militates against his perseverance in same.

Prognosis

Further episodes of mania (or depression) frequently occur, though there may be lengthy periods of remission.

Manic-depressive psychosis, circular type

In recent years, a new approach to classifying manic-depressive psychosis has emerged. This consists in distinguishing depressed patients with a history of manic episodes (bipolar group) from those who have only experienced recurrent depression and no manic episodes (unipolar group).

The rubric *manic-depressive psychosis, circular type* is used to describe the bipolar group, and, depending whether the sufferer is currently depressed or manic (or hypomanic), an addition of *but currently depressed* or *but currently manic* is added to the diagnosis.

Unipolar and bipolar depressions

At this point we shall digress to point out differences found between the unipolar and bipolar groups, some of which are relevant to management.

Firstly, the average age of onset of bipolar illness is 20 to 25 years, while that of unipolar illness is somewhat later, about 30 to 35 years.

Secondly, there is a higher frequency of positive family histories for the illness in the bipolar group as opposed to the unipolar group.

Thirdly, the following findings are relevant to decisions on the management of patients suffering from manic-depressive psychosis: the use of tricyclic antidepressants is more likely to lead to hypomania in the bipolar group than in the unipolar group; and the bipolar group responds better to lithium both as a prophylactic and a treatment measure. Also, recent evidence strongly suggests that bipolar patients with a family history of mania respond better to lithium than do bipolar patients with no such family history.

Management

The management of manic-depressive psychosis, circular type will depend on the phase currently present, and follows the management outlined for the depressed type and manic type of manic-depressive psychosis. Great care needs to be exercised in order not to precipitate the opposite mood state to that being managed.

Manic-depressive psychosis, circular type, mixed

This term is used to describe an affective psychosis in which manic and depressive symptoms are present at the same time. The state occurs in the transitional phase between swings of mood from depression to mania and vice versa, or it may appear in transitory fashion during what appears to be a purely depressive or manic attack. Only rarely does it occur de novo, that is, as an independent attack.

Involutional melancholia

No longer accorded a separate diagnostic category from manic-depressive psychosis, depressed type, but included under this rubric is a condition which was formerly termed ‘involutional melancholia’. The earlier separation was based on the clinical picture and on some evidence pointing to differences in hereditary factors. It was thought that there were more sufferers from schizophrenia among the relatives of these people than among the relatives of those showing a more typical picture of manic-depressive psychosis, depressed type. For all practical purposes there seems little point in separating the two categories, but for historical interest a brief comment will be made on what earlier writers said about involutional melancholia.

This condition is ‘an affective psychosis occurring approximately between the ages of 45 and 65 years (and in women, commonly at the menopause) in patients of both sexes without previous history of affective psychosis . . .’ Cases commonly present several of the following features:

1. The absence of a previous mental breakdown but the presence of an anankastic (obsessive-compulsive) pre-morbid personality.
2. Agitation, which may be marked. Mental and motor retardation is usually absent.
3. Hypochondriacal ideas reaching delusional intensity.
4. Morbid anxiety and apprehension, often accompanied by stereotyped depressive utterances and gesticulations of despair. For example, a patient may sit wringing his hands repeating 'My God, oh, my God . . .'.
5. Delusions of guilt and nihilistic delusions. The patient may believe wrongly that his family is dead or that persons or things normally dear to him have ceased to exist.
6. The onset tends to be gradual and, if untreated, the course prolonged.

As in any psychotic depressive state, remorse and suicidal impulses may be marked. Some cases are characterised by marked paranoid ideas. In such instances, the differentiation from paranoid schizophrenia or a paranoid state may be difficult. Patients suffering from involutional melancholia however, are more likely to have feelings of guilt, unworthiness and self-blame. The paranoid schizophrenic or sufferer from a paranoid state will tend to blame others or outside factors rather than himself.

Management

Management is as described for manic-depressive psychosis, depressed type. ECT is probably the treatment of choice, especially as patients over the age of fifty years, with first attacks of depression, generally respond well to ECT. The tricyclic antidepressants are also effective. In cases where there is a strong paranoid element, one would give phenothiazine derivatives along with ECT or with one of the tricyclic antidepressants. Leucotomy may be considered in intractable cases unresponsive to other forms of treatment.

OTHER NON ORGANIC PSYCHOSES

The diagnostic categories mentioned below 'should be restricted to the small group of psychotic conditions that are largely or entirely attributable to recent life experiences. They should not be used for the wider range of psychoses in which environmental factors play some (but not the *major*) part in aetiology.'

Depressive type

A depressive psychosis which can be similar in its symptoms to manic-depressive psychosis, depressed type but is apparently provoked by saddening stress such as a bereavement, or a severe disappointment or frustration. There may be less diurnal variation of symptoms than in manic-depressive psychosis, depressed type and the delusions are more often understandable in the context of the life experiences. There is usually a serious disturbance of behaviour, e.g. major suicidal attempt.

This condition, also known as reactive depressive psychosis or psychogenic depressive psychosis is differentiated from manic-depressive psychosis, depressed type, by the presence of environmental precipitating factors and the absence of a history of depressive episodes or of marked cyclothymic mood swings.

Management is identical to that of patients diagnosed as suffering from manic-depressive psychosis, depressed type.

Excitative type

An affective psychosis similar in its symptoms to manic-depressive psychosis, manic type, but apparently provoked by emotional stress.

The management is the same as that described under manic-depressive psychosis, manic type.

Reactive confusion

Mental disorders with clouded consciousness, disorientation (though less marked than in organic confusion) and diminished accessibility often accompanied by excessive activity and apparently provoked by emotional stress.

Acute paranoid reaction

Paranoid states apparently provoked by some emotional stress. The stress is often misconstrued as an attack or threat. Such states are particularly prone to occur in prisoners or as acute reactions to a strange and threatening environment, e.g. in immigrants.

Psychogenic paranoid psychosis

Psychogenic or reactive paranoid psychosis of any type which is more protracted than the acute reactions covered under the rubric 'acute paranoid reaction'.

Also included in this group of disorders are hysterical psychosis and psychogenic stupor.

14

NEUROTIC DISORDERS

The I.C.D. Glossary description of neurotic disorders (already quoted on page 83) is as follows:

> Neurotic disorders are mental disorders without any demonstrable organic basis in which the patient may have considerable insight and has unimpaired reality testing, in that he usually does not confuse his morbid subjective experiences and fantasies with external reality. Behaviour may be greatly affected although usually remaining within socially acceptable limits, but personality is not disorganised. The principal manifestations include excessive anxiety, hysterical symptoms, phobias, obsessional and compulsive symptoms, and depression.

The glossary points out that the distinction between neurosis and psychosis is difficult and remains subject to debate, but it has been maintained in view of its wide use. The author believes the distinction to be valid, for in contrast to patients with psychoses, patients suffering from neuroses do not present gross disorganisation of personality.

The neuroses may be seen as syndromes arising out of different ways people handle anxiety, through the various mental defense mechanisms, and the student at this point should refer to the sections on anxiety and unconscious motivation in Chapter 6. The most common mental or ego defence mechanisms that come into play in the development of neuroses are rationalisation, repression, reaction formation, dissociation (and isolation), displacement and conversion. The more pathogenic mechanisms of regression, denial, projection and introjection are invoked to a lesser extent.

There are all gradations of neurotic disturbances, from those which interfere little with the business of living to those which are grossly incapacitating.

Most of us, if not all, are neurotic in some respects, but are able in most areas to lead reasonably satisfying and productive lives. Other people may suffer as a result of our defensive manoeuvres to deal with our anxiety, and we certainly may be inhibited from developing our potentialities to the full, yet we can hardly be labelled as suffering from illnesses. This brings us to the point of asking 'At what stage can neurotic disturbances, so widely present in society, be classed as illnesses?'

One might say that neurotic disturbance achieves the status of an illness when the disturbance interferes to a marked extent with one's ability to work or to maintain harmonious interpersonal relationships, free from an undercurrent of conflict or hostility. On the other hand, one might take the criterion of illness to be the point at which a person seeks help from his doctor, his spiritual adviser, or even from the neighbour over the side fence. People differ however, in their help-seeking thresholds, so such a criterion is indeed a fluid one on which to make the assumption that a person is 'sick' or not. There are those who, in spite of marked neurotic mechanisms, will never see themselves as being abnormal in any way. Take, for example, the professional man involved in numerous club and service organisations, his time so taken up that his family suffers, deprived of his presence in the home. He may, indeed, be fleeing into such activities in order to cope with some feelings of inadequacy or other conflict within himself, yet he would hardly see himself as emotionally maladapted. Unless gambling or alcoholism, used in a vain attempt to obviate inner tensions or conflict, leads to gross financial or physical hardship, most compulsive gamblers or alcoholics would not regard themselves as poorly adapted.

We shall leave unanswered the question of when a neurotic disturbance should be classed as an illness, but the example of the compulsive gambler and drinker lead us to think of fairly widely-used concepts, namely, character neuroses and symptom neuroses.

A *symptom neurosis* is one in which the outstanding feature is a particular psychiatric symptom or group of symptoms, usually commencing at some point in time, and perhaps running a fluctuating course in response to stress situations which trigger off anxiety. These patients are handicapped in more or less specific ways. They may for example, have difficulty in travelling, have to wash their hands compulsively, develop bodily symptoms on the basis of the mechanism of conversion, experience free-floating anxiety (page 215), or they may experience more than one of these symptoms at the same time.

Taking a dynamic viewpoint, symptoms develop as a means of lessening the effects of inner conflict or anxiety, and the patient is able to function reasonably adequately in areas not directly related to his neurotic conflict which, at least in our culture, is usually related mainly to sexuality, aggression, or dependency needs.

In *character neurosis*, the individual lacks specific symptoms such as those mentioned above, but his whole character or life-style is abnormal to a greater or lesser degree. Some people are able to live with their characterological defects, recognised or unrecognised by themselves, without them becoming obvious to others, while in others there is an obvious disturbance of behaviour patterns. Such patterns of behaviour appear to have no clear point of onset and, frequently from a very early age, neurotic behaviour, that is, immature and highly defensive behaviour, has been in evidence. Some authorities subsume personality disorders, sexual deviation, alcoholism and drug dependence under the heading of character neuroses, but the I.C.D. appears to limit the term character neurosis to personality disorder.

An individual may frequently show features of both character neurosis and symptom neurosis, with one or other predominating at a point in time, for example, or the asthenic personality who develops various phobias. This is an instance of a symptom neurosis engrafted on to a long-standing character neurosis.

Patients with symptom neurosis are more likely to seek treatment than individuals with character neurosis, who tend to accept their life style, or don't even recognise in themselves any deviation from a 'normal pattern of living'.

In this chapter we shall deal with symptom neuroses only, leaving the disorders subsumed under the heading of 'character neuroses' to individual attention in a subsequent chapter.

It is well to note that the neuroses, as listed in most classifications, including the *Ninth Revision of the International Classification of Diseases*, are 'symptom neuroses' in the sense that this terminology has been used above. Before dealing with each neurotic disorder separately, brief comment will be made on aetiological factors and the overall incidence of neurosis.

Aetiology

Experiences and relationships in infancy and childhood (fundamentally the parent-child relationship) constitute the major predisposing factors in the later development of the neuroses. Conflicts arising within the personality in the realms of dependency, sexuality and aggression are important in this respect, and clinically the most important source of anxiety, at least with respect to sexuality and aggression, is guilt. These conflicts are dealt with in Chapter 10. Mention has been made earlier of the effects of maternal deprivation. Later stress factors such as are mentioned in Chapter 10, Fig. 4, including critical periods of normal life, marriage and parenthood, pregnancy, occupation, combat, bereavement and migration, serve to kindle or trigger off old unconscious conflicts, leading to anxiety which is dealt with by ego defence mechanisms, giving rise to the variety of clinical pictures termed the neuroses.

It must be most rare, if it ever occurs at all, for a single stress or disturbing incident to cause a neurotic illness. People generally are prone to lay the blame for their maladjustment on to a single cause, perhaps because of a need to blame something, or at least to satisfy an innate demand for an explanation of their state. Single events or particular stresses are merely precipitating factors, the stage having already been set for the development of a neurotic illness.

Sociocultural factors are important in the aetiology of the neuroses. Nowadays in western cultures, where close family ties have become somewhat attenuated, there is less emotional support available to the individual. This is added to by stresses arising out of the complexity of modern living. A relatively higher level of neurosis is noted in the higher social levels, attributed to ambivalence and status strivings present in the family environment of many middle-class families. One may see overt overprotection and smothering, behind which lurks feelings of hostility and rejection. The mother may be very authoritarian, and being the single focus of both authority and affection, the child finds it impossible to express rebellion in case it loses her affection. Acceptance and approval are contingent on conformity and submission, but at the same time, the child has pressures on him to be an independent individual.

Hereditary factors are stated by many to have very little place in the development of neurotic disorders. Even if one assumes however, that the fundamental aetiological factors lie at the feet of disturbed parent-child relationships, one still has to examine the determinants of such relationships. Looking at the infant alone, it would appear that there is strong evidence to support the contention that the infant's emergency emotions of fear and rage are genetically determined. A mother's frustration of the child's need for love, food, warmth and exploration which produces fear and/or rage, the degree of which is largely genetically determined, will to some extent determine the mother's reaction to the child's expressed frustration, in the direction of care or rejection. This is an example of the interwining of hereditary and environmental factors in the mother-child system.

To explain the development of different neurotic clinical syndromes dynamically, solely on the basis of inner conflict or anxiety from any cause would appear to be rather far-fetched. For example, why does one person suffer from compulsive phenomena, another from hysteria, another from phobias? Perhaps hereditary factors could account for these particular neurotic manifestations arising out of anxiety, which is the common factor. Mayer-Gross, Slater and Roth, after looking at available evidence, do in fact state, 'clinical classifications have some relationship to real genetic differences. . .'.

A theory that merits some attention arises out of the work of Pavlov and other learning theorists (see page 324). Socially acceptable or unacceptable modes of behaviour, and control of emotion or lack of it, may indeed be based on conditioning. The child learns habitual modes of response to a stimulus or group of stimuli presented in a recurrent fashion by parents, and these responses continue into adult life. Conditioning however, could never provide more than a part answer to the development of some clinical forms of neurosis.

Incidence

From earlier statements made in this chapter on the lack of definition as to when neurotic manifestations so common in society constitute an illness, it is impossible to give a precise figure for the incidence of these disorders. Figures are obtainable of numbers of patients in psychiatric and general hospitals, and of numbers attending outpatient clinics, but a very large number are treated privately by psychiatrists or general practitioners and these figures are difficult to obtain. It is probably reasonable to say, however, that the neuroses constitute the major proportion of psychiatric disorders. Among inpatients in a psychiatric hospital however, the nurse will see few examples of clear-cut neurotic syndromes. For example, at one of Sydney's admission centres, only 1 in 60 patients admitted in a six-month period was diagnosed as suffering from a neurotic disorder other than depressive neurosis, and there may have been a multiplicity of factors apart from the disorder itself which led to admission.

We shall now look at the clinical varieties of neurotic illness, or neurosis. One will find in practice that cases frequently do not fit into precise categories as delineated, there being an overlapping of symptomatology, governed largely by the defence mechanisms operating, and cases are diagnosed in terms of the most prominent clinical symptoms.

Anxiety states

These are described as

> various combinations of physical and mental manifestations of anxiety, not attributable to real danger and occurring either in attacks or as a persisting state. The anxiety is usually diffuse and may extend to panic. Other neurotic features such as obsessional or hysterical symptoms may be present but do not dominate the clinical picture.

Synonyms for these states include: anxiety neurosis, anxiety reaction, anxiety state (neurotic) or panic attack, panic disorder or panic state.

The illness may have an acute onset and be severe in intensity, appearing against a relatively normal background, or it may be of a chronic nature present since adolescence in mild degree, but fluctuating in severity according to current stress factors.

The anxiety is described as diffuse, or free-floating, not being attached to any object or situation such as occurs in the phobic state (page 222). It is as if no specific ego defence mechanisms control the anxiety as they do in other neurotic disorders.

The patient has a feeling of inner tension and anxious expectation, and there are usually bodily or somatic symptoms present as well, e.g. palpitations, pallor, sweating, goose flesh, dry mouth, anorexia, indigestion, diarrheoa, wide pupils, frequency of micturition etc. These somatic symptoms associated with anxiety are mediated through the autonomic nervous system and may involve one or all bodily systems. The anorexia which occurs may give rise to a loss in weight.

Emotional and physical preoccupation may lead to difficulty in concentration. There may be difficulty in getting off to sleep, which may be disturbed by anxious dreams or nightmares. Not infrequently the patient with anxiety neurosis expresses fears of insanity. Headache, sometimes described as 'a tight band around the head' or a 'queer sensation in the head', is present in many instances, and some patients have a terrifying feeling of impending death.

Overbreathing may occur in an acute anxiety state, and not uncommonly, in young women about the time of their menstrual periods. The rapid shallow breathing blows off carbon dioxide producing a state of relative alkalinity in the body. This leads to *tetany*, in which tingling in the extremities, dizziness, and muscle spasms involving the face, limbs, respiratory and abdominal musculature occur. Such muscle spasms may be excruciatingly painful. A simple remedy for this state of affairs is to get the person so affected to rebreathe into a paper bag, thus building up the carbon dioxide and hence carbonic acid in the blood, reversing the state of alkalinity.

One should repeat a warning given earlier of wrongly diagnosing a psychotic depressive illness as an anxiety neurosis in middle-aged agitated persons. Suicide is a real danger in the former, and one should look for the symptoms of such a psychotic depression.

Traumatic neurosis is the term applied to an anxiety neurosis that develops following what the patient sees as a serious threat to his life. Such trauma may range from serious accidents and combat stress to near misses or minor injuries, particularly to the head. Such patients, as well as having the clinical manifestations of an anxiety state already described, frequently experience terrifying dreams in which they relive the traumatic situation. They may develop conversion symptoms which are functional symptoms added to any physical disability that may be present. The condition then presents the hallmarks of hysteria, and if compensation is involved, it is graced with the appellation 'compensation neurosis' (Page 221).

Management

Most sufferers from anxiety neurosis do not require hospitalisation and are treated on an outpatient basis or in the consulting room. Treatment may be divided into measures aimed primarily at the relief of anxiety or symptomatic treatment, and measures whose goal is to change aspects of the patient's personality, referred to as 'causal treatment'.

Symptomatic treatment includes such measures as giving a minor tranquilliser, e.g. chlordiazepoxide, diazepam. In addition, physiotherapy and occupational therapy may be of value.

Of the measures aimed at modifying aspects of the patient's personality, one of the forms of insight psychotherapy is probably the treatment of choice. What might be termed more superficial psychotherapy has its place, the prime objectives being the development of 'insight into the more conscious conflicts with deliberate efforts at readjustment, goal modification, and the living up to existing creative potentialities' (Wolberg).

In some patients, it may be as well not to try to uncover serious conflicts as this may lead to a heightened state of anxiety. A more recent development is the use of cognitive therapy which involves, among other things, the correction of erroneous beliefs and faulty conceptions leading to the allaying of inappropriate emotional reactions.

Hysteria

The I.C.D. description will first be quoted, then embellished below:

> Mental disorders in which motives, of which the patient seems unaware, produce either a restriction of the field of consciousness or disturbances of motor or sensory function which may seem to have psychological advantage or symbolic value. It may be characterized by conversion phenomena or dissociative phenomena. In the conversion form the chief or only symptoms consist of psychogenic disturbance of function in some part of the body, e.g. paralysis, tremor, blindness, deafness, seizures. In the dissociative variety, the most prominent feature is a narrowing of the field of consciousness which seems to serve an unconscious purpose and is commonly accompanied or followed by a selective amnesia. There may be dramatic but essentially superficial changes of personality sometimes taking the form of a fugue (wandering state). Behaviour may mimic psychosis or, rather, the patient's idea of psychosis.

Aetiology

The word 'hysteria' means 'wandering of the uterus' and was used by the Greeks in the time of Pericles who recognised the relationship of the disorder to sexual disturbance. Various theories as to its causation have existed over the ages depending on the current views held about mental disorders at these times. During the Middle Ages, it was regarded as being due to possession by the Devil, and in the nineteenth century was commonly considered to be an organic disease.

Charcot challenged the organic theory and showed that emotional disturbance provoked the manifestations of the disease, and demonstrated the removal of such manifestations under hypnosis. Janet, who was a pupil of Charcot came to the conclusion that in hysteria one series of ideas becomes isolated from the general stream of consciousness in a process of dissociation, and he defined the condition as 'a malady of personal synthesis' which he attributed to an 'hereditary degeneration of the nervous system'.

Breuer and Freud (1893-5) presented evidence for their view that repression of ideas of a sexual nature disturbing to conscious awareness, was of major importance in the development of hysteria. They awakened emotionally charged memories often dating back to childhood, and encouraged patients to discuss the emotionally exciting situations giving verbal expression to the affect or emotion. The method of talking about emotionally charged, previously forgotten events was called 'mental catharsis', and the process of affording an outlet of the accompanying emotion through talking was called 'abreaction'. As this method of treatment helped some patients, it was concluded by Breuer and Freud that repression of memories traumatic to the psyche was the major causal factor in the development of hysteria. These two workers also showed that individual hysterical symptoms could be removed under hypnosis. Hypnosis was used initially as a method of lessening, or attempting to lessen, the patient's resistance to bringing such memories back into conscious awareness. Freud later gave up this practice and used his technique of 'free association' instead.

One theory on the development of hysteria is based on Freudian concepts. It is held that there occurs a fixation in early psychosexual development at the phallic or early genital phase, when the oedipal complex is present, with a failure to relinquish the incestuous tie to the loved parent. In the adult patient, conflict over the sexual drive (libido) exists as it retains its forbidden incestuous quality. The ego defence mechanism of repression, by relegating the sexual drive and associated conflict into the unconscious, reduces guilt. The energy from the repressed sexual drive is said to be converted into a physical symptom by the ego defence mechanism of conversion, which not only protects the patient from a conscious awareness of the drive, but also provides a symbolic representation of it, e.g. a daughter developing the symptoms of mother's last illness.

The precipitating cause of hysteria is usually an emotionally charged situation which the patient cannot face, and which presumably triggers off the old conflicts related to the oedipal stage. These conflicts, and sometimes the emotionally charged situation which activates oedipal conflict as well, become excluded from consciousness to be replaced by physical symptoms. Consequently there is little or no evidence of anxiety as such. This reduction in mental discomfort arising out of the formation of physical symptoms is known as the 'primary gain' of the illness. Once the symptom has developed, it in itself may bring certain advantages to the patient in terms of additional attention, compensation, removal from a difficult situation, and so forth. Such factors appear to maintain the presence of the developed symptom, and these secondary advantages constitute what is termed 'secondary gain'. Secondary gain may be a feature in any illness, and the term need not be restricted solely to hysteria.

The above comments make reference only to the formation of physical symptoms, and describe the development of what in an earlier classification was regarded as 'conversion reaction'. This same classification spoke of a 'dissociative reaction' in which mental dissociation, as distinct from the conversion of anxiety into bodily symptoms which themselves are then virtually ignored or dissociated from the patient's consciousness, is the major clinical feature. In our present classification, the results of conversion of anxiety into bodily symptoms and the outcome of mental dissociation fall into the one diagnostic category, hysteria, and are believed to be the result of similar aetiological factors.

The hysterical personality is one which uses attention-seeking behaviour and which overacts in a histrionic fashion. Further details of such a personality will be given later (page 235), but at this point it should be stressed that the pre-morbid personality of the person who develops hysteria is not necessarily hysterical, neither do all hysterical personalities develop hysteria.

Clinical Manifestations

In recent decades, there has been a decreased incidence of classical hysteria in urban western society, particularly of hysterical convulsions, blindness and severe paralyses. Such disorders are still stated to be common among the unsophisticated. Hysteria is manifest in many different forms, some of which may readily be confused with organic diseases. Indeed it has been stated that hysteria is one of the great imitators in medicine. This is a point in favour of making a positive diagnosis, rather than diagnosing hysteria by exclusion of all physical illnesses likely to lead to particular symptomatology. In brief, the clinical features in hysteria are:

1. A group of physical symptoms occurring in the absence of an organic lesion, or the presence of mental dissociation.
2. Complacency in the presence of gross objective disability (la belle indifference, described by Janet).

NOTE: In *chronic* hysterical conversion, anxiety may be pronounced.

We shall now study hysterical convulsions, paralysis, involuntary movements, sensory disturbances, affective disturbances, and dissociative phenomena in more detail.

CONVULSIONS

Hysterical convulsions may simulate the generalised convulsions occurring in epilepsy. The following are pointers to a possible hysterical basis rather than an organic one:

(a) Patient is not completely unconscious.

(b) Attacks occur in the presence of onlookers.
(c) Patient does not fall in a dangerous situation.
(d) Corneal, pupillary, and deep reflexes, are present.
(e) Patient does not bite his tongue nor micturate.
(f) Face becomes red rather than blue or white.
(g) Attempts to open the eyes are resisted.
(h) Pressure on the supra orbital notch causes withdrawal of the head.

PARALYSIS AND INVOLUNTARY MOVEMENTS

In some cases paralysis is more or less complete. There may also occur monoplegia (one limb), hemiplegia (essentially upper and lower limbs on one side), paraplegia (both lower extremities). Sometimes the paralysis is associated with tremors of the affected limbs. If the condition is long-standing, muscular contractures may develop.

Other symptoms in this group include astasia-abasia in which leg movements may be carried out when lying or sitting down, though standing and walking are impossible, bizarre gait, tics (habit spasms) and muscular spasms alone or with paresis, disturbances of speech amounting to aphonia, choreiform movements in children, spasmodic torticollis (twisting of the neck), and occupational cramp (e.g. writer's cramp).

SENSORY DISTURBANCES

Pain may occur anywhere. Some patients may experience pain in the top of the head as if a nail is being driven into the skull (clavus). Severe pain and hyperaesthesia of the scalp may be localised in the temporal or parietal regions.

Diminution in sensation is common, sometimes amounting to complete anaesthesia. The anaesthesias do not follow typical neural distributions, but involve, for example, a limb, or frequently the distal part of it in the fashion of a glove or stocking. In fact the name glove and stocking anaesthesia is used in such cases. Such anaesthesia may also be sharply limited by the midline to one half of the body.

The special senses may also be involved, giving rise to blindness, deafness and loss of smell (anosmia). The blindness may involve one eye only. Certain other sensory disturbances occur which have been designated as the hysterical stigmata. These may also arise from, or be accentuated by, iatrogenic suggestion, and include localised reduction in cutaneous sensation, pharyngeal anaesthesia, hyperaesthetic spots over the ovaries, absence of reflex closure of the eye on touching the cornea, concentric contraction of the field of vision (tubular vision), and the feeling of a lump in the throat (globus hystericus) which may be associated with difficulty in swallowing, a motor phenomenon.

AFFECTIVE DISTURBANCE

A normal person afflicted with such symptoms as are mentioned above would be expected to show some degree of perturbation. In hysteria however, the patient seems able to dissociate from what to the observer are gross abnormalities, and retains a detached calm (la belle indifference).

DISSOCIATIVE PHENOMENA

Dissociative phenomena represent a personality disorganisation, manifest by the following: aimless running or 'freezing', stupor, depersonalization and derealization, amnesia which is circumscribed, a fugue state, somnambulism (sleep walking), and the rare states of multiple personality, for example, Stephenson's literary fictional model of Dr Jekyll and Mr Hyde.

A patient was admitted to a London psychiatric hospital having been discovered in a Scottish loch. He was a transport driver who, for some time, had been faced with problems in the domestic situation which he could not resolve. One morning he set out from Southend to London, and completed his journey in Scotland, with complete amnesia for the intervening three days, during which time he was obviously able to wash, dress and shave himself, something that does not occur in complete amnesia from an organic cause. This was a circumscribed amnesia which gradually cleared in hospital, and eventually all details, including the stress factors which precipitated the fugue state, were remembered.

Another patient in her thirties named Ivy, who, under extra stress at the time of the anniversary of her father's death, developed a dissociative state and presented as a stammering, snivelling little girl, suddenly becoming Kathryn who was the epitome of her domineering mother named Catherine. As Kathryn, Ivy did not stammer, but stood up, became aggressive in manner, and motioning to the now empty chair, referred to 'that snivelling stammering Ivy'. This move from one personality to another lasted some weeks and recurred under stress 1-2 years later. After six years, having been seen every 1-3 months in the interim, Ivy commented that she felt she was developing into a more mature and realistic person namely Lorraine, which is her middle name. Feeling like Lorraine, she also did not stammer, an affliction that had commenced and been present since the age of 2-3 years. For the next ten years Ivy coped with a variety of stressful life events without further dissociative phenomena.

GANSER'S SYNDROME

Sometimes known as pseudo dementia, this is an hysterical disorder in which the patient talks past the point (paralogy). He gives approximate answers, for example 2 plus 2 equals 5, or when shown an object and asked to name it, gives an incorrect answer which is close enough to indicate that he really knows what the object is, but is giving the incorrect answer 'deliberately'.

So much for the clinical manifestations of hysteria. It should be pointed out again that a patient suffering from a neurotic illness does not necessarily show a pure text-book picture, and mixtures of neurotic manifestations may be present. A male patient in his early twenties, who was a compositor in a printing business, lost 'half touch' sensation on the tips of his fingers, this being part of an hysterical mechanism. As well as this he concurrently suffered a severe phobic neurosis, feeling he was going to fall down or go mad walking along a footpath whenever he neared the half way point between two intersections.

Management

Management will depend to a large extent on the circumstances surrounding the hysterical manifestation.

In general, early treatment is indicated before the added effects of multiple secondary gains increase the patient's difficulty in relinquishing the symptom. This was found to be particularly important when fear-provoking situations produced paralysis in soldiers in World War II. In such cases of recent onset, abreaction or narcoanalysis using I.V. thiopentone or I.V. sodium amylobarbitone enables the sufferer to relive the fear-producing episode which triggered off the anxiety, and the cathartic effect of this procedure hastens recovery. Methylphenidate (Ritalin) I.V. may be given initially and followed via the same needle by one of the barbiturates mentioned.

In many instances of conversion reactions following a severely stressful precipitating situation, simple supportive methods of psychotherapy often suffice for recovery.

Hypnosis, both as a means of uncovering areas of conflict, and as a means of suggestion, is used in suitable patients. The therapist, in using suggestion to remove a somatic conversion symptom, would, of course, be aware of the possibility that with the protection afforded by conversion symptoms removed, the patient may have his facade of indifference shattered and become depressed, anxious, confused, or may feel he is the subject of victimisation if there are paranoid traits in his personality.

Some authorities claim that conversion reactions are best treated by psychoanalysis. Such factors as advanced age, exceptionally great secondary gain, and a low level of intelligence would be definite contra-indications to this approach.

Compensation neurosis

Compensation neurosis is included as a manifestation of hysteria, and poses problems created by secondary gains, particularly when monetary settlement is protracted. This is indeed a factor, but money comprises only one aspect of secondary gain.

Let us assume that a man has suffered an injury at work, with resultant physical symptoms. He is seen by doctors and lawyers, and receives the sympathy of relatives and friends, and numerous tests may be undertaken. If this attention satisfies dependency needs, such a person could hardly wish for the situation to alter too abruptly, and in fact he may engage in the practice of malingering, particularly if he thinks prolongation of illness time will mean a judgement in his favour for greater monetary compensation. In some instances, the injury triggers off conflict or anxiety, and through the unconscious mechanism of conversion, symptoms become superadded to the initial physical ones. If this occurs, then we are dealing with a compensation neurosis, and all the factors satisfying dependency needs, including the prospect of monetary settlement, become secondary gain.

In any given case, there is probably a mixture of truly hysterical unconscious physical symptomatology and secondary gain factors, the latter being at least partly conscious, and either of these elements will serve to prolong the incapacity.

There are some writers who tend towards the belief that compensation neurosis (and the type of anxiety neurosis termed traumatic neurosis) is not an unconsciously motivated clinical entity, but that the injured person is malingering. It will frequently be found that such writers have never been able to grasp the concept of the unconscious and of unconscious motivation.

It is difficult at times to distinguish malingering from hysteria. As a guideline, malingerers generally show more inconsistencies in their histories as they are repeated to different people, and the patient consciously simulating physical disease often deliberately produces physical signs, which is a rare pattern of behaviour in hysterical patients.

Phobic state

These are

> neurotic states with abnormally intense dread of certain objects or specific situations which would not normally have that effect. If the anxiety tends to spread from a specified situation or object to a wider range of circumstances, it becomes akin to or identical with anxiety state, and should be classified as such.

Unlike the picture in an anxiety state, in which anxiety and the resultant emotion of fear are said to be free-floating, in phobic states fear becomes attached to specific objects or situations. These objects or situations are known by the patient not to be a source of real danger, and the patient is fully aware of the irrationality of his fear. The term 'phobia' is given to such an irrational fear, and though having insight into the irrationality of his behaviour the patient feels compelled to avoid those objects or situations which expose him to overpowering anxiety. In other words, he attempts to control his anxiety by avoiding the phobic object or situation. the concomitant physiological symptoms present in an anxiety state such as palpitations, pallor, sweating, etc. may likewise accompany an acute phobic state.

The phobias may be broadly grouped into those relating to objects such as animals, insects, dirt, syphilis, etc., and those relating to situations, for example, open spaces (agraphobia), closed spaces (claustrophobia), stage fright, fear of blushing in public (erythrophobia), heights (acrophobia), etc.

A practical classification described by Freud is:

1. Common phobias—an exaggerated fear of all those things that most people detest or fear to some extent, e.g. night, solitude, death, illness, snakes, etc.
2. Specific phobias—the fear of special circumstances that inspire no fear in the normal man, e.g. agraphobia and the other phobias of locomotion (travel phobias).

It seems that any object may become the object of a phobia, and a patient, having lost one phobia, may readily develop another.

A policeman in his twenties finally sought treatment when the delivering of a notice to a first floor apartment became an unbearable ordeal. He had a long history of phobias, developing while he was working on an oil tanker after a crew member fell from a mast. He found that climbing to heights, or down into the tanks to clean them, became paralysing experiences. Driving on autobahns in Germany next terrified him. It became necessary to speed across English bridges lest something happen to him there. Possessing a powerful motor cycle, he found the distance he could travel from his home becoming more and more limited, and a state of acute panic developed the further he travelled from home. It is an interesting sidelight that following his marriage, and knowing that heights terrified him, he chose to honeymoon near the edge of a virtual cliff, spent the first night in a state of panic, then moved elsewhere.

Another patient developed a phobia towards razor blades. This ceased, to be replaced by a phobia of travel on the tube railway, though buses were no real problem.

Aetiology

Freud's classical case of 'Little Hans' is mentioned earlier and it has been pointed out that aggression and dependency as well as sexuality may be involved in the development of a phobic state (page 98). Various mental defence mechanisms may be involved in the development of a phobic state, namely, repression, displacement, projection, identification and regression.

Dollard and Miller describe phobias as learned responses to painful experiences. They are common in children, and the following are suggested as causal dynamic factors: the little boy's castration fear (and in girls may be found a corresponding factor in phantasies of previous injury to the genitals), symbolic threat of sexual attack in girls, and in boys with passive homosexual tendencies.

Separation anxiety is also important in the pathogenesis of phobias, and this is especially so in the development of 'school phobia' where the necessary circumstances are stated to include:

1. A history of a poorly resolved dependency relationship between a child and its mother.
2. An acute anxiety in the child produced either by organic disease or some external situation, and,
3. A recent frustration or threat suffered by the mother, increasing her need to exploit the child's dependency needs, with the result that separation from mother when going to school becomes a traumatic experience.

It goes without saying that in investigating any particular case of 'school phobia', one must explore possible factors that could be operating at the time the child wakes up, en route to school, upon arrival at school, and in the classroom.

Management

Most can be treated on an outpatient basis but some patients become so restricted in their activities that inpatient treatment in a neurosis unit becomes necessary.

The most practical and probably most successful treatment is a form of behaviour therapy combined with the use of anxiolytic (anxiety reducing) drugs such as the minor tranquillisers. The patient is given an anxiolytic drug and encouraged to face the phobic situation or object through small but gradually increasing exposures.

It is necessary for a relative, a member of the therapeutic team, or the therapist to accompany the patient, giving encouragement and support. As the patient with the help of drugs, is able to faced phobic situations without accompanying anxiety and physiological symptoms, these symptoms cease to be associated with the previously feared situations. He is ultimately able to face such situations or objects on his own with the help of drugs, and finally, after gradual reduction of anxiolytics, without this pharmacological prop.

This type of management is particularly useful in phobias associated with travel, patients being able to effectively increase their radius of mobility.

It is important to remember however, that we should not simply try to treat a symptom in some mechanical fashion, for we are dealing with a person who probably has a number of 'hangups' or areas of conflict. Psychotherapeutic measures should be employed as well, with the object of helping total personality development, for the phobic symptomatology may indeed be the end result of a complex of unresolved conflicts in areas of sexuality, aggression and dependence.

Obsessive-compulsive disorders

The I.C.D. defines them as

> states in which the outstanding symptom is a feeling of subjective compulsion—which must be resisted—to carry out some action, to dwell on an idea, to recall an experience, or to ruminate on an abstract topic. Unwanted thoughts which intrude, the insistency of words or ideas, ruminations or trains of thought are perceived by the patient to be inappropriate or nonsensical. The obsessional urge or idea is recognized as alien to the personality but as coming from within the self. Obsessional actions may be quasiritual performances designed to relieve anxiety e.g. washing the hands to cope with contamination. Attempts to dispel the unwelcome thoughts or urges may lead to a severe inner struggle, with intense anxiety.

These disorders include anankastic neurosis and compulsive neurosis.

General note on obsessive-compulsive symptoms

Obsessive-compulsive symptoms can be found in normal people. If we recall our own childhood acquaintances, and perhaps our own actions, we may remember such activities as not stepping on cracks in the foot-path, or tapping every third paling on the fence. The superstitions of adults probably have a similar compulsive basis, for example, throwing a pinch of salt over the left shoulder if salt is split at table, making payment of a coin if one is given a cutting implement as a gift, etc.

Another common symptom in normal adults is the simple persistence of some thought or tune in the mind. Such episodes are more common when fatigued, and in hypnagogic states (between a state of wakefulness and sleep).

How many of us, when tired during a lecture, have compulsively estimated when the second hand of the clock on the wall will have traversed each 10 seconds?

Obsessive-compulsive symptoms may be unmasked by a depressive illness or they may precede or become interwoven in the symptoms of a schizophrenic illness. In this context, if the patient with obsessive-compulsive symptomatology appreciates the irrationality of his symptoms and tries to resist them, however unavailingly, he is most likely suffering from obsessive-compulsive neurosis. If he passively complies with them or feels they come from outside himself, the chances are he is suffering from a schizophrenic illness. Obsessive-compulsive symptoms are seen also in association with organic brain disorders, and particularly after encephalitis lethargica.

Most commonly, obsessive-compulsive symptoms are the major symptoms of an independent illness, namely obsessive-compulsive neurosis, which occurs in predisposed people. The term obsession is used in relation to thoughts, while a compulsion usually refers to an act.

Aetiology

There is strong evidence to suggest that hereditary factors play a large role. The age of onset is roughly the same in both sexes, approximately one third of patients showing symptoms by the age of 15 years. After twenty, the risk of developing obsessive-compulsive disorder decreases with increasing age, and it is rare for it to develop after the age of 40 years. Patients tend to be more gifted, energetic and intelligent than average, and this may account in part for its increasing prevalence as one proceeds up the social scale. The pre-morbid personality of most, but not all patients, who develop this form of neurosis is described as anankastic (page 235). (The commonest form of severe psychiatric disorder suffered by anankastic personalities is a psychotic depressive illness.) Personality factors in such people include rigidity, inflexibility, lack of adaptability, conscientiousness, love of order and discipline, persistence and endurance in the face of obstacles, dependability, reliability, puctuality, precision, scrupulousness in matters of morals, and the capacity for self-effacement. Underlying the prim and correct demeanour of these people, there is often found a crude, turbulent sexualism which is occasionally expressed in perversions. The surface traits may be regarded as an over-compensation for feelings of internal insecurity, and the anankastic personality is never completely free from tension and irritability.

Stresses of various kinds, for example, promotion involving extra responsibility and authority, or changing circumstances, lead to symptoms which reflect a weakness in the personality structure.

Obsessional ideas and fears arise out of the sense of insecurity engendered, and compulsive actions are said to represent expiation for feelings of failure and inadequacy.

In psychoanalytical theory, the anankastic personality is regarded as a person with an overdeveloped and savagely critical super-ego, this being associated with anal-erotic tendencies and a sadistic quality of personality.

Clinical picture

Three categories of symptoms are usually described:

1. Spells of doubting and brooding, in which the patient swings backwards and forwards between the same set of pros and cons without being able to reach a decision and act upon it. Doubts may invade a belief, a proposition, an observation, or a recollection. The patient has to check to make sure gas is off, lights are turned off, etc. This checking may be repeated many times. One female patient in her late twenties took 1-1½ hours to leave the office each evening after work having to repeatedly check whether some papers had fallen from the desk into the wastepaper basket. The term *folie de doute* (the 'doubting madness') is applied to this category of symptoms.

2. Bouts of ritual making, in which the patient executes a series of motor acts. This includes such things as hand washing, washing or cleaning wearing apparel, touching some objects and avoiding others, and the compulsion to count, for example, the number of parked cars, or the carrying out of various mathematical gymnastics with car registration numbers. Rituals may become complicated. One female patient in her early thirties found morning and afternoon teas quite lengthy procedures. To eat a biscuit she would break off a piece, then take a small portion of this piece, placing it on the edge of her plate, before committing the remainder of the piece to her mouth. By the time she had finished her tea break there would be what was apparently a defensive perimeter of small pieces of biscuit around the edge of her plate.

3. 'Fits of horrific temptation' in which the patient is suddenly beset by the idea or urge to kill someone (characteristically, a close or beloved relative). He recoils in horror from a temptation so alien to his entire being, and locks up knives and other possible weapons. The temptation being against the patient's will, is resisted, and it is doubtful whether any such morbid idea has ever been translated into action by a patient suffering from obsessive-compulsive disorder.

One must keep in mind, however, the fact that folk experiencing obsessional fears of or having obsessional impuses to harm someone may not be suffering from obsessive-compulsive disorder, but from a psychotic depressive illness for example. Depressed women, particularly in the puerperium, may express the fear of harming their children. Such fears are not infrequently translated into action, and separation of the mother from her children at this stage, probably by hospitalisation, is mandatory unless other water-tight precautions can be taken to protect the children. If the basic illness is schizophrenia with obsessive-compulsive symptoms such a tragedy may indeed occur. Where tension and anxiety rising to panic, associated with fits of horrific temptation are sustained, there is the possibility that the patient may suicide.

It must be stressed again that the clinical picture of obsessive-compulsive disorder may not necessarily appear in its pure form, but may be associated with other neurotic symptomatology, a not uncommon presentation being to have phobic symptoms also present in the patient suffering essentially from an obsessive-compulsive disorder.

Prognosis

The illness runs a fluctuating course with a general tendency to recovery. Sometimes the illness suddenly improves for no obvious reason.

Management

There is some evidence to suggest that in certain patients psychotherapy of an analytical type has an advantage over simple supportive management and other forms of psychotherapy in this illness. Avoidance of situations which appear to aggravate the obsessional tendency, and advice concerning sublimatory activities may be all that is required in some instances. Behaviour therapy techniques aimed specifically at symptom control have their advocates. Tranquillising drugs have a place in symptomatic treatment, and where there is an affective component in the illness, tricyclic antidepressants may prove useful. In severe intractable cases where great 'inner tension' is experienced by the patient, leucotomy may be beneficial.

Neurotic depression

This is

> A neurotic disorder characterized by disproportionate depression which has usually recognizably ensued on a distressing experience; it does not inlcude among its features delusions or hallucinations, and there is often preoccupation with the psychic trauma which preceded the illness, e.g. loss of a cherished person or possession. Anxiety is also frequently present and mixed states of anxiety and depression should be included here. The distinction between depressive neurosis and psychosis should be made not only upon the degree of depression but also on the presence or absence of other neurotic and psychotic characteristics and upon the degree of disturbance of the patient's behaviour.

The terms anxiety depression, depressive reaction, neurotic depressive state and reactive depression are also applied to this disorder.

In neurotic depression, the anxiety is allayed or partly relieved by depression and self-depreciation. The precipitating factor is some loss sustained by the patient, and is often associated with a feeling of guilt for past failures or deeds. It is perfectly normal to experience depression following stress involving loss such as bereavement. Depression becomes pathological when it is more marked and prolonged than is usual, and when the patient cannot overcome it by his own efforts.

Some authorities see depression in a neurotic depression, as a combination of sadness and pessimism. It is the patient's conscious or unconscious idea that what has happened to him now will always continue happening, or that the condition in which he finds himself now will never change. In many cases it would seem that such patients have been sensitised to the precipitating traumatic event by previous losses or insecurities, and by stressful situations occuring in childhood. The current situation of loss or disappointment, seen by the patient as loss of love, mobilises the old anxieties, and the patient's anxiety is reduced by the development of depression. The student should revise the section on the origin of depression in Chapter 8.

Clinical picture

The depression experienced by patients may range in degree from mild to severe, and in the more severe cases suicide is a distinct possibility, although the attempt may have a somewhat attention-seeking quality. Commonly, the mood may be lightened by a cheerful environment. Depression is usually felt to be worse in the later stages of the day and evening. Patients may cry, and if left to their own devices, show disinterest in things about them. Sleep is disturbed, and the usual pattern is difficulty in getting off to sleep. Appetite is frequently poor, though not so marked as in a psychotic depressive illness. Resultant weight loss is also usually less than in a psychotic depressive illness. Activity is limited, resulting more from disinterest than showing the hallmarks of the retardation experienced by the patient with psychotic depression.

The differences between the clinical pictures seen in psychotic depression and neurotic depression are summarised as follows:

Psychotic depression	*Neurotic depression*
1. Environmental changes have little or no effect on depression	Mood may lift in cheerful company
2. Sleep disturbance always severe. Early morning waking characteristic (delayed insomnia)	Sleep disturbances may or may not be present, if so there is difficulty getting off to sleep (initial insomnia)
3. Retardation of thought and action is common	No retardation in physiological sense, but may complain of fatigue
4. Speech slowed as part of process of retardation	Usually talkative, keen to discuss symptoms, and frequently complains a lot
5. Physical symptoms are marked. They include anorexia, weight loss, impotence, amenorrhoea and commonly constipation	Anorexia and weight loss less marked, and may even be absent. Impotence, amenorrhoea and constipation are not associated physiological symptoms
6. Delusions are commonly present	Delusions never present
7. Patient tends to blame himself for his state	Patient usually blames others or his environment for his state

Insight into the fact of illness is not a valid differential point. Both categories of patient are usually aware, and psychotic depressives painfully so, of the fact that all is not well with them. Comment might be made on 'anaclytic depression' described by Spitz. This condition occurs in young children, and is stated to result from severe emotional neglect. Clinical features include, loss of appetite (hence failure to gain in weight), apathy, lowering of mood level, frequent stools, and general progressive marasmus that may end in death.

Management

The management of neurotic depression may be summarised briefly as follows:

1. Hospitalisation is usually unnecessary but may be indicated in severe cases where suicide is a possibility and little or no support is available in the family or the community.
2. Psychotherapy in individual or group setting.

3. Electroconvulsive therapy is rarely needed and is probably contra-indicated in some patients as it adds to symptomatology, particularly a temporary small memory loss or a feeling of depersonalization, which gives the patient more to complain about.
4. Drugs
   (a) Antidepressant drugs which would include the tricyclids or the monoamine oxidase inhibitors, providing precautions are exercised in the use of the latter (see page 312).
   (b) Tranquillisers administered by day are probably a better proposition than sedatives by night as the patient comes to develop reliance on the magic pill and does not learn to fall asleep 'under his own steam'.

   In Forest House Neurosis Unit at Claybury Hospital run on therapeutic community lines, where a major plank in treatment consisted of group therapy, it was customary, except in very exceptional circumstances, never to give night sedation. Patients who were convinced they required sedative drugs to sleep and who in most instances had taken them for years before admission, were surprised to find that they could manage to sleep well without them within a few days. A hot drink and a chat with the nurses on night duty were all, if anything, that was required on the first night or so after admission to the unit.
5. If in hospital, occupational and recreational therapy in bright surroundings are of value.
6. Environmental changes may be indicated, for example, in the family and in the patient's work. The family may also be helped to adjust to the patient's illness and may themselves have to make some adjustments in attitudes for the present and future well-being of the patient.

Neurasthenia

Neurasthenia or nervous debility is

> a neurotic disorder characterized by fatigue, irritability, headache, depression, insomnia, difficulty in concentration, and lack of capacity for enjoyment (anhedonia). It may follow or accompany an infection or exhaustion, or arise from continued emotional stress . . .

Much disagreement is in evidence in literature through the years regarding the status of neurasthenia as a nosological entity. One must remember that these rather vague symptoms can be present in association with physical disease, and also in association with more specific psychiatric disorders such as depressive illneses and schizophrenia. Care must therefore be taken in making a diagnosis of neurasthenia.

Aetiology

This appears to be shrouded in mystery and there is little point in going into the numerous postulated hypotheses. The capacity to withstand stress whether physical or mental, varies between individuals, and varies at different times in the same individual according to circumstances. Some people show the features of neurasthenia more readily than others, succumbing relatively quickly to even minor stress, probably on the basis of a combination of inherited and early environmental factors. Precipitating factors are manifold, the state being the sequel to such things as having to accept extra responsibility, irksome working conditions, domestic upsets and frustration from any source. It may follow a psychiatric or physical illness.

There is a wide variety of symptoms, a prolonged feeling of weakness and fatigue, aches and pains in any region of the body, and strange bodily sensations, being most common. Insomnia and irritability, and weight loss, occur frequently. Headache, dyspepsia, flatulence and constipation may be complained of.

Palpitations, giddiness, sweats, pallor of skin and cold clammy extremities may form part of the picture, and hyperaesthesia may occur in the skin over one or more viscera. Muscle tone may be affected, with tremors occuring in eyelids, tongue and hands.

Patients lack attention and concentration and are unable to sustain mental or physical effort. Mood level is unstable and these people become easily upset, life becoming a series of 'crises'. Any physical or mental effort made may be accompanied by a complaint of fatigue or even exhaustion. It is not surprising that the neuraesthenic person tends to conserve his energies and withdraw from social life, and to indulge in attention-seeking behaviour, because he cannot achieve recognition through success in life's normal pursuits.

Management

The planning of treatment will depend on a proper assessment of the patient's ego resources and of the various stress factors present. If a patient has habitually adopted what might be termed a 'sick role' leading to satisfaction of his particular needs, then motivation to get well may be extremely low and therapeutic endeavour wasted.

One must, as always in psychiatric management, treat the whole person. Here we have a patient with both mental and physical debility, and so a two-pronged management programme is involved.

The physical condition should be dealt with along general medical lines, including the utilization of graduated exercises, games and even manual work to increase the patient's physical tolerance, and to give him something else to think about apart from himself. Hospitalisation may be necessary to provide a suitable programme.

Concurrently, some form of psychotherapy is indicated wherein the patient can discuss his conflicts and difficulties, and where the relationship between emotional factors and physical symptoms can be laid bare.

It may be necessary to bring about changes in the patient's work and family situation if he is ever to function even at a moderate level of efficiency.

Neurasthenic patients, when they are unwilling to give up the 'secondary gains' accruing from their 'illness', may prove an intolerable burden to relatives, never pulling their weight in domestic chores, but still able to walk to the pub on Friday to buy their week-end beer.

Hypochondriasis

Hypochondriasis is

> a neurotic disorder in which the conspicuous features are excessive concern with one's health in general or in the integrity and functioning of some part of one's body, or, less frequently, one's mind. It is usually associated with anxiety and depression. It may occur as a feature of severe mental disorder and in that case should not be classified here but in the corresponding major category.

The condition is not amenable to reassurance.

The hypochondriac may be seen as relating to his environment in a distorted way, in the sense that he fails to make meaningful relationships with others. He feels worthless and rejected and attempts to opt out of interpersonal relationships, becoming more preoccupied with his bodily functions.

Sometimes patients with hypochondriasis have some definite organic disorder, often of a minor kind, about which they show inordinate concern. Normal physiological reactions common to us all, but mostly ignored, become the overriding concern of these patients who believe themselves to be ill, and are forever complaining about their ailments to anybody who is prepared to listen.

In some, attention focusses on the bowels which must run like clockwork. Others become preoccupied with the heart rate. Others become 'cranks' about diet. The manifestations are legion.

Management

What has been said about the management in neurasthenia may well apply to the management of the patient who suffers from hypochondriasis. One must be a keen clinician to determine whether one is dealing with a neurotic disorder or whether the ideas have developed delusional intensity and are indicative of a schizophrenic illness. We have also learned that sufferers from psychotic depressive illness frequently manifest hypochondriacal ideas and even hypochondriacal delusions. Many are subject to a variety of physical investigations before the true nature of their illness is appreciated. Many other categories of psychiatric disorders may have hypochondriasis as part of the clinical picture.

As in neurasthenia, the patient who finds the 'sick role' a satisfactory compromise in the matter of living, will wish to grapple to his heart his beloved complaints with hoops of steel, and he becomes a difficult treatment proposition.

Depersonalization syndrome

The I.C.D. gives the following description:

> A neurotic disorder with an unpleasant state of disturbed perception in which external objects or parts of one's own body are experienced as changed in their quality, unreal, remote or automatized. The patient is aware of the subjective nature of the change he experiences. Depersonalization may occur as a feature of several mental disorders including depression, obsessional neurosis, anxiety and schizophrenia; in that case the condition should not be classified here but in the corresponding major category.

Such a condition may occur in association with a traumatic incident which takes the form of a real or symbolic emotional threat.

People have experienced depersonalization following a near traffic accident. Also, in these days of rapid global travel, overtired air passengers moving suddenly from one culture or place to another may become depersonalized.

15

PERSONALITY DISORDERS

We shall now describe groups of personality attributes which cannot readily be classified as psychiatric illness, but which can determine a person's attitudes to life and to a large extent influence behaviour.

When manifest behaviour, resulting from particular personality traits or attributes, assumes proportions which place it outside the broad limits of mental health, one can begin to think about personality disorders as opposed to personality characteristics, which are evident in each one of us.

Occasionally, certain organic brain disorders can lead to clinical pictures resembling personality disorders, but cannot be classified as such, as the clinical picture is due to organic insult, and not to developmental defects or pathological trends in the personality structure. Among organic brain insults which can lead to clinical pictures resembling personality disorders are epidemic encephalitis, head injury, Alzheimers's disease and cerebral vascular diseases.

Of personality disorders the I.C.D. has the following to say:

> Deeply ingrained maladaptive patterns of behaviour generally recognizable by the time of adolescence or earlier and continuing throughout most of adult life, although often becoming less obvious in middle or old age. The personality is abnormal either in the balance of its components, their quality and expression or in its total aspect. Because of this deviation or psychopathy the patient suffers or others have to suffer and there is an adverse effect upon the individual or on a society. It includes what is sometimes called psychopathic personality, but if this is determined primarily by malfunctioning of the brain, it should not be classified here but as one of the non-psychotic organic brain syndromes. When the patient exhibits an anomaly of personality directly related to his neurosis or psychosis, e.g. schizoid personality and schizophrenia or anankastic personality and obsessive compulsive neurosis, the relevant neurosis or psychosis which is in evidence should be diagnosed in addition.

As mentioned earlier the term 'character neurosis' is also applied to a personality disorder.

We shall now briefly describe the different types of personality disorders, remembering that the characteristics described are present to a greater or lesser extent in all of us, and that they can be regarded as abnormal, only when behaviour resulting from the possession of these attributes offends the particular tenets of one's society, or leads to unwarranted discomfort of fellow beings, or gross personal inconvenience.

Paranoid personality disorder

This is a

> personality disorder in which there is excessive sensitiveness to setbacks or to what are taken to be humiliations and rebuffs, a tendency to distort experience by misconstruing the neutral or friendly actions of others as hostile or contemptuous, and a combative and tenacious sense of personal rights. There may be a proneness to jealousy or excessive self-importance. Such persons may feel helplessly humiliated and put upon; others, likewise excessively sensitive, are aggressive and insistent. In all cases there is excessive self-reference.

'Self-reference' in this description simply refers to the overwhelming tendency in the paranoid personality to see everything in his surroundings as referring or relating to himself.

Affective personality disorder

Such personalities are

> characterized by lifelong predominance of a pronounced mood which may be persistently depressive, persistently elated, or alternately one then the other. During periods of elation there is unshakable optimism and an enhanced zest for life and activity, whereas periods of depression are marked by worry, pessimism, low output of energy and a sense of futility.

Cycloid or cyclothymic personality and depressive personality fall within this category.

Individuals who are persistently elated are seen by some authorities as representing an extreme degree of extraversion.

Jung first described the characteristics of extraversion, describing the extravert as the man of action, the person who displays a positive movement of subjective interest towards an object in such a way that no doubt can exist regarding his positive dependence upon the object.

Schizoid personality disorder

This name is given to

> personality disorders in which there is withdrawal from affectional, social and other contacts, with autistic preference for fantasy and introspective reserve. Behaviour may be slightly eccentric or indicate avoidance of competitive situations. Apparent coolness and detachment may mask an incapacity to express feeling.

Such personalities, in childhood, are usually quiet, shy, obedient, sensitive and retiring. At puberty, they frequently become more withdrawn, manifesting the aggregate of personality traits described by Jung as introversion, namely quietness, seclusiveness and unsociability, often with eccentricity.

At this point, comment on the concept of autism will be made.

Bleuler regarded *autism* as 'detachment from reality, together with the relative and absolute predominance of the inner life'. Autistic processes characterise schizophrenia but are also present in normal persons, and to a larger extent in persons of schizoid personality. One's autistic experience includes the store of private meanings, reveries, emotions and formulations of experience, which are difficult to communicate to other persons. When one is absorbed in autistic processes, communication with the outside world is diminished in proportion to the degree of absorption.

There are fundamental differences in the autistic experiences of 'normal' persons including those with schizoid personalities, and schizophrenics. The normal and schizoid personalities can, by an act of will resume communication with the outside world; can translate autistic experiences into comprehensible form; can work out a balance between their autistic life and their relationship with the outside world. The severely disturbed schizophrenic cannot.

Explosive personality disorder

This disorder is

> characterized by instability of mood with liability to intemperate outbursts of anger, hate, violence or affection. Aggression may be expressed in words or in physical violence. The outbursts cannot readily be controlled by the affected persons who are not otherwise prone to antisocial behaviour.

Between outbursts their affective relationships to their fellow men may be excellent.

Anankastic personality disorder

Into this category fall individuals who experience

> feelings of personal insecurity, doubt and incompleteness leading to excessive conscientiousness, checking, stubbornness and caution. There may be insistent and unwelcome thoughts or impulses which do not attain the severity of an obsessional neurosis. There is perfectionism and meticulous accuracy and a need to check repeatedly in an attempt to ensure this. Rigidity and excessive doubt may be conspicuous.

Obsessional and compulsive personalities are included here, 'obsessional' emphasising more the ideational aspects and 'compulsive' referring more to the executive or action functions. These people lack a normal capacity for relaxation, and their chronic tension may precede neurotic illness, but this is not an invariable consequence. When obsessive-compulsive disorder develops, it may appear as a persistence of an adolescent pattern of behaviour in the anankastic personality. On the other hand, it may be the result of regression from a mature level of functioning, when the person is under stress.

Hysterical personality disorder

This personality disorder is

> characterized by shallow, labile affectivity, dependence on others, craving for appreciation and attention, suggestibility and theatricality. There is often sexual immaturity, e.g. frigidity and over-responsiveness to stimuli. Under stress, hysterical symptoms (neurosis) may develop.

Synonyms for the disorder are histrionic personality and psychoinfantile personality.

Jaspers writes of the hysterical personality in the following way:

> Instead of contenting himself with his endowments and potentialities as they are, the hysterical personality needs to appear in his own eyes and those of others, more than he actually is, to experience more than he is capable of

> experiencing. In place of genuine, spontaneous experience, naturally expressed, there appears a spurious, theatrical and forced experience, not consciously so, but arising from his ability, the true hysterical attribute, of living on his own stage and for the moment identifying himself entirely with his role, so that the whole act acquires an apparently genuine stamp. From this, all other hysterical traits can be understandably derived. The hysterical personality seems to have lost its core and to consist entirely of a series of shifting masks.

This description is difficult to better. Such personalities are usually attention-seeking and manipulating in their behaviour.

Asthenic personality disorder

The asthenic personality disorder is

> characterized by passive compliance with the wishes of elders and others and a weak inadequate response to the demands of daily life. Lack of vigour may show itself in the intellectual or emotional spheres; there is little capacity for enjoyment.

The terms dependent personality, inadequate personality and passive personality are included under this category.

Personality disorders with predominantly sociopathic or asocial manifestations

This appellation is given to a

> personality disorder characterized by disregard for social obligations, lack of feeling for others, and impetuous violence or callous unconcern. There is a gross disparity between behaviour and the prevailing social norms. Behaviour is not readily modifiable by experience, including punishment. People with this personality are often affectively cold and may be abnormally aggressive or irresponsible. Their tolerance to frustration is low; they blame others or offer plausible rationalizations for the behaviour which brings them into conflict with society.

Other terms applied in this category of disorder are amoral, antisocial or asocial personality.

Aetiology

The problem of sociopathic or antisocial behaviour has been studied by many professional groups in an effort to determine causative factors. A number of theories of causation have been proposed.

Arising out of adoption studies on adult psychopathy and criminality, there seems little doubt that genetic factors play a part. Electroencephalographic studies show bilateral slow wave activity in the E.E.G.s of adult criminals and antisocial personalities similar to that found in childhood. This is suggestive of slow cortical maturation in these people, which may account for some antisocial behaviour arising out of poor impulse control and slow development of social maturity. Other studies show that criminal tendencies are associated with slowness of social learning; also that antisocial personalities do not learn conditioned fear responses as readily as other people, and therefore have more difficulty in learning responses motivated by fear or anxiety, which leads to a certain recklessness and failure to learn from the untoward outcomes of deviant actions.

In addition to the biological evidence presented above, there is evidence that non-genetic parental influence is also important. Studies have concerned themselves with early deprivation, parental separation, parental rejection and parental deviance, and as yet, the particular environmental influences relevant to the development of antisocial personality disorder have not been satisfactorily elucidated.

Management of personality disorders

At the risk of appearing to be therapeutically nihilistic, there is little that the doctor or nurse can do to alter basic personality characteristics. Claims are made for the efficacy of various forms of psychotherapy, including psychoanalysis. Recidivist criminals, who would fall within the antisocial personality disorder group, are said to have become more socially adapted as a result of LSD therapy combined with group therapy, carried out within the umbrella of a therapeutic community.

Drugs are of little value except as temporary symptomatic measures, when stresses give rise to behaviour fairly characteristic of each personality disorder.

There are many who favour a group approach rather than an individual psychotherapeutic one. In the former, the patient's similarities and differences from others are emphasised, and he is given the opportunity to form relationships; in short, to learn to live with others by modifying at least his behaviour, if not his attitudes. Other group procedures involving for example, therapeutic social clubs, or conjoint family therapy have their advocates.

The therapist, if he undertakes to help patients with some of the above personality disorders, is committed to long term frustration and disappointment, and exposed to the manipulative endeavours of his patients. Perhaps the main attributes the therapist must have, are flexibility and patience, and the ability to remain a consistent model.

From the point of view of nurses, and, in fact, of all workers in psychiatry, it is worthwhile knowing that little can be achieved in a short time. If there is any group of patients who bring home to the therapist or nurse the fact that he is not the Almighty, but a weak instrument, it is this group of patients. One must however, maintain an optimistic and flexible attitude within a fairly broad limit-setting frame.

As the antisocial personality who finds his way into a treatment setting, usually unmotivated to make an effort to modify his attitudes, can behave like the proverbial cat among pigeons, a separate note will be made on the management of people with antisocial personality disorder.

At the outset, one must say that the usual hospital or psychiatric milieu is unsatisfactory for these people, as insufficient external controls can be established. There is also evidence supporting the uselessness of traditional out-patient therapy.

If one views the antisocial person as one who has failed in the process of socialisation which is associated with lack of adequate inhibition over unacceptable social behaviour, he is hardly likely to fit into the society of the hospital which merely reflects the outside world, a place with which he has already shown himself to be behaviourally incompatible, and in an enduring manner unlike most other inpatients.

For the antisocial person's management, an inpatient treatment setting which can enforce limit-setting behaviour would appear mandatory. Within such a setting providing external controls, involving the use of authority and maybe even forms of punishment at times, the antisocial person may slowly develop his own inner controls over his behaviour. Some positive claims are made for such regimes. Possibly because of biological maturation enabling social learning to proceed, the untoward behaviour of many antisocial personalities settles down in middle life.

One sees few 'psychopaths' over the age of forty. This may partly be due to the maturation suggested above but also, in the view of some authorities, to the fact that many die either at their own or others' hands.

Other personality disorders are the eccentric and 'haltlose' type personality, and the immature, passive-aggressive and psychoneurotic personalities. The term *passive-aggressive* refers to a personality disorder in which aggressive feelings are manifested in various ways especially through mild obstructionism, procrastination and stubbornness.

'Haltlose' which is rarely if ever used in Australian psychiatry is derived from the German *haltlos* meaning unstable, unsteady, vain, unprincipled, without support, or rootless.

16

SEXUAL DEVIATIONS AND DISORDERS

The I.C.D. refers to sexual deviations and disorders as

> abnormal sexual inclinations or behaviour which are part of a referral problem. The limits and features of normal sexual inclination and behaviour have not been stated absolutely in different societies and cultures but are broadly such as serve approved social and biological purposes. The sexual activity of affected persons is directed primarily either towards people not of the opposite sex, or towards sexual acts not associated with coitus normally, or towards coitus performed under abnormal circumstances. If the anomalous behaviour becomes manifest only during psychosis or other mental illness the condition should be classified under the major illness. It is common for more than one anomaly to occur together in the same individual; in that case the predominant deviation is classified. It is preferable not to include in this category individuals who perform deviant sexual acts when normal sexual outlets are not available to them.*

Normal sexual behaviour

There is a tendency to eschew the terms 'normal' and 'abnormal' in relation to sexual practices, and indeed as inferred above normal sexual inclination and behaviour differ in different societies and cultures. What is considered normal by a particular society or culture may be seen as abnormal by another. Also accepted attitudes within a particular society or culture may alter over a period of time. For example, there are currently strong moves (and countermoves) in many western societies to add legislative blessing to homosexual acts occurring between consenting adults in private, something undreamed of in past decades.

Apart from differing and changing cultural norms, the range of sexual activity in people one would consider well-adjusted is very wide.

Before looking more closely at the question of sexual deviation, it would be well to consider what is generally accepted to be normal sexual practice, remembering that 'normal' or 'abnormal' has no significant meaning except in terms of cultural or social background. At one point in time, what is considered normal in one culture or society may be considered abnormal in another, and accepted attitudes may change over a period of time within a particular culture.

Apart from the differences in sexual norms existing between different

* The term 'sexual perversion' with its moralistic overtones was once used to denote what is now called 'sexual deviation'.

cultures, in our western culture for example, the range of sexual activity in people one would consider well-adjusted is very wide. Kinsey, in the United States of America, found that such practices as cunnilingus, fellatio, intercourse per rectum, were not at all uncommon. It also appeared that certain practices were more common at particular social levels.

It is obvious that divergent views must exist regarding normal sexuality, particularly as many such practices, socially frowned upon and often considered seriously deviant, are so commonly engaged in without any apparent deleterious effects, that they can hardly be regarded as being of psychiatric importance.

With our lack of precise knowledge of sexual practices in this country one must, in a sense, duck the issue of defining average or 'normal' sexual behaviour, and make the following broad statement: normal sexual behaviour consists of being able, without fear or guilt, to engage in a heterosexual relationship wherein sexual intercourse (penile-vaginal intercourse) constitutes the ultimate in sexual pleasure and satisfaction. This does not mean that obtaining pleasure from a variety of activities, such as those associated with sexual foreplay, is in any way abnormal, providing such activities do not consistently constitute the major means of sexual gratification.

Two areas of sexual activity about which erroneous and guilt-producing views are commonly held are masturbation and sexual intercourse after the menopause. Firstly, it can be categorically stated that masturbation itself does not have any bad after-effects. It can be considered normal during puberty and adolescence in a society in which marriage does not take place until a good many years after the attainment of physical sexual maturity.

Masturbation has been termed a comfort habit, and when there are no other sexual outlets available the activity cannot in general be considered morbid or abnormal. When it becomes a prevailing habit it is very likely that there exists emotional deprivation and marked frustration of activity. Some of the older members of our society raise their hands in horror when middle-aged females, particularly after the menopause, still show interest in sexual matters, as if this were something quite abnormal or perverse. It is not.

Aetiology of sexual deviation

The causes of sexual deviation are difficult to unravel. The sexual instinct or drive becomes distorted in such a way that the deviant person behaves wrongly towards the right sexual object, or chooses the wrong object to achieve sexual gratification.

Developmental factors

With the exception of male homosexuality, where there appears to be evidence that hereditary factors may have at least some part to play, deviance would appear to be determined by developmental and environmental factors.

If we follow the Freudian concept of normal psychosexual development (page 43ff.), we see that the developing child passes normally through various phases: the oral, wherein he derives pleasure first by sucking and later by biting; the anal, characterised first by an aim initially to expel and later to retain faeces; the phallic phase, wherein interest becomes centered on his own phallus and body, and sexual satisfaction if obtained from the primary sex organ, the phallus or penis. Interest also centres on others in his environment, and eventually enough emotion is directed towards a sexual object, normally a person of the opposite sex, and the adult capacity to love is developed. A fixation at, or in other words, a failure to develop past a particular phase, is said to give rise to certain attributes peculiar to that phase. For example, a great deal of hate is associated with the oral biting (oral sadistic) stage, and if fixation occurs at this level then the person will continue to derive pleasure from sadistic activities. Freud believed that the sexual practices in homosexual relationships symbolised regression to fixation points in libidinal development. His formulations will not be dealt with here.

Whether or not such fixations are environmental or genetically determined does not seem to be clear. Looked at in another way it is still not certain to what extent the individual develops spontaneously through these various phases and to what extent environment plays a part. The position will probably never be clarified as it is impossible to bring up a child normally without others in his environment.

Environmental factors

Here we shall look briefly at conditioning, fear, guilt and feelings of sexual inferiority.

Pavlov, the Russian scientist, found that it was possible to link a stimulus with a reflex or instinctual action: dogs salivate at the sight or smell of food. If a stimulus such as a bell ringing is associated in time with the production of food, the dog will become conditioned to salivate (a reflex action) on hearing the sound of a bell even in the absence of food, this being termed classical conditioning (see page 324). Human beings can be conditioned by events that become attached to their sexual responses. Thus, repeated sexual assaults can influence a child's sexuality, the original emotions of fear or guilt associated with the assault later being triggered off by subsequent sexual acts. Leaving aside such flagrant sexual trauma, which must be relatively rare, there is much in the environment to produce fear or guilt associated with the sexual act in the developing child. Such guilt or fear may arise through the process of conditioning, in this instance instrumental or operant conditioning (see page 324).

Probably the most powerful influence determining a child's attitude towards his erotic feelings is the attitude toward sex expressed or implied by parents. The parent as well as the child, at least in western civilization, is influenced by the attitude of a society that is far less tolerant of sexuality than are many cultures. In these days, even though parents may not condemn the developing sexual interests and behaviour of their children as much as in the past, their reticence about speaking of sex as a positive pleasurable activity and the pinnacle of communication, still puts it in the taboo class for the child, something not quite proper, and about which the child cannot help feeling a degree of guilt.

The sexual act is an expression of love, in fact, the ultimate in communication and expression of this relationship. In terms of incest taboos, in most societies a child can never, without concomitant guilt, even consider the possibility of fulfilling such a close relationship with an opposite sexed parent. This unfulfilled state remains until such times as the young adult finds a suitable mate. In some instances, if marked guilt exists over the development of a close relationship with a parent, the young adult will avoid sexual relationships with people reminiscent of parents on the basis of so-called incest taboo. In the case of the young male this could possibly mean turning to a female quite different from mother, in fact someone seen in the same light as a prostitute, or to more deviant behaviour. The young woman may be so guilty about a close sexual relationship with someone reminiscent of her father, that she may turn to prostitution where numerous relationships having no depth are experienced.

For whatever reasons fear and guilt exist over normal heterosexual intercourse, the general thesis is that they may lead a person to seek deviant ways of achieving sexual gratification. For example, in the case of homosexuality, sexual gratification is preserved, but fear is avoided by renunciation of heterosexuality. The sexual masochist must be punished for guilt associated with heterosexual gratification, and so engages in painful activities in association with heterosexual experiences.

Feelings of sexual inferiority and lack of confidence that one is loveable or loved for oneself, are found in many people suffering from sexual deviation.

Sexual inferiority consists in the feeling that one does not match up to the particular sexual role that society demands. If the man is not the doyen of masculinity, and the woman not the acme of feminine perfection with all the attributes demanded by society, then repeated reassurances may be sought, and deviant ways of achieving sexual gratification may be entered into. This feeling of sexual inadequacy affects men more than women, and the majority of types of sexually deviant behaviour are found in the male.

Lack of confidence that one is lovable may often be attributed to an early failure in the relationship between child and mother. One sees many instances however, where this difficulty in relationship would appear to result from constitutional or inherited personality attributes of the child rather than from any mismanagement by the mother. Again, this lack of conviction that one is lovable, and so is unable to function in a socalled mature sexual relationship, is a pressure that may turn one towards deviant sexual practices.

This is but a brief overview of some of the factors considered to be of importance in the aetiology of sexual deviation. Enough has been said to indicate that moral judgments are inappropriate in many cases of sexual deviation. Many deviants are indeed not filthy, perverse individuals, but people with particular crosses to bear who feel acutely their differences from the social norm.

It is on this point that conflicting views may rear their heads between psychiatrists and upholders of the law. Laws as they exist must be upheld, but punishment in terms of incarceration, apart from segregating from society people who may harm society, itself a reasonable objective, is in no way helpful as a curative measure. A great deal is yet to be learned about the aetiology and therefore the effectual management of sexual deviance. On this rather sobering note, we shall look at some of the types of sexually deviant behaviour that are seen clinically.

Homosexuality

The term homosexuality is derived from the Greek prefix *homo* meaning 'the same as', and so the term homosexual may strictly be applied to both males and females who are exclusively or predominantly attracted to persons of the same sex with or without physical relationship. In common parlance, 'homosexuality' is applied to such deviance in the male, and 'lesbianism' to that in the female.

Female homosexuality

Statistically, homosexual relationships between women are less common than those between men, and society's attitude is such that homosexual attachments between women cause less comment and are less associated with guilt than those between men. Relatively few cases of women soliciting homosexually or seducing minors are recorded. The female homosexual relationship is often confined at a psychological level, but as affection and sex go hand in hand, such relationships, even though commenced for the sake of companionship only, may develop sexual components.

Every girl probably experiences some attraction towards members of her own sex during her development, and the frequent existence of crushes wherein the preadolescent girl tries to model herself on an older female is virtually a homosexual phase of development. These attractions are usually more marked and intense when the relationship between mother and daughter has been defective. A defective relationship or absent mother will create insecurity in the daughter, and, because she does not have a good model with whom to identify, she will not readily develop her own identity as a woman.

Marked insecurity and a failure to realise their feminity are characteristic of the female homosexual, the insecurity leading to the strong dependency that usually exists between female homosexual couples. It would seem that two major areas of need are partly served in a lesbian relationship, the need for a sexual partner, and the need for a mother and/or to mother someone.

In some female homosexual relationships, one of the pair assumes a dominant masculine role rather than a maternal one. The development of such identification with the male can often be seen throughout childhood in the playing of male games, taking part in activities usually reserved for males, and eschewing feminine clothing. It is quite common for girls to pass through this tomboy stage, and such behaviour in the preadolescent girl should not alarm parents. Arising out of a variety of interacting dynamic factors however, some girls maintain this male identification along with an abhorrence or even loathing of males whom they are, in a sense, copying.

Lesbian relationships are probably more lasting and satisfying than their male counterparts.

Male homosexuality

Male homosexuality is probably developmental in origin, arising out of the emotional influences to which the sufferer was exposed in early childhood. There are, nevertheless, those authorities who claim homosexuality to be an inherited constitutional abnormality.

It is stated that male homosexuals tend to be born of elderly mothers, and to arrive later in the family than unaffected brothers and sisters. This is used as an argument that some chromosomal abnormality, which is not really an inherited genetic factor but which has developed in the ageing ovum, is responsible for this form of deviance.

Whether or not genetic factors or chromosomal abnormalities play a part in male homosexuality, evidence would strongly support the proposition that homosexuals are made and not born, and that sexual preference in adulthood is largely determined by early environmental influences.

Within every male there is the potential for homosexual behaviour. Kinsey, in the populations studied by him in the United States of America, found that 37% of males had some homosexual experience. In some tolerant cultures it has been found that one hundred percent of males freely engage in homosexual as well as heterosexual activities. Where males are isolated from females, as in schools, prisons, or in some aspects of service life, homosexuality is relatively common.

The male who remains exclusively homosexual is found to have failed to pass a normal milestone in sexual development and may be regarded as immature in this respect in the same way as his female counterpart.

Certain patterns of family life appear with great frequency in families of male homosexuals. The most common pattern is a father who is detached from and who shows little affection for, or is openly hostile to his son, together with an over-emotional and intimate mother. The close emotional tie that develops with mother tends to arouse premature eroticism in her son. His sexual drive cannot be fulfilled with her, and he is destinated to be frustrated. Such a male frequently has difficulty in forming a close relationship with other women, for he may see all women as seductresses like his mother, arousing him sexually and depriving him of sexual fulfilment, thus taking his masculinity from him. In adult life, male homosexuals may have relatively satisfactory platonic relationships with women, but become alarmed when the possibility of sexual involvement looms on the horizon.

Rado states that a homosexual adaptation is the result of 'hidden but incapacitating fears of the opposite sex'.

Another facet of development of homosexual orientation lies in the fact that a son is unable to identify with an indifferent or hostile father. The boy sees attributes in other men which are not in his father, and comes to hero-worship them; they may be older boys, schoolmasters, sportsmen, or even fictional television characters.

For some reason, the homosexual adult does not grow out of what can be considered a normal phase of hero-worshipping, analogous to the crushes that girls have on other females, and never really assumes his own masculine identity. Male figures remain important to him, and he does not cease to be attracted by men, while shunning females.

For choice of a partner most homosexual males are said to seek a rugged tough male, while a minority show a preference for young men or youths conforming more in appearance to the feminine stereotype.

Male homosexual relationships are, in general, not as enduring as lesbian relationships, and the male in his restless searching for a suitable mate, changes partners more frequently.

There would appear to be a continuum from homosexuality to heterosexuality, and many men cannot be designated in a clear cut way as either homosexual or heterosexual. Many homosexual offences, in countries where homosexual practices constitute an offence, are committed by married men.

This brief overview of male homosexuality should indicate that many homosexual men are indeed sufferers in the true sense, and abysmally lonely. The male who solicits in public toilets may indeed be a lecherous self-gratifying individual, but he may also be driven by unhappiness and loneliness to make contact with others in the only way open to him, even though he deplores his own actions, especially in the light of legal and social strictures.

Fetishism

The word fetish is applied to an 'inanimate object worshipped by savages for its magical powers or as being inhabited by a spirit' (*The Concise Oxford Dictionary*). It connotes something 'irrationally reverenced'.

Fetishism more commonly described in males, is the name applied to the form of sexual deviation in which a person feels a compulsive and irrational sexual attraction towards an inanimate object usually representative of or belonging to a person of the opposite sex. The attraction may also involve a fascination for any part of the body other than the genitals, such as hair or breast. The male who is attracted by hair or female breasts, a normal enough attraction, is not a fetishist unless these parts substitute totally for the person.

Fetishists are usually heterosexual in their orientation, but homosexual fetishism also exists.

Practically any item of wearing apparel, especially female underwear, parts of the body, and the many decorative objects worn by women can be fetishes. These fetishes arouse the same feelings which, in the ordinary man, are aroused by the female genitals.

The presence of the fetish is necessary before some males can achieve erection, or if not present, some males phantasise the fetish in order to achieve erection. This may be necessary as a prelude to or during penile-vaginal intercourse, serving the purpose of fully arousing the male so that he will be potent enough to function in a satisfactory fashion. One would not see this as a severe degree of fetishism, nor as a true deviation; in fact, such a state of affairs is probably relatively common. Witness the husband's requests for a particular nightdress or a particular brand of perfume to be worn. The true deviant at the other end of the continuum is the male who is able to gratify sexual desires only through masturbatory activity and only while gazing upon or utilizing the article or object. In this instance, the fetish has become a substitute for the whole female.

There are a number of dynamic explanations put forward for the development of fetishism. In broad terms it may be said that the fetish becomes established as a sexual stimulus in early life, and as a result of fear or guilt associated with heterosexual contact there is a halt in emotional sexual development, with the fetish remaining the main or only sexually stimulating object for the person concerned.

The desire for a fetish may provoke stealing, for example women's undergarments from a clothesline. Fetishists are usually timid withdrawn people, who keep much to themselves and do not have a proclivity for violence.

Paedophilia

In this fortunately uncommon deviation a man or woman is exclusively attracted to children.

The sexual advances made to children usually take the form of verbal approaches or genital display, without physical contact. On the other hand, the child may be encouraged to handle the sexual organs of the seducer or seductress, and the child's sexual organs may constitute erotic playthings for the adult. In rare cases, the perpetrator being a male, actual intercourse is attempted or engaged in, sometimes with disastrous results to the child. If for a moment we discount physical trauma, some authorities hold that more emotional trauma is caused by the attitudes of, and the sensationalism created by the general public and those investigating the assault, than by the assault itself.

The seduction of female children by adults is generally regarded with horror, possibly because of the high value that sections of society place on female virginity; possibly and more generally because there is something sadistic and grossly inappropriate in an adult with his physical and intellectual advantages, forcing his attention on a child. It would seem however, that the reason for such sexual seductions lies not so much in the adult's preference for children, but in his or her inability to find sexual satisfaction in an adult relationship. He is not the 'oversexed monster' that many would label him, but somebody unable to make contact with contemporaries because of his immature sexuality.

Paedophilia occurs in people who are either of heterosexual or homosexual orientation.

Certain groups of people may exhibit paedophilic behaviour without being true paedophiliacs. The libertine, tired of his multiplicity of conquests, may seek new pastures in the hope of restoring flagging sexual appetite, and the virginal girl may prove attractive inasmuch as the male is traversing new ground devoid of competition from other men. Apparently, erstwhile normal men suffering from sexual deprivation may, under the effects of alcohol or other organic brain syndromes, lose judgment and self-control and make sexual advances towards children.

Transvestism

The term transvestism, also called 'transvestitism' is derived from the Latin prefix *trans* meaning across and the noun *vestis*, a garment. It applies to the act of dressing in clothing appropriate to the opposite sex. Transvestites are found in most cultures and are predominantly males.

Transvestism occuring in the male is believed to be largely the result of a failure to make a normal male identification, resulting from the absence of father, or the presence of an unsatisfactory or inadequate father or male figure in early years, together with subtle, perhaps unconscious, pressures from the mother to be like her. The transvestite thus makes a feminine identification.

The I.C.D. defines transvestism as

> sexual deviation in which sexual pleasure is derived from dressing in clothes of the opposite sex

and points out that 'there is no consistent attempt to take on the identity or behaviour of the opposite sex'.

There is some confusion in the literature concerning the motivation for cross-dressing. Buhrich (1978) reviewed the literature and reported his own findings which may be summarised as follows:

> The most frequent and sustained sensation reported by transvestite subjects was a feeling of comfort or ease and relief of stress or tension . . . Almost half the transvestite subjects reported that while cross-dressed they felt relieved of current responsibilities or of normal masculine demands.

The compulsive nature of transvestite urges and the narcissistic aspects were also highlighted.

Narcissistic aspects are measured by time required for make-up and cross-dressing, time spent in parading before a mirror, and number of photographs the subject has of himself when cross-dressed. Though not a high percentage (12%) was apparent in this particular series of transvestites, fetishistic sexual arousal does appear to play a significant role in cross-dressing.

Transvestism may appear as a symptom of psychotic or neurotic illness or be present in association with organic brain disorders. Presumably these states merely trigger off a latent tendency for cross-dressing.

Trans-sexualism

Opinions vary as to the relationship between transvestism and trans-sexualism there being some points in common between the two conditions, for example cross-dressing. However other features would appear to indicate that transvestism and trans-sexualism are separate clinical entities. In a summary of another study by Buhrich he states:

> In comparison to the transvestite subjects, significantly more transsexuals were younger, were single, cross-dressed fully, and reported homosexual interest, a feminine gender identity, and a desire for sex-change surgery. In comparison to the transsexual subjects, significantly more transvestites reported heterosexual interest, cross-dressed partially, and had shown fetishistic arousal.

The I.C.D. makes a clear distinction between transvestism and trans-sexualism and gives the following description of the latter:

Sexual deviation centred around fixed beliefs that the overt bodily sex is wrong. The resulting behaviour is directed towards either changing the sexual organs by operation, or completely concealing the bodily sex by adopting both the dress and behaviour of the opposite sex.

It should be pointed out that there is no anatomical abnormality in the trans-sexual such as is seen in hermaphrodism where genital components of both sexes are present.

Exhibitionism

Exhibitionism is a 'sexual deviation in which the main sexual pleasure and gratification is derived from exposure of the genitals to a person of the opposite sex'. It is exclusively a male deviation and it provides some sexual gratification. An extremely primitive way of displaying masculinity, exhibitionism is engaged in by males who are weak and insecure in their sexual role. The author recalls the instance of a man suddenly opening the door of his parked car displaying his erect penis to a young girl walking along the footpath. Possibly horror, disgust or excitement in the female are the desired effects, as the display of some sort of emotion in a female reassures the male that, even if he cannot command love from a female, he is powerful enough to produce a reaction other than indifference.

Such an exposure may be followed by masturbatory activity. Exhibitionists, in the main, have no intention of seeking a physical relationship with the female to whom they display their genitalia. The act may be in the nature of a compulsion, in which case it frequently recurs in spite of penalties and treatment.

In other instances, an adult male may engage in a single exhibitionistic act during his lifetime as a regressive substitute in a situation where sexual gratification is not possible.

It is probable that some men displace their desire for display on to their female partners requiring them to dress better than any other female in order to show them off. The urge to display one's virility, especially in men who doubt it, is evidenced in their penchant for powerful motor bikes or expensive cars.

Some authorities believe this deviance to be so common that every school girl should be forewarned of its existence, and reassured that exhibitionism is a nuisance rather than a menace to them.

Disorders of psychosexual identity

Also known as gender-role disorder this refers to 'behaviour occurring in preadolescents of immature psychosexuality which is similar to that shown in the sexual deviations described under transvestism and trans-sexualism. Cross-dressing is intermittent, although it may be frequent, and identification with the behaviour and appearance of the opposite sex is not yet fixed. The commonest form is feminism in boys'.

Frigidity and impotence

The I.C.D. gives the following definitions:

Frigidity—dislike of or aversion to sexual intercourse, of psychological origin, of sufficient intensity to lead, if not to active avoidance, to marked anxiety, discomfort or pain when normal sexual intercourse takes place. Less severe degrees of this disorder that also give rise to consultation should also be classified here.

Impotence—sustained inability, due to psychological causes, to maintain an erection which will allow normal heterosexual penetration and ejaculation to take place.

As well as being of psychogenic origin, frigidity and impotence may be symptomatic of other conditions and the importance of looking for and ruling out organic or even mechanical causative factors cannot be overemphasised.

Other sexual deviations

Brief mention will be made of frotteurism, voyeurism, buggery, bestiality, sadism and masochism.

Frotteurism is the practice of rubbing the genitals against another person, particularly in a crowd. Also known as frottage, it appears to be due to a persistence of the infantile love of being rubbed and cuddled. There must be very few men with a heterosexual orientation who have not experienced the urge to engage in such body pressing behaviour in crowded lifts, trains or buses. A frotteur is truly deviant when he engages in this activity only and avoids coitus.

Voyeurism, also known as scopophilia, is another way of obtaining sexual gratification without entering into a personal relationship with someone of the opposite sex. It consists in witnessing sexual scenes or naked bodies, especially genital organs, and deriving sexual pleasure from this. The desire is so widespread that it can hardly be regarded as a deviation unless utilised for sexual gratification to the exclusion of conventional methods.

Buggery refers to anal intercourse, and in some countries it is a crime to insert the penis into the anal orifice of man or woman, even if the woman is one's spouse, in which case both husband and wife are equally liable. The term sodomy is also applied to this practice in humans. The term bestiality applies to sexual or anal intercourse with animals.

Sexual sadism is the obtaining of sexual pleasure from acts of cruelty. Sadism ranges from cruelty seemingly unassociated with sexuality to the deriving of frank sexual pleasure from cruel acts. Probably the most horrific expression of sexual sadism is seen in the activities of the so-called lust-murderer who usually behaves normally until an 'outbreak' occurs, in which cutting and stabbing of the breasts or genitalia are among some of the appalling practices accompanied by intense sexual pleasure and excitement. Such a sadist, if not apprehended, almost invariably repeats his behaviour.

Masochism is the obtaining of pleasure by being hurt, humiliated, dominated, bound or degraded. Masochism and sadism do not appear in pure form, and in any one individual with either of these proclivities, the other is also found to some degree.

Management

It is beyond the scope of this volume to detail the management of sexual deviations and disorders. A considerable literature has been built up over the past two decades.

In terms of deviance from the norms of sexual inclination and behaviour, whatever these may be, there is at present a sound tendency not to tamper with those people who do not request change but rather to help them adapt to the business of living with the gender orientation they have. It is found, for example, that attempts to change a homosexual preference on a long-term basis are replete with failure.

For those requesting change in sexual preference, often a request that is probably engendered by society's punitive and critical attitudes towards homosexuality, some authorities claim that approximately one-third can achieve some change.

The main therapeutic method is long-term psychotherapy. The deviant person may first lose the feelings of guilt and inferiority associated with deviance, and, through long association with a stable therapist, learn to develop an adult emotional relationship. Physical treatments and drug therapy are of little or no avail.

Aversion therapy or deconditioning techniques can extinguish responses by the homosexual person to homosexual cues, but long-term follow up frequently shows disappointing results.

Comment has already been made on the potentially conflicting views of the psychiatrist and upholders of the law on the question of the management of sexual deviation, and as stated earlier a great deal has yet to be learned about the management of the sexually deviant, including those measures proscribed by law.

In the management of erectile dysfunction, ejaculatory incompetence, general sexual dysfunction and orgasmic dysfunction due to psychological causes, a form of behaviour therapy known as in vivo desensitization (page 323) has proved effective. Different behavioural techniques are employed in the management of premature ejaculation and vaginismus and interested students are referred to larger texts on the subject.

17

ALCOHOLISM AND DRUG DEPENDENCE

We have dealt, in Chapter 12, with organic and physiological effects of some drugs of dependence. Our object now is to study this phenomenon of dependence, and to look more closely at these and other drugs which are implicated.

Although the I.C.D. separates the Alcohol dependence syndrome from Drug dependence (See Appendix I) they will largely be dealt with together in this chapter as there seems to be little difference in the factors leading to both, save social or cultural ones and the availability of these agents. Alcohol is indeed just another drug, but in certain contexts will be mentioned separately as it has become traditional to do so.

Drug use and abuse

Before looking at the question of dependence, it must be remembered that drugs have what might be termed a normal social use. This has been so throughout history. For example, the Sumerians (3000 B.C.) described on clay tablets, techniques of cultivation and preparation of opium which was mainly used for religious purposes. Similarly, marihuana, cocaine and mushroom hallucinogens have been utilised for religious purposes, and throughout the ages in a variety of cultures, in the preparation of warriors for battle. Opium was known and used in China under traditional social and administrative controls from the ninth century until the time of the opium wars, while alcohol use was widely established before recorded history.

Traditionally, the social use of drugs including alcohol, involves their intake in group situations. The solitary use of a drug is generally censured. As indicated above, some primitive cultures restrict the use of drugs to religious occasions, while others utilise them to inflame hatred against other external groups. Most commonly however, drugs are used to reduce inhibitions at social gatherings, and so facilitate interpersonal communication and bonhomie. At what point does the use of drugs, including alcohol, become an abuse? There is no easy answer to this question. With alcohol, for example, one finds a continuum starting with the non-drinker who, acting on conviction, does not drink, perhaps even believing it to be a sin. Another person will drink moderately and only on social occasions. Others, due to personality deficiencies that make social contacts difficult, drink to feel less inhibited in a social setting. When a person comes to depend on alcohol to enable him to cope with living, including his work or pleasure, or finds himself drinking alone, he may well have progressed to the far end of the continuum, the full-blown chronic alcoholic. The patient is often the last person to judge whether he has gone past the stage of 'social drinking'. He may admit to minimal drinking only, and produce a host of rationalisations for his drinking practices.

Similarly, when does the use of other drugs become an abuse? This is an extremely complicated issue, as most of the other drugs used for a psychological effect have legal strictures placed upon them, and in a legal sense presumably, any use of most of these drugs, unless under medical direction, could constitute abuse. Leaving aside legal considerations, for whatever reason a person commences taking drugs, whether it be because friends do, because of the thrill, or to feel better, the same comments may be made about them as about alcohol. In essence, it may be said that when a person resorts to self-prescribed drugs in order to cope with living, then abuse exists. There is a greater problem with some drugs than with alcohol, in terms of physiological dependence and withdrawal symptoms, to be mentioned later, which lead to more frequent administration of certain drugs in order to avoid an unpleasant state of withdrawal.

It might be argued that a patient who takes drugs prescribed by a doctor to help with the business of living is in fact engaged in drug abuse. The author believes this to be essentially different from self administration, but there is little point in pursuing a philosophical argument here. A warning should be sounded however, that doctors have indeed produced dependence on drugs in patients by their failure to supervise their patients' taking of prescribed drugs, and by giving symptomatic remedies, potentially addictive, without looking for and dealing with psychiatric disorders and problem areas in the patients' lives which produce the symptoms for which such drugs are given.

Incidence of alcoholism and drug dependence

The incidence of alcohol and other drug dependence varies greatly from country to country, from culture to culture, and from occupation to occupation, making it extremely difficult to obtain accurate incidence figures. Alcoholism is probably most common in France, Scandinavia and the United States of America, and is said to be least common among Japanese and Jewish peoples. From 2-5 adults in every hundred are quoted as being alcoholics. Publicans, brewery workers, commercial travellers and those people who conduct their business in pubs, and seamen, appear to provide more than the average percentage of alcoholics. Doctors and other workers in situations where drugs are utilised, obviously are at risk in terms of drug dependence, and recorded figures would appear to bear this out.

Alcoholism is said to be 4 or 5 times more common among males than females, but some authorities now cast doubt on these figures. It could well be that drinking patterns are changing in Western countries, including Australia. In a survey of 654 consecutive patients* admitted to a metropolitan admission centre in New South Wales, 125 (19%) of admissions had a primary diagnosis of chronic alcoholism, and the ratio of males to females was 2:1. Among the 57 patients (9% of admissions) admitted during the same period suffering from drug dependence the ratio of males to females was 1:2, a reversal of ratio. In the population studied, there was no significant difference in admission rates for alcoholism and drug dependence between the social status groups represented. Contrary to popular belief, possibly arising out of press reports, it is not the youth of today who comprise the bulk of drug dependent people in our culture, the most frequently involved decade being 41-50 years, many of these being middle aged housewives dependent on bromides and bromureides, or barbiturates.

It is an extremely difficult undertaking to give an accurate estimate of the extent of dependence on alcohol and other drugs, as the criteria of dependence vary, as figures from doctors in private practice, numbers of admissions to private hospitals, and of dependent persons who have not sought medical assistance, are not universally obtainable.

Dependence and tolerance

There are two types of dependence described. The first and most important is *psychological dependence*, which refers to the overwhelming repetitive need to seek whatever ease, pleasure or stimulus is provided by a drug. Psychological dependence is common to all drugs of dependence even though the physiological effects of different drugs may be quite dissimilar. For example, some stimulate, some sedate, some relieve pain and some have markedly discomforting side effects, such as the constipation associated with the taking of opium. Some drugs on which psychological dependence develops may have virtually no physiological effects.

Physical dependence relates to the pharmacology of a drug. In the course of repeated administration of certain drugs, the body's metabolic processes adapt themselves to these drugs. If such a drug is suddenly withdrawn, the metabolic balance achieved is upset, and as the concentration of the drug in the body falls without a comparable quick re-adaption of metabolic processes within the cells of the body, withdrawal or abstinence symptoms occur. Any drug, the sudden stoppage of which leads to withdrawal symptoms, may be said to have produced a state of physical dependence. Withdrawal or abstinence symptoms are due in the main, to hyperactivity of those functions previously depressed by the drug. Examples of withdrawal symptoms are convulsions and/or delirium tremens following the rapid withdrawal of barbiturates or alcohol, and vomiting, diarrhoea, lachrymation, sweating, sneezing and marked restlessness that occur following the abrupt cessation of a sufficiently large morphine intake.

Tolerance has been defined as a diminishing response to repeated doses of a drug. This simply means that with each subsequent administration of

* The figure of 654 excluded patients re-admitted within the survey period of six months.

a drug its effects are less noticeable. For the addict this means that increasing amounts of a drug are taken at each dose to produce the same desired effect experienced in the earlier stages of drug abuse.

Aetiology of drug dependence

There is no conclusive evidence that drug and alcohol dependence are due to physical or organic factors, either inherited or acquired.

The feature common to all forms of drug dependence is the phenomenon of psychological dependence. The fact that withdrawal from drugs producing physical dependence gives rise to unpleasant symptoms, and that these are ameliorated by giving the drug involved, is not an argument that the withdrawal state has any aetiological significance, neither does it explain why the dependent person started taking the drug in the first place. It is also a fact that repeated doses of a drug must be taken before the symptoms of withdrawal are possible, for example, it usually requires a two-week period of administration of 15-20 mg of morphine four times daily, before its sudden withdrawal will cause clear-cut, yet mild abstinence symptoms.

What is the basis of psychological dependence which seems to be the central aetiological factor?

Bell, the author of a *Current Affairs Bulletin* entitled *Drugs and Addiction*, concluded that 'addiction is usually precipitated by a stressful change in the lives of disturbed individuals, creating circumstances that thrust them into a new and more demanding role. Crises such as these are known as critical role transitions and are recognised as being a time of life in which there is an increased risk of mental illness'.

Among role transitions that may precipitate drug dependence are the change inherent in undertaking more mature and responsible heterosexual activities, the change from childhood to adult status involving areas of adolescent adjustment, and the changes necessitated by the loss of a companion or sexual partner.

Persons predisposed to dependence on drugs and alcohol usually show some personality abnormality, though it is doubtful whether any specific personality type is implicated. If hereditary factors play a part, then it is probably through their effect on personality development. Usually there has existed a disturbed childhood environment with such factors as parental discord or separation and overt or covert rejection of the child who later becomes drug or alcohol dependent.

There appears to be a disproportionately high incidence of drug dependence among parents of children so afflicted, for example, an alcoholic father or a 'pilltaking' mother. On the other hand, where teetotal parents forbid any alcohol in the house and constantly decry the evils of drink, a general interest in alcohol rather than an aversion may be generated in the children, and such a family appears to provide more than its share of alcoholics.

Some parents derive vicarious satisfaction from the misdemeanours of their children, and children are therefore encouraged in subtle ways to engage in antisocial activity into which parents themselves are unable to enter. This could apply to activities that foster drug dependency.

The taking of alcohol or other drugs may be symptomatic of a wide range of psychiatric disorders. If it is found that taking drugs or alcohol relieves tension, a pattern of relieving tension may be established using these agents.

It has been pointed out earlier that numerous drugs have their social use in a variety of cultures. Such cultures embody rules that attempt to control drug abuse, and in the main these are effective. If, for example, a culture is disrupted by a conquering civilisation, as in the case of the Spanish conquest of the Inca civilisation in Peru, such controls break down and the abuse of drugs increases. In this example, the abuse of coca leaves was implicated. The introduction of any drug to a community may lead initially to an epidemic of abuse, as the use and control of the drug takes time to be incorporated into the culture concerned.

Another self-evident factor in the aetiology of drug dependency is the availability of the drugs concerned, which to a large extent determines the variation in addictive experience seen in different cultures.

Following this brief overview of a very complex problem, we shall look at a number of individual syndromes and drugs.

Alcohol dependence syndrome

The I.C.D. describes this as

> a state, psychic and usually physical, resulting from taking alcohol, characterized by behavioural and other responses that always include a compulsion to take alcohol on a continuous or periodic basis in order to experience its psychic effects, and sometimes to avoid the discomfort of its absence; tolerance may or may not be present. A person may be dependent on alcohol and other drugs.

Three subcategories are described, namely acute drunkenness in alcoholism, dipsomania, and chronic alcoholism.

Dipsomania is the term used to describe a periodic craving for alcohol. In many cases this appears to be associated with obsessive-compulsive disorder, the depressed phase of a manic-depressive psychosis or episodes of increased irritability having an epileptic basis. The treatment is that of the underlying condition if present.

Clinical descriptions of the chronic alcoholic disorders are given in Chapter 12 and the student should study these in conjunction with the present chapter.

Management

GENERAL

Treatment is carried out more easily in hospital than at home. If the patient has been drinking recently, alcohol is rapidly or gradually withdrawn according to the patient's ability to co-operate, and to his physical state. In most hospitals however, the giving of alcohol in reducing doses is not an accepted form of treatment for the good reasons that, the duration of its action is relatively short, the margin of safety between toxic cumulative doses and doses sufficient to produce a gradual lowering of blood alcohol level is quite narrow, and the drug provides calories devoid of other appreciable nutrition which may enhance fatty changes in the liver. It is important to stimulate the appetite and give a well balanced diet supplemented by Vitamin B preparations, and perhaps glucose.

PSYCHOTHERAPY

Psychotherapy, either individual or in a group setting, has an important part to play. It should be pointed out that supervision following discharge from hospital is of paramount importance. A relationship commenced as an inpatient should not be denied the alcoholic patient once he leaves hospital. He needs fairly long-term encouragement and support.

DRUGS

Modified insulin treatment may be used to stimulate appetite. Drugs used during alcohol withdrawal are discussed in Chapter 12.

SPECIAL TECHNIQUES

Deconditioning based on Pavlovian principles may be attempted. The patient is given apomorphine hydrochloride by intramuscular injection along with alcohol by mouth. Apomorphine is a powerful emetic and the nausea and vomiting resulting from its administration becomes associated with the use of alcohol. In this way it is hoped to build up an aversion or disgust for alcohol.

Various regimes may be followed in this form of aversion therapy, though patients must be in reasonably good physical condition, as cardiovascular collapse may complicate some regimes. Careful observation of temperature, pulse, respiration, and fluid balance especially urinary output, are essential.

Antabuse (or sulfiram) interferes with the metabolism of alcohol and causes a marked increase in acetaldehyde in the blood. Acetaldehyde has the effect of producing unpleasant symptoms, namely congestion of face and conjunctiva, sweating, tachycardia, giddiness, headache and a feeling of general distress. These symptoms are frequently followed by drowsiness, and sometimes by nausea and vomiting.

Treatment is best commenced in hospital or similar situations where blood pressure and patient's general condition can be closely observed, as symptoms of peripheral cardiovascular failure have occurred on giving a test dose of alcohol. Should this happen, 50 mg of ascorbic acid I.V. should be given immediately, the usual methods of combating shock being implemented in addition.

The procedure consists of giving the patient 0.5 G–1.5 G Antabuse daily for a few days, after which a test dose of 1 fl oz or more of whisky or gin is given. If flushing or other above-mentioned symptoms occur, the patient is ready to go into the world with his Antabuse tablets and instructions to take 0.25 G every morning.

A variant of the technique is to give 0.5 G once or twice followed by an alcoholic drink. This procedure is repeated several times with a view to conditioning the patient against his craving. On discharge the patient is again instructed to take 0.25 G each morning (tablets are manufactured in strengths of 250 mg and 500 mg).

The co-operation of the patient is obviously essential, as is supportive follow-up, for he simply has to leave off his daily medication in order to drink without unpleasant effects.

A contra-indication to Antabuse therapy is diabetes mellitus, and great care should be exercised if the patient suffers from cardiac disease, nephritis, epilepsy or cirrhosis of the liver.

Attention should be given to domestic and environmental conditions.

Spouses and other family members frequently require counselling, and may usefully enter into group therapy with patients.

The moral and suggestive influences of societies such as Alcoholics Anonymous (A.A.) as well as religious organisations, prove helpful to a large number of patients. Al-Anon is an organisation that came into existence for the assistance of spouses and families of alcoholics.

Many failures in therapeutic endeavours to manage the problem of alcoholism are probably the result of inadequate follow-up, leaving the patient 'on his own' before he is ready.

The Withdrawal and Motivational Unit*

With the recent awareness that long-stay 'treatment' of alcoholic people offers no advantage over short-stay treatments, and that the model for treatment existing in psychiatric admission units is not specifically geared to treat alcoholics, special units have developed to meet the needs of this group. At one such unit, 'McKinnon', at The Rozelle Hospital, people are admitted if they meet the criteria of being intoxicated or in acute withdrawal and if they wish to do something about their problem. Medical observation is strict, and should a person be developing delirium tremens or withdrawal fits, appropriate medical treatment is implemented. The crisis of withdrawal is the best time to aid motivation in alcoholic people, and nursing staff, who remain at the bedside as long as necessary, establish a rapport with the patient and explain that the basic choice for each is whether to continue to drink (or take drugs) or to attempt a new life without alcohol. The rapport established at this time is a vital component in the development of trust and the ultimate recovery of the patient.

As soon as possible, patients attend some group meetings which are directive and informative, and others which deal with the steps and principles of the Alcoholics Anonymous programme. A close link with Alcoholics Anonymous is established while in hospital, and families of alcoholic patients are referred to Al-Anon or Alateen where they learn about themselves and the alcoholic person, and share their experiences, strengths and hopes with other people in similar circumstances.

This new look on the problem of alcoholism is encouraging, and one awaits with interest the long term results of this rational and enthusiastic endeavour.

It should be pointed out that these outlines of management follow the medical model treating alcoholic and other drug dependent persons as if they were suffering from diseases. There is in fact considerable debate as to whether these states should rightly be labelled diseases, and perhaps a major rationale for the disease concept is that it is acceptable to mobilise social support and rehabilitation for deviant behaviour only if the deviant is also labelled 'sick'. Another alternative way of dealing with deviant behaviour is by punishment, even to the extent of executing recidividist addicts as is reported to have occurred in one large socialist country in

* The author is indebted to Dr M. Chegwidden, past-Director, 'McKinnon', Rozelle Hospital, New South Wales, for information regarding this unit.

our time. Countries which still place value on individual freedom of action would find this ultimate cure somewhat difficult to countenance.

While health professionals must use the tools at their disposal for the perceived betterment of the affected individual, his family, or society, this is tackling but one aspect of an enormous problem, a large part of which must surely have its roots in a person's perception of his effectiveness within his social system. Maybe the major thrust towards minimising drug dependence and alcoholism should now be directed at factors existing in the broader social context.

Drug dependence

The I.C.D. definition of drug dependence differs little from that of the alcohol dependence syndrome but will be quoted for the sake of completeness:

> A state, psychic and sometimes also physical, resulting from taking a drug, characterized by behavioural and other responses that always include a compulsion to take a drug on a continuous or periodic basis in order to experience its psychic effects, and sometimes to avoid the discomfort of its absence. Tolerance may or may not be present. A person may be dependent on more than one drug.

Morphine type

Drugs of the opiate group (morphine type) which both relieve pain and produce sleep are known as narcotics. Dependence on morphine and other opiates is relatively rare in Western countries, but is becoming more of a problem as the facilities of modern transport become more widespread and while law breakers and other interested parties wish to make big money. It is an interesting fact that crude opium grown in Laos, converted into opium bricks in Bangkok, refined as heroin in Hong Kong and sold on the Western market, appreciates in value some 640 times weight for weight. In other words the poppy growers receive, say, $25.00 for one pound of crude opium, while the final pusher collects $1,000.00 for one ounce* of refined heroin derived from this amount of opium.

Until recently, in Western countries, dependence on the opiates was largely confined to people who had ready access to these drugs, namely, pharmacists, doctors and nurses.

Morphine has the property of tolerance and also leads to physical dependence. Tolerance develops rapidly, depending to a large extent on the frequency of administration. Some addicts have been known to take as much as 2,000-5,000 mg per day in order to try to recapture the original effects of the drug.

When one considers that 16-20 mg of morphine by injection has a powerful analgesic action and frequently leads to somnolence or even deep sleep, one gets some idea of the tremendous tolerance that can develop to this drug.

There are few signs of morphine addiction in the person who is able to maintain regular administration of the drug. Slight drowsiness may or

* These figures were relevant before 1968. Illegal heroin was being sold in Australia in 1972 for $3,000-$4,000 per ounce.

may not be present, meiosis (constriction of the pupils) may be marked, the term 'pin-point pupils' being applied to this state; and multiple small scars may be seen on areas of the anatomy where self-administration using a needle and syringe can be carried out, notably the arms, abdomen and thighs. Bluish scars and needle marks in the region of the veins in the antecubital fossa or forearm may be present if the drug has been 'mainlined'. If, however, the drug or suitable substitute is not available, withdrawal symptoms commence some 12-16 hours after the last dose. They comprise yawning, rhinorrhea, lachrymation, pupillary dilation, sweating, piloerection and restlessness. This state is followed later by muscular aches and twitches, abdominal cramps, anorexia, vomiting, diarrhoea, hypertension, sleeplessness, agitation, profuse sweating and weight loss. Spontaneous seminal emissions may occur in the male and menstrual bleeding in the female. Abstinence phenomena reach their greatest intensity on the second or third day after the last dose of morphine, and subside rapidly over the next week. Complete stabilisation may not occur however, for 6 months or more.

An injection of morphine given during the abstinence syndrome will abort the symptoms but they reappear within 4-6 hours. The giving of a morphine antagonist such as nalorphine to a person dependent on morphine will precipitate withdrawal symptoms which may appear in a matter of minutes, depending on the route of administration. Nalorphine may be used to demonstrate physical dependence on opiates when obvious symptoms and signs are absent. A subcutaneous injection of 3 mg is given, and if this produces the typical withdrawal symptoms it can be assumed that physical dependence on opiates, of one sort or another exists. If there is no reaction in 20 minutes a second injection of 5 mg is given. If this produces no signs after a further 20 minutes, a third and final injection of 7 mg is given. In the absence of signs after the third dose, the test is considered negative.

Other common drugs in this particular group, of which morphine is described as the main example, are, opium itself, heroin (diamorphine) and codeine. Opium is prepared from the sap of the poppy seed capsule, Papaver somniferum. The dried sap takes the form of a brown powder which has a characteristic smell. Opium contains morphine, codeine, papaverine and many other alkaloids, its narcotic action being mainly due to morphine. Opium, used as a drug of addiction, is commonly smoked, but due to the significant aroma produced during its preparation and use, and to the fact that it requires equipment which is not readily disposed of in an emergency, many addicts have turned to heroin which requires a minimum of equipment and which may be inhaled, smoked or injected. Heroin is prepared from morphine and has a similar though 2-3 times more potent action. It causes more respiratory depression and less gastric disturbance and constipation than morphine. Codeine is not as powerful as morphine and is stated to have only one twelfth of morphine's analgesic properties when injected subcutaneously. It has a depressant action on the cough centre and is used as a cough suppressant (linctus codeine). Its use as an analgesic is in the form of codeine phospate, and in association with other mild analgesics, it is used in a range of proprietary preparations.

Synthetics with morphine-like effects

Meperidine (Pethidine) has certain of the properties of both morphine and atropine, having analgesic, antispasmodic and sedative actions. Its analgesic effect is approximately one-eighth that of morphine, and it is widely used in obstetric practice as an analgesic in the second stage of labour.

Methadone (Physeptone) is roughly equivalent to morphine in analgesic activity but has less sedative and euphoric potency, while the analgesic potency of dextropropoxyphene (Doloxene) is about the same as that of codeine.

Opiate poisoning

Opiate poisoning by any of the opiates, their alkaloids or derivatives gives rise to unresponsiveness, slow or periodic breathing, pinpoint pupils, bradycardia (slow pulse), hypotension and hypothermia. In severe cases of opiate poisoning the pupils may be dilated, and the reflexes including the corneal reflex, may be absent. The patient may be cyanotic and have a rapid pulse of poor amplitude. Such patients may require intubation with a cuffed tracheal airway and artifical respiration. One of the morphine antagonists such as nalorphine (Lethidrone) given intravenously in a dose of 3-5 mg will rapidly increase respiration, raise the blood pressure and reduce meiosis. The dose may need to be repeated as required until vital signs remain at acceptable levels. The restoration of consciousness is less readily effected and should not be the primary aim of treatment as one runs the risk of overdosage of the morphine antagonist.

Nalorphine is also used to combat the effects of overdosage of the synthetic analgesics with morphine-like effects mentioned above.

Management of opiate dependence

The management of a patient dependent on the opiates or on the morphine-like synthetic analgesics will probably involve: (1) Drug withdrawal in a drug-controlled institution which can be by rapid reduction over a period of 5-10 days, substituting codeine at a later stage, or by stabilising the patient on methadone and progressively reducing the dose over 3-10 days. (2) General supportive therapy including intravenous infusions of 5% glucose in saline solution where necessary, acetylsalicylic acid for aches and pains, barbiturates or other sedative for sleep, and a good dietary intake. (3) Social and milieu therapy, psychotherapy, counselling with respect to employment and place of residence. (4) A stay of several months in a drug-controlled environment is considered necessary in view of the fact that withdrawal phenomena may continue for as long as 6 months. (5) Follow-up is essential, and there is evidence to suggest that some form of probation for a number of years is a sound policy in this extremely difficult treatment group, whose continued dependence is largely related to deficits in personality. The same may be said for any of the drugs of dependence.

Methadone maintenance

A relatively recent development is that of methadone maintenance clinics where opiate, and particularly heroin addicted persons may attend at prescribed intervals to obtain methadone which is used on the basis that it produces less euphoriant effects than heroin or morphine. The hope is that the addicted person will gradually be able to reduce the dose of methadone until he is drug free. One must remember however, that methadone is also a drug of dependence capable of producing an unpleasant abstinence syndrome on withdrawal. In summing up its value it would seem that it provides a legal substitute for illegal drugs and enables a person to function relatively guiltlessly in society without being preoccupied with the ways and means of obtaining an illegal form of opiate.

Acupuncture

A quite revolutionary form of management of opiate withdrawal symptoms, first described by Wen* and Cheung in Hong Kong in 1973, is to insert acupuncture needles into the lung points in both ears and to pass a 10-volt current at 125 cycles-per-second for 30-40 minutes. A number of treatments is required. Acupuncture needles are not necessary for this procedure, and Dr Margaret Patterson in London has used blunt electrodes with good results. An interesting feature of this method is that some dependent persons lose the craving for opiates at least during the period of treatment and usually for some time afterwards. There would appear to be some merit in this regime which does not require the substitution of another drug of dependence.

Barbiturates

There are a number of barbiturate sedatives with a varying duration of action. Examples of long-acting barbiturates (10-12 hours) are phenobarbitone and barbitone. Amylobarbitone is a medium acting drug (6-8 hours), while pentobarbitone (Nembutal) has a short duration of sedative action (4-6 hours). A person may become dependent on any of the barbiturate sedatives. As with all drugs of dependence, psychic dependence is a feature, and some degree of tolerance develops as does physical dependence. The abstinence syndrome produced by cessation of the drug and its management is described in Chapter 12. Withdrawal symptoms occur on rapid reduction of barbiturates, regardless of their duration of action. The author has observed status epilepticus and delirium tremens precipitated by a doctor in a general practice taking a firm line with a female patient, and abruptly stopping her intake of phenobarbitone, a long acting barbiturate. Convulsions usually appear fifteen or more hours after withdrawal with a peak at thirty hours, though seizures may not occur until the fourth or fifth day.

---

* Wen (1977) has developed a faster technique to detoxify heroin addicts. He uses acupuncture and electrical stimulation (5-10 volts at 125 cycles per second) in combination with a short-acting opiate antagonist, naloxone, which displaces opiates from receptor sites in the brain. The technique does not provide a cure, and Wen advocates psycho social rehabilitation in addition.

Other hypnotics and sedatives or 'tranquillisers'

The bromides and bromureides have been mentioned in Chapter 12. Meprobamate, paraldehyde, chlordiazepoxide and diazepam are misused by some patients, and become drugs of dependence. Some authorities speak of the possibility of amitriptyline leading to dependence, but this has not been the author's experience in his use of this drug.

Cocaine

Cocaine is the alkaloid obtained from coca leaves. In medicine it has been used as a local anaesthetic, either injected or applied topically. Owing to its variable toxic properties it has largely been replaced by safer compounds, but cocaine hydrochloride still has a place in ophthalmology where it is used to produce local anaesthesia, and to dilate the pupil for long periods of time. It also has its use as a local application in oto-rhinolaryngology (E N & T work).

In South America, the chewing of coca leaves dates back to the Inca civilisation. To reduce fatigue and hunger whilst carrying packs over the mountainous tracks, the Andean Indians chewed cuds of coca leaves mixed with lime. Cocaine in its purified form can be taken orally, by injection, or as snuff. Taken for its exhilarating effect, it aids and abets psychic dependence. Tolerance and physical dependence do not occur, therefore no abstinence syndrome occurs on its abrupt withdrawal. Symptoms of cocaine dependence include apprehension and tremulousness. The patient may develop tachycardia, hypertension, mydriasis (dilated pupils), and needle marks over veins may be in evidence.

If large amounts are taken, psychotic symptoms including visual and auditory hallucinations are likely to develop. Tactile hallucinations, which seem to the patient to be insects crawling under the skin (formication), are not uncommon. Delusions of a paranoid nature may develop, contributing to the sometimes violent behaviour of cocaine abusers. Withdrawal is easily accomplished with a co-operative patient as an abstinence syndrome does not occur.

Cannabis (hashish*, marihuana, hemp)

The cannabis plant grows readily in many parts of the world and is seen in places as divergent as South East Asia and New South Wales. It may be seen in its abundance on sale in many village markets in South Vietnam and grows in its wild state in the Hunter River Valley in New South Wales. The North American name for the drug is 'pot' and this is also its common appellation in Australia. Drug subcultures develop their own terminologies and while a 'reefer' was the common name for a cigarette made from the dried blossoms and top leaves of cannabis sativa, the current 'in-word' would appear to be a 'joint'.

The effects of smoking marihuana seem to depend on a variety of factors, the common ones being disorientation, a loss of sense of time, and hallucinations. Smokers may show drowsiness, tremor, ataxia and

* Hashish is largely made from the resin of the Cannabis sativa or Indian Hemp plant which contains the active constituents. It is several times more potent than preparations made for smoking.

nystagmus, and increased sensitivity to pain and touch. Overdosage may give rise to tachycardia, diarrhoea, vomiting and sweating, and may produce depression or obvious psychotic experiences.

Tolerance to marihuana is not developed, neither is physical dependence, and hence cessation of its use does not lead to withdrawal phenomena. The main active constituent of cannabis, namely tetrahydrocannabinol (THC) appears to accumulate in the fat the same way as does DDT and long term deleterious effects of the drug appear to be a possibility. It is also not known whether the offspring of a pot-smoking mother are affected, though evidence from its experimental use in rodents would suggest this is a possibility.

Not a great deal is known yet about the pharmacology of marihuana, and it is a foolish man who proclaims it to be a safe drug at this stage of knowledge. Thalidomide was an excellent hypnotic and sedative, and was an acceptable drug in medicine for some time before its drastic effects on unborn babies became known.

Amphetamine type and other psychostimulants

Included in this category of drugs are amphetamine (Benzedrine), dexamphetamine (Dexedrine, Phetadex), methylamphetamine (Methedrine), phenmetrazine (Preludin, Anorex), diethylpropion (Tenuate), chlorphentermine (Lucofen), and a more recently introduced drug, fenfluramine (Ponderax).

The last-mentioned drug is claimed to have no central nervous stimulating properties, a claim also made for diethylpropion, but the chemical structure of all these drugs is so similar that it seems premature to make such claims before they have been widely used clinically.

The older of these drugs have had considerable use in medicine as appetite suppressants for obesity, and some doctors prescribed them for 'mild depression' and 'states of fatigue'. The rapid development of tolerance wherein larger and larger doses are required to reproduce the initial anorexic and euphoric effects make them of little clinical use in the management of obesity and of depressive illnesses. Added to this is the fact that, when medication ceases, some patients feel 'let down' and experience depression. As a result of the great propensity for abuse of the amphetamine group of drugs, a number of them have been restricted to use in specific conditions only.

The degree of central nervous stimulation varies from one member of this group of drugs to another, depending on the side chain attached to the basic chemical structure. The following comments refer mainly to amphetamine, dextroamphetamine and methylamphetamine, drugs which, to date, have been most commonly abused, though it should be remembered that the other drugs mentioned would appear to have the same propensity for abuse.

Abuse may commence following the use of these drugs in the treatment of obesity, or it may develop from a group experience where young people experiment together to get a 'thrill'. Students and truck drivers who initially wish to stay awake may become dependent. The contents of Benzedrine inhalers, used to alleviate nasal congestion, were chewed before the contents of such apparatus was changed. Amphetamines are mainly taken as pills, and enormous quantities can be taken in a day, due to the rapid tolerance that develops. In recent years large quantities of phenmetrazine in Sweden, and methylamphetamine (speed, crystal, meth) in psychedelic ghettos in the United States of America have been injected intravenously ('mainlined') in a cyclical fashion.

Amphetamine abusers may first use the oral route, later 'snorting' crystalline methylamphetamine, finally seeking the 'rush' or 'flash' which follows immediately upon intravenous injection. A 'speed run' continues for a number of days, the addict 'mainlining' increasing doses 3-5 times daily, the increase being necessitated by rapidly developing tolerance. Such addicts have been called 'speedfreaks'. During a 'binge', death may occur from a paranoid miscalculation of the environment, or by injection of adulterated or contaminated material. Some users may develop homicidal rages. The 'speed run' is followed by a severe apathetic depression which may lead to suicide.

Dr Sidney Cohen who described the 'speedfreak' phenomenon, has the following to say,' . . . the disorganisation of personality, the disintegration of judgment, the deterioration of health, leaves the speedfreak in a limbo, neither psychically alive nor physically dead'.

Physical dependence does not occur with amphetamine use and so no characteristic abstinence symptoms develop. As indicated above however, on cessation of the drug the person may feel 'let down' and depressed.

Mention has already been made of the psychotic state resembling paranoid schizophrenia that may be associated with amphetamine abuse. Methylphenidate (Ritalin), though having a different chemical formula from the amphetamine group of drugs, also has a stimulant effect on the central nervous system. It has a place, as has methedrine, in certain abreactive techniques, where it is given by intravenous injection. It is also obtainable in tablet form. In some countries, legislative restrictions have been placed on this drug owing to the potential for its abuse.

Mixtures of drugs such as dexamphetamine and amylobarbitone have been produced in single tablet form. Drinamyl (purple hearts) is one such preparation and carries with it the same dangers as its individual constituents.

Brief mention will be made of the habit of sniffing. Glue containing toluene has had a vogue. Ether, petrol and lighter fluid have also been sniffed to produce some sort of exhilaration or to alleviate anxiety. At times other organic solvents, for example, paint thinners have been used by various subjects.

Hallucinogens

Included in this group are such drugs as mescaline and lysergic acid diethylamide (LSD_{25}).

tory of Mescaline and LSD_{25}

effects of mescaline (3,4,5-trimethoxyphenylethlamine) were pro-
wn to Aztec medicine before the conquest of the country by

Cortez (1485-1547). In the early sixteenth century, the 'prophetic' qualities of peyoth, the native name of a cactus preparation, were described. A pharmacologist named Lewin found that peyoth was in wide use among Red Indian tribes in Mexico and in North America near the Mexican border, particularly the Mexcalero Apaches who developed the cult of peyotism, and after whom the preparation is named. Indians used to chew mescal buttons (Peyoth) which Lewin (1888) discovered were part of a cactus plant.

It is said to take some hours of chewing before the mescal buttons produce symptoms which include visual hallucinations, depersonalization, and distortions of time. Elaborate ceremonies were associated with the gathering, preparing and the taking of the preparation by the Indians. In about 1900, the use of the drug spread to several Indian tribes in the reservations of North America. The use of mescal was originally associated with pagan rites in which peyoth was regarded as god-like. The Indian tribes to the north had been converted to Christianity, and the chewing of mescal buttons became customary among these converts at religious festival gatherings. The practice still exists among some Indian tribes in the south-west corner of the United States of America.

The preparation found its way to Europe, and various quite well-known men of science tried the effect of the drug on themselves in the late nineteenth and early twentieth centuries.

Lysergic Acid Diethylamide (LSD_{25}) was discovered by chance by a Swiss chemist, A. Hoffman, while he and a colleague, A. Stoll, were investigating the constitution of ergot in 1943. The actions of the drug in humans was first described by W.A. Stoll in 1947.

Clinical use

Mescaline appears to have been little-used clinically, but there was a vogue in the 1960s using LSD_{25} as an adjunct to individual or group psychotherapy mainly in the treatment of neurotic and personality disorders. In some patients it appeared to free the expression of thoughts and emotions connected with events of the past. This implies an increased ability to remember past events, and some patients would appear to experience the same intensity and quality of emotions that were present at the time of the remembered experiences.

There is no evidence that the clinical use of lysergic acid diethylamide has any advantage over other forms of therapy, and in view of this and its inherent dangers as well as the inordinate use of staff time entailed in maintaining constant observation, it is difficult to justify its continuance.

What follows, though largely of historical interest only, will give an idea of some of the effects of LSD on users.

For clinical use, LSD_{25} was prepared in ampoules of 1 ml containing 100 microgrammes. The clear solution was ingested orally, given subcutaneously, intramuscularly or intravenously.

Depending on the route of administration, physiological symptoms occur from ½-1 hour after taking the drug, and they include dilated pupils, slight increase in pulse rate, sensations of cold, numbness and paraesthesiae of the extremities, dizziness and nausea (*cf.* motion sickness) which is rarely followed by vomiting.

Psychic disturbances commence ½-1½ hours after administration, again depending on the route. These include blurring of vision followed by visual illusions, bright lights, patterns, floating colours. Distortion of body image of self and others is not uncommon. (One young woman with problems relating to her aggression, while under the effects of LSD saw her hands as enormous and destructive.) Impairment of pain sensation and spatial discrimination, inability to complete sentences, confusion and thought block, disorientation for time and place, depersonalization and stimulation of memory for past events, all form part of the 'drug psychosis' produced.

The state of psychic disturbance fluctuates in intensity, and the patient passes in and out of it, retaining insight into the fact that his sometimes very bizarre symptoms are due to the LSD administered.

Such insight however, does not minimise the anxiety felt by some people, and it is quite common for a person taking LSD to become depressed and even suicidal. Such symptoms no doubt depend on the individual's personality, on current difficulties, and on other factors in his background. The author has seen one young man in a state of severe depression precipitated by lysergic acid, decide that the only logical thing to do was to throw himself in the path of a moving bus. He, in fact, had to be restrained from carrying out his intention. On the other hand, LSD may produce a feeling of euphoria.

The commencing dose is low, e.g. 50 microgrammes, and is increased at subsequent sessions up to 400 microgrammes, depending on the patient's response. Too large a dose may lead to coma and even death.

Once over the initial physical and early psychic disturbances caused by LSD, the patient will usually talk freely of incidents and feelings, the most productive period often being about three hours after administration of the drug.

The effects of LSD may last several hours if not terminated by chlorpromazine 50-100 mg orally, or 50 mg I.M., or by amylobarbitone 150-300 mg orally.

Certain post-LSD symptoms such as prolonged feelings of euphoria followed by depression, or protracted depression of suicidal intensity may occur. A return of the symptoms experienced initially may occur a week or so later, and in addition, a psychotic episode may be precipitated.

The possibility exists that large doses of LSD_{25} may damage chromosomes.

What has been said about the effects of lysergic acid diethylamide under the anachronistic heading 'Clinical use' applies to those who misuse it, and, in some bizarre fashion, appear to become dependent on it. In this latter setting, the language changes and one speaks of 'acid' and 'trips' or 'acid drop-ins' when referring to parties with 'acid' on the menu.

Management of drug dependence

No special comment has been made on the management of dependence on each particular drug, but the factors in the aetiology require elucidation and management where possible, and the principles outlined in the management of alcoholism and of dependence on opium and its related compounds should be followed where applicable.

Terminology

In this chapter, the terms 'addict' or 'addiction' have been used as shorthand synonymous with 'drug dependent person' or 'state of drug dependency'. Terminology surrounding this subject is confusing, and one sees terms such as habituation, abuse and dependency used interchangeably. At one time, 'addiction' was used to refer to only those drugs which produced a state of physical dependence and hence abstinence phenomena, while 'habituation' or 'psychic dependence' referred to recurrent use of those drugs which did not lead to physical dependence. Surely however, one can be said to be habituated to those drugs that cause physical dependence, hence 'habituation' and 'addiction' are not mutually exclusive.

To clarify a confused area of terminology and to modify the prejudiced and punitive attitudes of society and the law to the concept of 'addiction', an Expert Committee of the World Health Organisation was responsible for the elimination of the terms 'addiction' and 'habituation' from the *Eighth* and *Ninth Revisions of the International Classification of Diseases* the latter of which we are following. The term proposed to replace both 'drug addiction' and 'drug habituation' was 'drug dependence'. Its characteristics will vary with the agent involved, and this must be made clear by designating the particular type of drug of dependence in each specific case—for example, drug dependence of morphine type, of cocaine type, of cannabis type, of barbiturate type, of amphetamine type, etc'.

The author of the *Current Affairs Bulletin* entitled *Drugs and Addiction*, referred to earlier in this chapter, has chosen not to talk about 'drug dependence' but to use the term 'addiction', which he defines as 'the abuse of drugs to the extent that the health, family or social life, or the occupation of the individual is harmed'.

Some text books still use specific terms for dependence on particular drugs such as morphinism and cocainism. One wonders whether dependence on cannabis could be referred to as 'cannab(al)ism'!

NOTE: Though the terms 'addiction' and 'abuse' have been used somewhat loosely in this chapter, it is emphasized that for recording purposes, the term to be used is 'drug dependence'.

Nondependent abuse of drugs

The I.C.D gives nondependent abuse of drugs a special coding and

> includes cases where a person, for whom no other diagnosis is possible, has come under medical care because of the maladaptive effect of a drug on which he is not dependent and that he has taken on his own initiative to the detriment of his health or social functioning.

Nondependent abuse of drugs may be secondary to psychiatric disorder. The student is invited to turn to Appendix I for glossary descriptions of nondependent abuse of drugs.

18

PSYCHOSOMATIC DISORDERS

Introduction

Although the relationship between mind (psyche) and body (soma) has fascinated man for centuries it is only since the 1920s that the discipline we know as psychosomatic medicine came into being. Prior to this the relationship between mind and body exercised the minds of philosophers only. Early studies into this branch of medicine tended to be philosophical and anecdotal. In the last two decades however, increasingly more stringent research methodology is helping to define more clearly what is fact and what is fiction in the many hypotheses that have been propounded to explain the relationship between mind and body.

Psychosomatic medicine concerned itself initially with a limited number of physical diseases in the genesis of which psychological factors appeared to play an important part, but the concept of psychosomatic medicine has widened immensely during the past few decades. It is now appreciated that all illnesses have psychological aspects that influence their cause, precipitation, manifestation, course and outcome, and all illnesses, both mental and physical, have psychological and somatic components. Furthermore, man is part of a social environment, and this environment, as we have seen earlier in our section dealing with factors in the causation of mental illness, exerts a variety of forces upon him.

Nowadays, psychosomatic medicine, rather than concerning itself with discrete disease entities, is seen as a particular approach to illness which studies the interrelationships of psychological, organic and social factors. Sheehan and Hackett of Harvard Medical School elegantly define psychosomatic medicine as 'the study of the reciprocal relationship among sociological, psychological and biological factors in maintaining health and in influencing the onset and course of disease'.

Difficulties have existed and still do exist in the definition of boundaries of this branch of medicine, as evidenced in the many differing titles given to it in a variety of illness classifications. The present I.C.D. makes no reference to psychosomatic disorders as such but covers the majority of states considered as being psychosomatic disorders under two separate headings. The first of these is *Physiological malfunction arising from mental factors*, under which conditions not associated with tissue damage are grouped; and the second is entitled *Psychic factors associated with diseases classified elsewhere.* In this second group of disorders tissue damage has occurred.

Examples of conditions falling under the first rubric are: psychogenic torticollis, hyperventilation, cardiac neurosis, psychogenic pruritus, aerophagy (air swallowing), and psychogenic dysmenorrhoea.

In the second group such examples as psychogenic asthma, dermatitis, peptic ulcer, and ulcerative colitis are included. Students are invited to turn to Appendix I (pages 383, 388) for the glossary notes describing these two groups of disorders.

In describing some representative conditions usually included among the psychosomatic disorders no attempt will be made to place them in either category of disorder described in the I.C.D. and mentioned above. It is left to the student to undertake this. Before describing these conditions under the headings of the systems affected, a brief look will be taken at the anatomical and physiological substrates through which the mind may influence the body.

Aetiology

It has never been demonstrated that emotional or psychological factors alone can produce a psychosomatic disorder. The evidence points to some physiological vulnerability in a specific organ (or organs), probably constitutionally determined, causing or allowing it to be affected by psychological or emotional factors.

It is normal for bodily or somatic changes to occur when one experiences such emotions as grief, rage or anxiety. When the emotion has passed, the body's homeostatic mechanisms cause a normal state of equilibrium in the healthy person to be resumed.

There are certain individuals however, who are organically vulnerable to emotional arousal, and if the arousal is sufficiently strong or protracted and a normal state of equilibrium is not achieved, pathological lesions develop in the vulnerable organs.

In summary, it may be stated that psychosomatic diseases are due to a chronic exaggerated state of the normal physiological expression of emotion, affecting a particular constitutionally-determined vulnerable system or organ. If long-continued, the emotional reactions may lead to structural damage of the organs. Among the systems and organs affected are: the respiratory system giving rise to asthma, various parts of the gastro-intestinal system leading to duodenal ulcer or ulcerative colitis, the skin, etc. These are dealt with more fully below.

We now know that both continued psychological disturbances, and organ or system vulnerability are crucial factors in the development of psychosomatic disease. The psychological disturbance or emotional arousal is dependent on a variety of stress factors, both internal and external.

Referring to our earlier chapter dealing with factors in the causation of psychiatric illness (Chapter 10), and to the variety of psychiatric disorders already covered, it becomes evident that emotional conflict or anxiety can lead to a variety of clinical manifestations. Why should it lead to psychosomatic disorders and not for example, to neurotic illnesses in some people? Is it due to the fact that the defence mechanisms leading to neurotic symptomatology have failed, or is it due to some inherited or constitutional factor which determines the type of clinical manifestation that will occur? There is really no answer to this question in our present state of knowledge, but one would tend to favour the latter proposition. People with psychosomatic illness can concurrently display neurotic symptomatology, as indeed we all can.

What is said above does not do justice to the many theories developed and investigations carried out that are producing a clearer picture of the aetiology of these disorders. One should mention the work of Thomas Holmes who showed that life events or life changes require physical adaptation, and the greater the adaptation required in a particular time the more likely is a broad range of physical or psychiatric illnesses to ensue, including those initially narrowly designated as psychosomatic. Some hypotheses do not postulate a state of anxiety or conflict as being necessary for the development of these disorders. A person's mode of coping with stressful stimuli, itself influenced by his psychological structure, has a bearing on the development or otherwise of these disorders. It has been found that body image perception bears a relationship to the site in which symptoms develop. The field is indeed a complex one and the interested student is referred to more comprehensive texts.

With regard to organ vulnerability or susceptibility, one might ask what makes a particular organ vulnerable? Apart from some constitutional or inherited weakness, such factors as physical trauma, infection, or state of nutrition of the organ may be predisposing factors. Also it has been shown that the action of the automonic nervous system can to some extent be conditioned, which raises the question of early 'pathological' conditioning in determining the organ or site affected. Certain conditions such as asthma may have a largely allergic basis, but attacks may develop in the absence of the usual precipitating allergens, for example, when a patient develops an asthma attack in the presence of artificial flowers bearing no pollen.

Certain features present in sufferers from psychosomatic disorders warrant attention, for they are of aetiological significance. Among these are, firstly, the psychological stress situation that provokes the reaction is usually characteristic and repetitive for the same patient; and secondly, the emotional conflict that develops as a result of the stress situation is usually characteristic for a particular patient and reflects weak points in his emotional make-up.

Anatomical and physiological considerations

A consideration of the functions of anatomical pathways involved in psychosomatic disorders will serve to underline the intimate relationship existing between mind and body. Indeed, mind and body would appear to be but two avenues of expression of the functioning of the human organism. The hypothalamus and limbic system (Fig. 12) are concerned with emotion, and discharge from the hypothalamic nuclei occurs simultaneously upwards to the higher centres giving rise to the subjective aspect of emotions, and downwards via the autonomic nervous system (sympathetic and parasympathetic) to produce the external aspects of emotion, that is, the symptoms and signs associated with emotion apart from the subjective feelings.

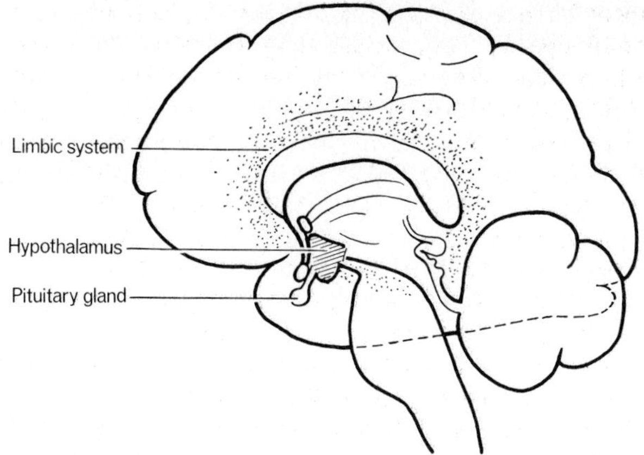

Fig. 12. Hypothalamus, limbic system and related structures

Also, the hypothalamus exerts control over the anterior pituitary gland, probably by adrenergic secretions passing to the gland via the vascular portal system. In turn, the secretions of the anterior pituitary gland, or pituitary hormones, play a part in regulating the secretions of the other endocrine glands, for example, the adrenals, thyroid and sex glands.

These other endocrine glands have a 'feed-back' regulatory effect on the anterior pituitary.

The hypothalamus influences, and is influenced by, the neocortex which is concerned with symbolic or ideational functions. It bears a similar relationship to the limbic system, or visceral brain concerned with feelings, to the reticular activating system, and to the various endocrine systems, and it discharges impulses via the autonomic nervous system.

These are the various complicated pathways through which psychosomatic disorders are probably produced. For example, during an attack of asthma precipated essentially by emotional factors, the parasympathetic activity on the lungs mediated through the vagus nerve causes constriction of the bronchioles and increased bronchial secretion. In the early stages of hypertensive vascular disease, the rise in blood pressure is thought to be due to activity of the sympathetic nervous system causing constriction of arterioles. In addition, noradrenaline which also constricts arterioles, is produced due to the stimulation of the andrenal medulla via the sympathetic nervous system.

With this background of the mechanisms involved in their production, we shall now look at some of the diagnostic categories subsumed under the term 'psychosomatic disorders'.

Skin

The skin, existing as it does at the interface of the individual and the environment, is an important factor in the maintenance of bodily homeostasis, particularly through mechanisms of heat and fluid regulation. It also readily reflects emotional changes, and for many centuries such descriptions as pale with fear, or white or crimson with rage have been in common use, though psychosomatic skin disorders are not due to psychogenic factors alone. They are multicausal and determined by a combination of constitutional and acquired factors, emotion being but one. Allergy for example, has a large part to play in the origin of many skin disorders, while systemic or local infections, an excess or deficiency of sunlight, damp, cold, local irritations, etc., are implicated in the development of others.

No specific personality type or unconscious conflict has been found to be related to particular skin conditions, and the exacerbations of skin disorders follows a wide variety of psychological stresses, particularly loss. Neurodermatitis and flare-ups of psoriasis may be preceded by psychological stresses, as may pruritus and urticaria.

Musculo-skeletal system

Included in this group of disorders are conditions due to muscle spasm or cramps, leading to back-ache or 'fibrositis' and other myalgias including some cases of tension headaches. Tremor, apparent paralysis and torticollis may occur. Joint disorders, presumably arising from abnormal muscular tension, are described. Rheumatoid arthritis is regarded by many as a psychosomatic condition.

An interesting patient was referred to the author following observation for possible peptic ulcer. He was an army artillery sergeant who, while on active service, developed marked epigastric cramping pain. On examination, the muscles in this area (upper half of rectus abdominus muscles) were in spasm. He exhibited obsessive-compulsive personality characteristics, had been under some pressure and was angry with his superiors because for some time his gun crew was working short-handed. When rested and given an opportunity to ventilate his unhappy position, the spasm gradually subsided and he resumed duty.

Respiratory system

The main clinical disorder in which psychogenic factors affect the respiratory system is asthma. Hyperventilation which may lead to tetany, vasomotor rhinitis, sighing respirations, and hiccoughs may also have emotional factors in their aetiology.

Asthma

The symptoms of asthma, which may be defined as dyspnoea with wheezing, are due to bronchial obstruction mainly caused by bronchospasm and bronchial oedema. Mucous plugs also form, adding to respiratory difficulty.

Among the factors implicated in asthma for which there is clinical and experimental evidence are allergy, infection, physical agents, and emotional factors. One or more of these may precipitate an attack.

Arguments have been put forward in the past contending that specific emotional factors cause psychological asthma. For example, it has been stated that asthma represents a suppressed cry for help; it occurs when there is a separation or threat of separation from the mother; it results from suppressed aggression, etc. Though these specific factors apply in some cases, they certainly do not in all. Professor W. Linford Rees (London, 1958) studied a group of 800 asthmatics and found that stressful life situations preceded the initial attack in 12% of asthmatic children, 36% of asthmatics between 16 and 45 years of age and 45% of those having onset over 45 years. The types of life situations associated with subsequent attacks were similar to those associated with the initial attack.

Potentially stressful psychosocial situations relevant to the development of asthma varied according to the age of the individual, and Professor Rees found the following relevant factors in people studied by him:

Children—parental lack, faulty parental attitudes, particularly those of rejection, overprotection or perfectionism.

Elderly—adjustment difficulties following retirement or the death of a spouse were of particular importance.

While working as a senior registrar in an English general hospital, the author saw out-patients for a consultant who was away. Among these was a young lady who frequently developed asthma attacks when she was with her fiance. From the history it appeared that there was a large emotional factor in the precipitation of her attacks, so a subsequent appointment was made for her to see the consultant to whom she had been referred. At her next attendance, the consultant was again away, and the young lady, free from wheezing when she arrived at the Outpatients' Department, developed a severe asthma attack as she entered the consulting room and saw the author and not the expected consultant. She was angry at seeing 'the boy' once again and not a consultant. After being given the opportunity to express her feelings of anger, her attack abated and she left without a wheeze. This is one example where emotional factors predominated, and many similar cases are seen by physicians and psychiatrists.

Management

In the management of the asthmatic, each possible factor must be carefully weighed and appropriately treated. In such multicausal conditions the co-operative efforts of at least the physician and psychiatrist may well be indicated. As a nurse or doctor, one must never lose sight of the fact that patients are indeed people with worries and conflicts that they may wish to ventilate, and even in a busy hospital situation they should be given the opportunity to relate in some way to one or more members of the staff. In some instances this may do more for the patient than drugs, as evidenced by the following anecdote.

A middle-aged male patient in a general hospital was in status asthmaticus and was currently being administered a cortisone preparation by intravenous drip, having run the gamut of other then-used drugs. His general condition had deteriorated and a consultant psychiatrist was asked to see him. For the first time, in hospital at least, he had the opportunity to talk to someone about the multitude of things that concerned him, with the result that before many hours had passed his breathing was easier, and drug therapy was able to be discontinued.

This brief description of asthma and its management concentrates on psychological factors. The condition however, requires the expertise of a number of subspecialties in medicine for the elucidation of causal factors and for a rational management programme.

Cardiovascular system

Included among the diagnostic entities subsumed under psychosomatic disorders of the cardiovascular system are a number of different forms of cardiac arrhythmia, the effort syndrome or 'cardiac neurosis' (also known as neurocirculatory asthenia or Da Costa's syndrome), vasodepressor syncope, essential hypertension, and migraine.

The exact role of psychological factors in the aetiology of coronary arterial disease is unclear, though emotional factors are known to contribute to functional coronary insufficiency in patients with established coronary arteriosclerosis. Type A personalities described by Friedman and Rosenman have a higher incidence of first attacks of coronary artery disease than do their counterparts, Type B personalities. Type A personalities exhibit competitive drive, ambition, an inclination to multiple commitments, a chronic sense of urgency and an acute awareness of time pressures or deadlines. Whether this coronary personality profile (Type A personality) is causative or whether environmental stress leading to Type A behaviour is the major factor still requires elucidation.

Overactivity of the vasoconstrictor nerves under the influence of emotions, would certainly appear to be one of the factors in the production of Raynaud's phenomenon in which recurrent symmetrical vasospasm occurs in the extremities, affecting the hands in particular.

The clinical features of 'cardiac neurosis' or effort syndrome include breathlessness, fatigue, left mammary pain, dizziness, headache, and sweating. The breathlessness is out of all proportion to the amount of exertion undertaken.

There is a sensation of inability to take a satisfactory breath, and a deep sighing type of respiration is characteristic. The pulse is rapid, and sweating, flushing and tremor are usually present.

So-called vasodepressor syncope or fainting, is due to acute peripheral circulatory inadequacy occurring for example, under conditions of pain, anxiety or shock. The theory of causation proposed by Engel is that the individual lacks the freedom to take appropriate action against his fear or anxiety. In response to fear, there occurs increased muscle blood flow in preparation for flight or fight. If no action ensues, there is no reflex increase in cardiac output, no contraction of muscles to redistribute blood, and no vasoconstriction in other parts of the vascular bed, thus leaving the blood pooled in the muscle masses of the extremities producing a relative ischaemia and anoxia of the brain, which in turn leads to blurred vision, light-headedness, loss of consciousness and falling. This type of syncope is seen in some people awaiting medical procedures such as a venipuncture or injection. The assumption of a horizontal position during premonitory symptoms of sweating, nausea, restlessness, muscle weakness and pallor will usually avert syncope.

Essential hypertension is the term used to refer to the sustained elevation of systolic and diastolic arterial blood pressure in the absence of specific pathology producing such a rise. The emotions exert an influence on the clinical course of essential hypertension, but the mechanism and role of psychological factors in the aetiology of the disease are not clearly understood. Mention has been made above of possible mechanisms (page 270ff).

Migraine

The migraine syndrome consists of headaches, unilateral or bilateral (in one third of cases), which are frequently accompanied by nausea and vomiting, photophobia, and scalp tenderness. About half the patients suffer from symptoms such as aphasia, paraesthesiae and visual disturbances (flashing lights, zig-zag fortification sprectra, blind spots or loss of half the field of vision) either before or during an attack. In a small proportion of cases, weakness or paraesthesia of half of the body may be experienced. The migraine headache occurs more commonly in women, and persists for less than 24 hours in about two-thirds of sufferers. It would appear to bear no primary relationship to epilepsy or allergy. The vasoconstrictive phase of migraine however, may precipitate epileptic phenomena in people with low fit thresholds, and it is also possible that allergic disturbances may trigger a migraine attack.

Evidence would suggest that migraine is largely due to an hereditary paroxysmal vascular instability, each episode of which comprises a phase of arterial vasoconstriction which is mainly intracranial, and a phase of arterial vasodilation which is mainly extracranial.

The intracranial vasoconstriction, along with other factors, is responsible for the neurological symptoms mentioned above, while the actual pain of the migraine headache results from dilatation of arteries, particularly extracranial or scalp vessels, but also to some extent from dilatation of cranial vessels. In addition to the distension of arteries and increased blood flow, a 'sterile inflammation' of the arterial wall occurs.

The importance of personality and stress factors in the genesis of migraine headaches appears to vary, whether seen through the eyes of the neurologist or psychiatrist. A broad spectrum of personality profiles and specific conflicts have been found in migraine sufferers. Emotional stress, or the relaxation that occurs after such stress, precipitates attacks in vulnerable individuals. Psychotherapy or some form of relaxation therapy with or without hypnotic induction may be of value in this group.

Haemic and lymphatic system

Emotional factors appear to have some effect on the clotting mechanisms of blood, and they may increase the red blood cell count and blood volume due to contraction of the spleen.

Gastro-intestinal system

In this group of disorders are included such conditions as duodenal ulcer, ulcerative colitis, irritable colon (spastic colon, mucous colitis), constipation and diarrhoea (without organic causes). Anorexia nervosa and some types of obesity are included among the psychosomatic disorders in some classifications, but in the glossary followed in this book they fall under the title of our next chapter, 'Special symptoms'. As an example of factors operating in the production of psychosomatic disorders of the gastrointestinal system, we shall look a little more closely at duodenal ulcer.

Duodenal ulcer

A duodenal ulcer, which is a break in the integrity of the duodenal mucosa, only occurs in the presence of acid and pepsin, both of which are secreted by the parietal cell mass of the stomach lining. A duodenal ulcer is one of the peptic ulcers, so-called because they develop in areas of intestinal mucosa which come into contact with the digestive agent, pepsin. From a physiological point of view, the development of a duodenal ulcer is dependent on the balance between the digestive properties of acid plus pepsin, and the resistance of the duodenal mucosa. The intra-intestinal factors which affect mucosal resistance include mucus, nutrition, blood supply and hormonal factors. Patients who suffer from duodenal ulcer have a very high gastric acid and pepsin concentration in the stomach, the level of which is controlled by genetic influences.*

Evidence that emotions play a part in gastric secretions was published in 1943, in an article on human gastric function by S. Wolf and H. G. Wolff. Wolf and Wolff described the case of a patient, Tom, who had a gastric fistula through which they were able to observe the gastric mucosa and its secretions. Tom's feelings were correlated with his gastric secretions, gastric motility, and vascularity. It was found that these functions were depressed when he was sad or frightened, and increased when he felt angry, resentful or anxious.

Other evidence for the relationship between emotions and peptic ulcer, was shown by French *et al.*, in 1954, when they described the production of peptic ulcers in monkeys by electrical sitimulation of the hypothalamus, an area known to be intimately related to emotional states.

Alexander has shown that most patients with peptic ulcers wish to remain in a dependent, infantile situation where they can be cared for. Such a wish, productive of low self-esteem, is in conflict with the adult ego's pride and aspiration for independence and is therefore denied and repressed. Sufferers compensate by aggression, hard work and ambition, and become chronically anxious and angry. The connection between such emotions and high gastric acidity and pepsin level is difficult to ascertain but still very probable.

Also, the 'adult' model used does not make it easy to understand why children sometimes develop duodenal ulcers. Presumably though, the early incorporation of parental attitudes and standards of behaviour could produce the same end result.

Apart from hypersecretion of acid and pepsin, and the particular conflict over dependency and the striving to be independent, there is usually some external stress factor that mobilises the dependency-independency conflict precipitating the development of a break in the integrity of the duodenal mucosa, giving rise to the clinical picture of

---

* Further evidence of genetic factors lies in the fact that peptic ulcer occurs more commonly in people of blood group O than in people of other blood groups.

duodenal ulcer summed up in the description of 'periodic, post-prandial pain, relieved by powders, pabulum and pewking'.

To summarise the factors leading to duodenal ulcer, it would appear that the following are necessary:

1. A sustained rate of gastric hypersecretion of hydrochloric acid and pepsins, probably genetically determined.
2. The presence of a conflict related to the persistence of strong infantile wishes to be loved and cared for, and the repudiation of these wishes by the adult ego.
3. Exposure to an environmental situation which mobilises conflict and induces psychic tension.

Much is yet to be learned about coping and defence mechanisms of duodenal ulcer patients when they are under stress, and perhaps the elucidation of these could lead to greater understanding and more refined management of these patients.

Genito-urinary system

The genito-urinary system has both urinary and reproductive functions. Symptoms or conditions of the urinary system which may arise on the basis of psychogenic factors, and which are included in our classification as psychosomatic disorders, include frequency of micturition and retention of urine.

Conditions affecting the male reproductive system are premature ejaculation and impotence, while females may exhibit a number of symptoms including frigidity, pseudocyesis (false pregnancy), amenorrhoea, metrorrhagia, dysmenorrhoea, dyspareunia, vaginismus, and mastalgia.

The artificiality of splitting the body into discrete systems is exemplified by the fact that impotence, amenorrhoea and metrorrhagia, as symptoms of psychosomatic disorders, may well have endocrine factors implicated, the latter themselves being affected by psychogenic influences.

Endocrine system

Under the sub-heading 'anatomical and physiological considerations,' we have mentioned the complicated interrelationships between the limbic system, the anterior pituitary, thyroid, adrenals and sex glands, and one cannot without a great deal of conjecture go much further than to say that these anatomical and biochemical pathways are doubtlessly involved in the maintenance of bodily homeostasis, an upset in which may lead to disordered function.

Management

It will have been noted that the majority of conditions mentioned have multiple factors in their causation, and a variety of physical presentations. These facts underscore the necessity for having a co-operative approach in management, involving both medical and psychiatric services.

Physical treatments used in other psychiatric disorders have little or no place in the management programme unless other more specific indications are concurrently present. Sedatives and tranquillisers may well afford symptomatic relief.

In caring for these patients, first class physical nursing is important, and a warning should be given that probing into aspects of the personal life of patients with psychosomatic disorders will do little good, and may in fact be quite harmful. The patient is a person, and not 'the ulcer in Bed 6'. The nurse's most useful role, psychologically speaking, is to provide the accepting emotional climate in which the patient is best able to express his feelings.

19

SPECIAL SYMPTOMS; STRESS AND ADJUSTMENT REACTIONS; DISTURBANCES OF CONDUCT

SPECIAL SYMPTOMS OR SYNDROMES

These may be described as

> conditions in which an outstanding symptom or group of symptoms is not manifestly part of a more classifiable condition.

They are neither associated with nor secondary to organic or functional mental disorders.

There is not complete agreement that all the conditions to be described should fall under this rubric. For example there are those who would classify anorexia nervosa as a psychosomatic disorder.

Stammering and stuttering

These are

> disorders in the rhythm of speech, in which the individual knows precisely what he wishes to say, but at the time is unable to say it because of an involuntary, repetitive prolongation or cessation of a sound.

Stammering is characterised by spasmodic, halting or hesitant speech. In its severe form, in which there is a more explosive quality based on violent expulsive respiratory movements, it is known as stuttering. In the adult these symptoms are usually associated with emotional conflict of some sort, and in a sense, form part of the ego's defence system. For example, a woman unable to express tremendously aggressive feelings towards her husband may stammer or stutter when speaking about him, but be able to speak normally on neutral topics. Under hypnosis these symptoms may completely disappear. Many people have long periods free from stammering and stuttering, to find they return at each crisis in life. Behaviour therapy may play an important part in management.

Anorexia nervosa

Some psychiatrists regard anorexia nervosa as a symptom of a number of psychiatric disorders, and not as a disorder or syndrome in its own right. The weight of evidence is against this view, and in this description we shall consider it as a particular syndrome which may or may not be accompanied by hysterical, phobic, anankastic or depressive symptoms depending on the psychopathology of the affected individual. Its causal dynamics vary greatly, and apart from dynamic factors giving rise to any of the above-mentioned symptoms, it may for example, arise out of a fear of poisoning, a phobic dread of food, an unpleasant symbolic significance of food, or in connection with an 'asceticism at puberty'.

It is an interesting fact that anorexia, or lack of appetite, is not present in patients exhibiting this syndrome, except when they are in extremis.

Typically, the age of onset of anorexia nervosa is puberty or post-puberty. It is estimated that 90% of patients are females.

The patient's upbringing is frequently at the hands of a dominant and restrictive mother and a passive father. Girls, at least, are usually of high intelligence, and frequently have exhibited childhood personality traits of athleticism and obsessionality. In post-puberty they are still mother-dependent, and they display irritability, lack of humour, paranoid sensitivity, withdrawal, and marked obsessionality.

The reduction in nutritional intake is psychically determined and occurs not infrequently following dieting for slimming, or after an emotional upset. The reason for slimming in some instances is an unwillingness for female patients to develop womanly characteristics, both physical and emotional, with their attendant expectations and responsibilities. A post-pubertal disgust for sexual thought and development is indeed common. Many other dynamic configurations are found, and most can be traced back to an ambivalent relationship with mother. Patients dislike proximity and physical contact.

In boys, it has been postulated that there is an entanglement of sexual and aggressive instincts with the concept of food intake. Basically immature, these youngsters fear growing up. Eating is said to become a destructive oral aggressive act, one that also has sexual connotations. Unconsciously, to eat is to grow bigger, more aggressive and more sexual. In warding off aggressive and sexual impulses, perceived as dangerous by the child, he also wards off eating. Spontaneous or self-induced vomiting occurs, usually in secret. In females, who form the bulk of patients, amenorrhoea (usually but not invariably) forms part of the syndrome. If amenorrhoea occurs it may take up to three years after the assumption of normal eating for menstruation to resume. Constipation and the marked physical effects of undernourishment are the other main features.

Weight loss is the outstanding physical outcome, extreme cases appearing like skeletons clad with skin. Often the loss of weight is accompanied by an increase of lanugo hair, which is hormonally determined, on the chin and upper lip, trunk and extremities. Body temperature, blood pressure, breathing and basal metabolism are all reduced, and peripheral circulation is poor, leading to cold hands and feet which may appear blue.

Even after prolonged wasting, it is remarkable how alert and even energetic these patients remain. Secondary anaemias, avitaminosis, chemical changes in the body, and intercurrent infections may occur, and untreated, anorexia nervosa has a disquieting mortality rate.

The I.C.D. description of anorexia nervosa appears in Appendix I (page 382).

Management

That the patient must be moved from her home environment is probably the only aspect of management about which there is almost universal agreement. Most therapists would take whatever emergency steps are necessary to halt the starvation cachexia, then institute psychotherapy as soon as possible. The condition may last for years even with the most understanding and expert treatment.

A whole gamut of drugs, including hormonal preparations, have been tried with brief success and later found wanting. Feeding by means of a Ryle's tube in initial stages has probably proved life-saving in some instances. Occasionally however, it appears to have provoked suicide attempts. The value of modified insulin therapy, which is used in other conditions to increase appetite, is doubtful, as insulin does not overcome the psychological barrier that prevents these patients from eating. There is also a tendency towards hypoglycaemia in patients with anorexia nervosa, and due to increased sensitivity to insulin, its use is such cases may lead to hypoglycaemic coma.

Chlorpromazine in syrup form given 8th hourly (and gradually increased to 400-600 mg per day) combined with psychotherapy will often enable patients to eat, leading to substantial weight gain in several weeks. This immediate response however, is not necessarily indicative of the permanent achievement of a normal pattern of eating behaviour and adequate heterosexual and social adjustment.

The treatment that shows most promise, at least in the production of weight gain, is behaviour therapy. One method is to restrict walking and to make mobility contingent upon weight gain. Predictable weight gain occurs but little evidence has been forthcoming to indicate the long-term benefit of such regimes used on their own.

Tics

The I.C.D. describes tics as

> disorders of no known organic origin in which the outstanding feature consists of quick, involuntary, apparently purposeless, and frequently repeated movements which are not due to any neurological condition. Any part of the body may be involved but the face is most frequently affected. Only one form of tic may be present, or there may be a combination of tics which are carried out simultaneously, alternatively or consecutively. Gilles de la Tourette's syndrome refers to a rare disorder occurring in individuals of any level of intelligence in which facial tics and tic-like throat noises become more marked and more generalized and in which later, whole words or short sentences (often with an obscene content) are ejaculated spasmodically and involuntarily. There is some overlap with other varieties of tic.

Initially, tics (habit spasms) seem to accompany emotions such as embarrassment, rage, anxiety and grief, or an emotion associated with sex. Later, they occur with no conscious awareness of the original emotion or affect that accompanied them. They may show exacerbation under emotional stress. The term coprolalia is applied to the utterance of obscene words or sentences that occur in Gilles de la Tourette's syndrome, the most effective treatment for which at the present time appears to be haloperidol.

Stereotyped repetitive movements

These are described in the I.C.D. as

> disorders in which voluntary repetitive stereotyped movements, which are not due to any psychiatric or neurological condition, constitute the main feature. Includes headbanging, spasmus nutans, rocking, twirling, finger-flicking mannerisms and eye-poking. Such movements are particularly common in cases of mental retardation with sensory impairment or with environmental monotony.

Specific disorders of sleep

Disorders are placed in this diagnostic category when a more precise medical or psychiatric diagnosis cannot be made and when no organic basis can be found. Included are: hypersomnia, insomnia, inversion of sleep rhythm, nightmares, night terrors and sleepwalking. Their meanings are self-evident and no further description will be given.

Other and unspecified disorders of eating

Again, this diagnostic category is used only when a more precise medical or psychiatric diagnosis cannot be made and when no organic basis for the symptoms are present. Disorders specified are: infantile feeding disturbance, loss of appetite (anorexia), overeating, pica, and psychogenic vomiting.

The term 'pica' refers to an abnormal craving to eat substances which are not recognised as foodstuffs (e.g. wood, chalk, lead pencils, paint).

Obesity

Obesity is characterised by an excessive accumulation of fat in the body. A person is said to be obese when body weight exceeds by 20% the average weight for a particular height. This does not constitute a reliable assessment of obesity however, as other tissues of variable mass, particularly muscle, contribute to body weight.

There are a number of factors involved in the development of obesity, the major final determinant being an excess of calorie intake over and above the energy requirements of the body, in other words more food and calorie-containing drink than is required to meet the body's need for energy.

One factor that may lead to obesity is therefore a decrease in physical activity. While the expenditure of increasing amounts of energy leads to increasing appetite, below a minimal level of activity appetite does not fall proportionately, so that very inactive people, in general, eat more than they require.

Socioeconomic factors play a part. In some cultures, obesity features more in privileged groups, while in others, an increase in socioeconomic status is associated with a decreasing incidence. From an epidemiological point of view age is also important, as the prevalence of obesity doubles between the ages of 20 and 50 years.

Genetic factors, probably through their influence on the body's metabolism, have been demonstrated to be related to obesity in lower animals, and probably play a part in obesity occuring in humans.

Emotional factors are important. Overeating is common when people are under stress, and neurotic traits and symptoms are found in obese people to a greater extent than in the non-obese.

Neither a particular personality type nor a specific psychodynamic conflict has been found to be associated with obesity.

Management

Management is difficult. Loss of weight can be achieved fairly readily if a person is admitted to hospital and placed on a strict dietary regime. Such loss of weight is usually short-lived once the patient returns to his customary environment.

Perhaps the most useful form of treatment for those patients who over-eat as a response to stress, is psychotherapy. Many quack remedies and expensive living-in programmes are available to the little men and women living inside large bodies from which they crave to be free. One rather questionable practice is the injection of diuretics, which by virtue of loss of fluid from the body produces rapid weight loss of a temporary nature. Such temporary weight loss is well known to boxers who dry out before weighing in for a bout.

Mention has been made of the appetite-suppressant effects of amphetamines in Chapter 17, where the point is made that tolerance to such drugs develops rapidly, thus rendering them unsuitable for long term use.

Enuresis

Enuresis is the term applied to the inappropriate and involuntary passing of urine. It can be defined as bed wetting or clothes wetting in persons over the age of three or four years who fail to inhibit the reflex to pass urine when awake, and/or fail to rouse from sleep in response to bladder sensations preceding the act of micturition.

The condition has no geographical boundaries, but tends to be more prevalent in socio-culturally deprived individuals. Males are affected twice as frequently as females, and about one enuretic in 1,000 is stated to suffer from an associated encopresis (involuntary passage of faeces).

Organic, intrapsychic, and social factors may be involved individually or concurrently in enuresis. The enuretic child is found to sleep very soundly.

Most children are dry by the age of ten years, but the distressing symptoms may persist well into the teens or into adult life, with attendant gross inconvenience or the shattering of any prospects of leading a full life, including marriage. A male member of one of the armed services managed to conceal frequently occurring nocturnal enuresis during twelve years of service life. Though functioning very satisfactorily in his job, the question arose of his being sent home from an overseas posting because of his enuresis. This man deserved a medal rather than admonition.

Some adults, enuretic in childhood but dry for years, may under emotional stress, have a re-exacerbation of this condition.

The I.C.D. definition appears in Appendix I (page 383).

Management

The treatment of enuresis is not simple and should be commenced by excluding any possible organic causes. The therapist, as in the management of any illness, must strive to promote trust and confidence in the patient and so develop good rapport with him. The patient on his part must wish to correct the problem. Parents, particularly mothers, may need psychotherapeutic support.

In attempting to help the patient, a number of methods are worth considering. Psychotherapy may well be helpful, and drug therapy has its advocates. Drugs that have been tried are many and variable in their action, and include central nervous stimulants to lighten sleep, tranquillising drugs to lessen anxiety, anticholinergic drugs to minimise parasympathetic nervous impulses involved in bladder tone and sphincter relaxation, antidiuretics, hormones and antihistamines. Of more recent use, are the tricyclic antidepressants such as amitriptyline and imipramine, for example 25 mg or 50 mg before retiring. Reports on the value of the tricyclids are conflicting, but even though it is difficult to separate the value of the therapeutic intervention from the effects of the tricyclids themselves, it would seem that in some patients these drugs reduce the number of wet nights.

Among what might be regarded as special techniques are: a conditioning device which wakens the patient by means of a buzzer or small electric shock the moment the first drop of urine contacts a wire pad on which he sleeps, bladder training in which the person forces fluids and waits as long as possible before voiding in an effort to increase bladder capacity, and hypnosis.

There are times when, irrespective of what is done, nothing except some change in the enuretic's life situation ameliorates the condition, as evidenced by a teenage boy in a boarding school, who, armed with a waterproof sheet, suffered for two years from nocturnal enuresis. He resorted to rising early to wash sheets and pyjamas, returning to bed in order to keep the dreadful secret from his school fellows. In his third year, being a student and sportsman of some consequence among his peers, he was made a school prefect in charge of a dormitory of more junior boys. During the first night of his prefectorial state his habit persisted, and in spite of all precautions his washed sheet was noted in the morning by one of the junior boys, so exposing him to possible ridicule. On the next night he remained dry, and has not had a recurrence of nocturnal enuresis in many years.

In the great majority of cases, parents can be reassured that their children will grow out of this condition. The degree of intervention entered into often appears to be governed by the attitudes displayed by parents towards their child's enuresis.

Encopresis

Encopresis is

> a disorder in which the main manifestation is the persistent voluntary or involuntary passage of formed motions of normal or near-normal consistency into places not intended for that purpose in the individual's own sociocultural setting . . .

The condition is not usually diagnosed under the age of four years. It may be a manifestation of failure to attain bowel control, or the encopretic person may have attained control only to lose it again. Associated psychiatric symptoms and smearing of faeces may be observed in some cases.

Psychalgia

Into this diagnostic category fall cases in which there are pains essentially of mental or psychological origin. The category includes tension headache and psychogenic backache.

ACUTE REACTION TO STRESS

Certain individuals who have shown no previous evidence of mental disorder may develop transient disorders in response to exceptional physical or mental stress such as accompanies natural disasters or combat situations.

These disorders, which usually subside within hours or days, may predominantly affect:

1. emotions (panic states, excitability, fear, depression and anxiety),
2. consciousness (fugue states), or
3. psychomotor functions (agitation, stupor).

Stress reactions may include mixtures of the above. Terms which fall under the rubric acute reaction to stress include, catastrophic stress, combat fatigue, exhaustion delirium and acute situational disturbance.

ADJUSTMENT REACTION

The term adjustment reaction is applied to

> mild or transient disorders lasting longer than acute stress reactions which occur in individuals of any age without any apparent pre-existing mental disorder. Such disorders are often relatively circumscribed or situation-specific, are generally reversible, and usually last only a few months. They are usually closely related in time and content to stresses such as bereavement, migration or separation experiences. Reactions to major stress that last longer than a few days are also included here . . .

These disorders do not lead to any significant distortion of development in the child.

A number of adjustment reactions are described.

The *brief depressive reaction* refers to states of depression not specifiable as manic-depressive, psychotic or neurotic which are generally transient and in which the depressive symptoms are usually closely related in time and content to some stressful event. The so-called 'grief reaction' falls in this category.

The *prolonged depressive reaction* differs from the above only in that it is long-lasting and usually develops in association with prolonged exposure to a stressful situation.

A third adjustment reaction occurs in which the main symptoms are emotional in type (e.g. anxiety, fear, worry etc.) but not specifically depressive, and this is termed *adjustment reaction, with predominant disturbance of other emotions*. An *adjustment reaction with predominant disturbance of conduct* is also described. An adolescent grief reaction resulting in aggressive or antisocial behaviour is an example of such a reaction.

A separate label is given to those adjustment reactions in which both emotional disturbance and disturbance of conduct are prominent features.

DISTURBANCES OF CONDUCT

Under the rubric 'disturbances of conduct not elsewhere classified', the I.C.D. has the following to say:

> Disorders mainly involving agressive and destructive behaviour and disorders involving delinquency. [The diagnosis] should be used for abnormal behaviour, in individuals of any age, which gives rise to social disapproval but which is not part of any other psychiatric condition. Minor emotional disturbances may also be present . . . the behaviour—as judged by its frequency, severity and type of associations with other symptoms—[is] abnormal in its context. Disturbances of conduct are distinguished from an adjustment reaction by a longer duration and by a lack of close relationship in time and content to some stress. They differ from personality disorder by the absence of deeply ingrained maladaptive patterns of behaviour present from adolescence or earlier.

An unsocialized disturbance of conduct is characterised by behaviours such as defiance, disobedience, quarrelsomeness, aggression, destructive behaviour, tantrums, solitary stealing, lying, teasing, bullying and disturbed relationships with others. The defiance may sometimes take the form of sexual misconduct.

Socialized disturbance of conduct refers to disorders in individuals who have acquired the values or behaviour of a delinquent peer group to whom they are loyal and with whom they characteristically steal, play truant, and stay out late at night. Promiscuity may also occur. The term group delinquency is relevant.

A *compusive conduct disorder* is a disorder of conduct or delinquent act which is specifically compulsive in origin, an example being kleptomania.

Lastly there occurs a *mixed disturbance of conduct and emotions* in which behaviours mentioned above occur in association with considerable emotional disturbance e.g. anxiety, misery or obsessive manifestations. The term neurotic delinquency may be applied to this category.

Only a little thought is required to see how the presenting symptoms of these disturbances of conduct are similar to those occurring in certain personality disorders, and even with a thorough psychiatric history it may prove difficult to distinguish between the two groups of disorders.

20

TREATMENT IN PSYCHIATRY

The management of patients suffering from particular clinical syndromes has received attention in the appropriate sections. This chapter will serve to overview treatment modalities in psychiatry.

In the management of any patient the following have to be considered:

1. Psychotherapy, individual and group.
2. Group techniques.
3. Drug therapy (psychopharmacology).
4. Physical treatments.
5. Social and milieu therapy.
6. Special techniques.
7. The nursing approach.
8. Rehabilitation techniques.
9. Community measures.

Some of these categories overlap and more than one approach is frequently used with the individual patient.

INDIVIDUAL PSYCHOTHERAPY

Psychotherapy literally means treatment of the mind, and therefore the term could logically be applied to any treatment method designed to cure or ameliorate mental illness. In practice however, the term is used to describe a method of treatment relying for its effect upon an exchange of ideas and feelings between a patient and therapist. It is aimed at influencing a patient's feelings and behaviour in the direction of relieving distress, promoting efficiency of mind and improving the patient's adaptation to the group in which he lives, to their mutual benefit. Psychotherapy is not solely the province of the doctor. With experience, staff of all disciplines are able to carry out psychotherapy at some level. Some highly specialised forms of psychotherapy do in fact require years of training, but this should not cause one to assume that nothing can be achieved by realistic counselling by staff who do not have such special training.

There are a number of differing forms of psychotherapy practised, and the various approaches are based to a large extent on the psychotherapists' theoretical orientation towards the development of personality and towards the development of illness. Some of these forms will be described briefly.

Psychoanalysis

Where it appears that a patient's problems emanate from past unresolved difficulties, be they triggered off by current situations or not, psychoanalysis may be the treatment of choice. Considerable judgment is required in the selection of patients, and such factors as a capacity for logical thought, age, ego-strength and analysability must be assessed. This form of psychotherapy could involve patient and therapist in four or more sessions a week, extending over a period of two to five years, or even more, and it may prove stressful for the patient, who is encouraged to regress and work through early painful experiences.

The psychoanalytic situation has changed little from the model established by Freud. The patient lies on a couch or sofa with the analyst sitting out of direct vision, usually behind him, and intruding minimally into the patient's thought processes. The fundamental rule in psychoanalysis is that the patient produces out aloud and without suppression or selection of any kind, all his thoughts and feelings about whatever comes into his mind, a process known as *free association.* A second rule is that the patient should be prepared to endure delay of instinctual gratifications so that optimal frustration will operate, thus facilitating communication about instinctual wishes with the therapist. Ignoring for a moment the state of consciousness, one might liken the treatment setting to the patient lying on the operating table while the surgeon explores and carries out his specific skilled functions; and just as the surgeon has ample opportunity pre- and post-operatively to develop a real relationship with his patient, so has the analyst. This relationship is of extreme importance, being something the patient can hold onto while passing through the many emotional traumas that may beset him on the way. Apart from these face-to-face transactions before and after a session, the analyst gives of himself in his timely interpretations during treatment sessions and remains anything but a faceless being.

Three phases of the analytic process are described. The first involves the initiation and consolidation of the analytical situation, during which occurs the development of the therapeutic alliance. Both patient and therapist develop a relationship contributed to by their real personality characteristics. Without the development of a substratum of basic trust at this stage, treatment must inevitably fail.

The second naturally-occurring phase relates to regression to what is termed transference neurosis. At this time, unresolved oedipal conflicts are focussed on the person of the therapist through the process of transference (page 30). Usually more marked in this second phase than in the other two phases of the analytic process is the phenomenon of *resistance* which has many manifestations, the one concerning the therapist in the analytic situation being the patient's inability to express everything that comes into his mind in spite of conscientious efforts to do so. This resistance is an unconscious defensive manoeuvre which militates against the regression to a transference neurosis; and as the material expressed in the transference neurosis is what the patient is gaining insight into and is being helped to work through, the analyst often spends much time in this second phase carefully interpreting and drawing the patient's attention to these resistances in order to re-establish the transference neurosis.

The satisfactory working through of oedipal conflict material using the therapist as a substitute for people in the patient's past, leads on to the third phase of the analytical process which involves preparation for and the ultimate separation of patient and analyst. The patient who, early in analysis, has passive and dependent wishes fulfilled must virtually renounce the fulfiller, cope with the mourning involved in the resultant separation, and take an independent stance in life.

Quite obviously all phases of psychoanalysis which has as its goal the reorganisation of character structure with an emphasis on understanding rather than symptom removal require handling by a well-trained and stable expert, one who has himself undergone the rigorous self-discipline involved in a training analysis (page 20).

Psychoanalytic psychotherapy

The term psychoanalytic psychotherapy has come to refer to a number of psychotherapies, based as is psychoanalysis, on psychoanalytical theory, but differing in their goals and techniques. These forms of psychotherapy are referred to as *insight therapy, relationship therapy* and *supportive therapy.* Some authorities limit the term psychoanalytic psychotherapy to insight therapy, and quite obviously the term insight therapy may properly be applied to psychotherapy based on psychological theories other than psychoanalytical theory.

While all psychotherapy may be concerned with insight, relationship, and support, a different emphasis is placed on these aspects in the modes of therapy to be described, and the use of a particular approach is based on an understanding of the particular patient to be treated.

In *insight therapy,* instead of attempting a total reorganisation of personality structure, involving also the correction of developmental lags as occurs in psychoanalysis, one aims at the resolution of specific conflicts and limited removal of pathological defenses. A greater emphasis is placed on interpersonal events and the patient's transferences on to other persons, and less on the interpretation of transference relationships to the therapist, though this latter may usefully occur. A couch is rarely used.

Relationship therapy aims to foster the growth of the relatively immature personality. The healthy relationship with the therapist, who becomes a helpful parental figure, is seen to offset the neurotogenic effects of earlier significant but unsatisfactory relationships. There occurs discussion and clarification of interpersonal events and a couch is contraindicated.

Supportive therapy is of value for relatively mature persons with limited symptoms who may be in a temporary state of disequilibrium arising, for example, out of environmental stress, and for persons who, having made a relatively good adjustment in life, are going through what appears to be a temporary period of pressure, indecision or anxiety. The goal of therapy is to restore prior equilibrium, to reduce fear and anxiety in new situations and to assist the patient to tolerate unalterable situations. The therapist actively intervenes, advises and fosters discussion and the direction it will take. This active role of the therapist is at the opposite pole to that of the psychoanalyst, who, comparatively speaking, takes a watching and listening brief on the patient's free associations and makes timely interpretations of transference and resistance.

Brief psychotherapy

All the above psychotherapies may be of long duration, and partly to offset this, and because less time-consuming procedures may be more advantageous in dealing with certain people and their problems, a distinct treatment modality known as brief psychotherapy had developed. The techniques used are based largely on psychoanalytical concepts and methods. However, the therapist does not necessarily restrict his attention to the patient alone as in psychoanalysis and may have some contact with relatives. He also takes a fairly active role in focussing on areas for discussion.

Following initial interview wherein problem areas are identified, the therapist and patient agree on a limited number of treatment sessions, usually 10 to 15, and then commence work on the circumscribed areas of emotional conflict underlying the patient's symptoms. The therapist relies on and capitalises on the patient's personality assets and adaptive resources while fostering problem-solving in those areas initially identified as targets for therapy. When the patient has mastered the circumscribed problem(s), therapy terminates.

Client-centred psychotherapy

Carl Rogers conceived of this form of therapy and developed its techniques between 1938 and 1950. Initially regarded as being a non-directive form of counselling or psychotherapy, the concept has been broadened and is now seen as an approach to all human relationships. Its principles are applicable in many groups and institutional settings, and in the broad field of education.

The term 'client' was chosen instead of 'patient' in order to underline the fact that the approach does not follow the medical prescriptive model of therapist treating a patient, and the individual coming for help is seen as a responsible client, capable of human growth in a setting or atmosphere which facilitates such growth. The atmosphere conducive to human growth is produced by the therapist (called in some situations, the facilitator).

Rogers sees the essential attitudes or conditions for success in therapy as: (1) the therapist's genuineness or congruence; (2) the therapist's complete acceptance of, or unconditional positive regard for his client; and (3) a sensitive and accurately emphatic understanding of the client by the therapist. A basic assumption of this approach is that in the human organism there is a fundamental tendency for human growth, or a self-actualising quality, and this quality constitutes the motivating force in therapy.

Rogers describes seven stages of maturation of the human organism, ranging from a person with rigid fixity of attitudes and perceptions through to the 'fully functioning person'. The seven stages are referred to as a process continuum, and reliable rating scales based on these stages have been developed which signify the effectiveness of therapy.

Extensive research and evaluation has gone hand in hand with the utilisation of client-centred therapy, and three aspects of research having a bearing on the conditions of therapy are summarised by Truax and Mitchell (1971) as follows:

> These studies taken together suggest that therapists or counsellors who are accurately empathic, nonpossessively warm in attitude, and genuine, are indeed effective. Also, these findings seem to hold with a wide variety of therapists and counsellors, regardless of their training or theoretic orientation, and with a wide variety of clients or patients, including college underachievers, juvenile delinquents, hospitalised schizophrenics, college counsellees, mild to severe outpatient neurotics, and the mixed variety of hospital patients. Further, the evidence suggests that these findings hold in a variety of contexts and in both individual and group psychotherapy or counselling.

From this statement it would certainly appear that in any of the psychotherapy treatment situations described above, the quality of the relationship between patient and therapist is at least a very important factor contributing to a successful outcome or otherwise.

Group psychotherapy will be described within the general framework of the next section dealing with group techniques.

GROUP TECHNIQUES

Group techniques in a psychiatric setting may be defined as ways in which people working in psychiatry use specialised skills to the benefit of individual patients who form a group. 'Benefit' here implies a more sound adjustment to the vicissitudes of life and less inner tension, in short, a move towards mental health. It should be emphasised that one is not treating an impersonal thing, the group, but is treating individual persons in a group setting. The very fact of having a number of people together, that is, the group setting itself, facilitates the process of helping the individual.

Historical perspective

In the year 1905, Dr J. H. Pratt, a Boston physician who is generally accepted as the father of modern group psychotherapy, assembled together groups of patients suffering from tuberculosis. He explained to these people the nature of their illness, pointed out the necessary therapeutic measures, and encouraged them in the regime of treatment they were to follow. Pratt was impressed by the effect on the patients of them actually seeing one another and being in each other's presence, and he made the following comment: 'The favourable cases that are making rapid progress towards recovery infuse a spirit of hope in all'.

The Russians claim that one of their physicians, Viazemskii, was the first to use group methods. In 1904, this physician used 'group' hypnotherapy in the treatment of alcoholism, hypnotising patients in turn. The mutual influence of the patients upon one another reinforced suggestibility, rendering subsequent subjects more readily hypnotisable. The systematic application of collective hypnotism for alcoholism however, does not appear to have been placed on a firm footing in Russia until Bekhterev accumulated clinical observations between 1910 and 1914.

The year 1908 saw the American physician Emerson begin his work with groups of children suffering from loss of appetite, by bringing together daily, groups of children with their parents. Netkachev, in St Petersburg in 1909, published a monograph on the 'group therapy of stuttering', while in 1911, J. L. Moreno, working with children in Viennese parks, devised a game situation that represented the foundation of his method of psychodrama.

In 1909, L. C. Marsh, in the United States of America began to accumulate material on community centre activities within a psychiatric hospital. Meetings attended by as many as 500 patients and hospital personnel, were conducted after the fashion of certain religious gatherings, with choral singing, reading aloud, and the reading of letters of gratitude from people who had recovered. Marsh published his conclusions in 1931, the year that the terms 'group therapy' and 'group psychotherapy' first came on the scene.

It is interesting to note that the forerunners of group psychotherapy were doctors of medicine or physicians, and not psychiatrists. Most studies in what came to be known as group psychotherapy published before 1917 posed a specific practical goal, that of employing the combination of patients in a group for the purpose of increasing the influence of the physician in the direction of a more conscious adherence by patients to the prescribed therapy. These types of groups would mainly fall into the category of the supportive-inspirational group, or as some would name them, the good-example-setting type of group.

The language of psychoanalysis emanating from Freud, with concepts like id, ego, superego, the oedipus complex, and the various ego defence mechanisms, were not introduced into group therapy until 1936-1945.

What has happened to group therapy since the early use of supportive-inspirational groups? This type of group first devised by Pratt is still used in psychiatry, and in addition, a different type of therapy has been developed. A purely supportive type of therapy designed to fill some need in a patient would be necessary as long as the need persisted in the patient. This time could be interminable if the patient did not develop in personality. Arising out of this self-evident truth, attention was directed towards a type of therapy that might do more than merely fill a need, a therapy, that, properly managed, would promote personality growth and thus enable a more efficient personality to function with a greater degree of autonomy than before. To this end, a type of therapy was developed that did not only take cognizance of factors or needs in the patient's conscious awareness, but encouraged observation, introspection and relatively free verbal expression restricted only by some consideration for the feelings of others in the group situation. In this way group members learned from the past as well as from the present, and from others as well as from themselves, and then applied their new knowledge to remedy some of the mistakes or misconceptions of the past. These groups fall into the category termed 'free interaction groups'.

This is an important development wherein groups, as well as providing support and suggestion, aid the process of self-understanding. The patient makes adjustments in behaviour and modifies attitudes within the therapeutic group. This therapeutic group is representative of the outside community, and if the patient can adjust in such a group, then the chances are he will be able to carry such attitude changes over into the day-to-day world of interpersonal relationships in the outside community.

Types of group therapy

The numerous forms of group activities occurring in a psychiatric setting certainly cannot all be subsumed under the title 'group therapy'. Though certain goals may be similar, it is not customary to include for example, activity groups, training groups, patient government groups, ward meetings, industrial therapy groups *per se* as forms of group therapy. Group techniques have been applied to a multitude of clinical conditions and to numerous domestic, social and occupational problems, both in inpatient and extra-hospital settings. The generally accepted types of group therapy will now be described briefly, there being obvious overlapping between some of these categories.

1. *Didactic groups* are based on educational material presented by the group leader as a basis for guided discussion.
2. *Therapeutic social clubs* are run along parliamentary lines. Patients elect their own officers and arrange their own programmes, the leader (psychiatrist, nurse, social worker, etc.) remaining intentionally in the background. Such clubs are especially useful for patients after discharge from hospital.
3. *Repressive-inspirational groups* lay chief stress upon building morale through strong group identification and the arousal of positive group emotions. One could perhaps place A.A. meetings in this category.
4. *Free interaction groups* are given a variety of names, for example, group psychotherapy, intensive group therapy, group centred psychotherapy, and group analysis. The details of conducting these groups and the type of content emphasised vary largely according to the therapist's theoretical orientation, particularly with the amount of attention paid to the unconscious meanings of patients' behaviour. All forms encourage interaction in an atmosphere conducive to a free and honest expression of feeling. The interactions are discussed by both patients and therapist with a view to exposing and correcting neurotic attitudes and achieving more mature ways of functioning.
5. *Psychodrama* is a method whereby members of the group produce and act out scenes from daily life or past experiences which have a particular significance for an individual in the group. One member plays his own role, while other members of the group play the parts of others in his life. This may be varied by giving a theoretical situation to a group of patients and encouraging them to ad lib on the theme. Such performances are followed by discussion involving both players and spectators.

To complicate matters a little, group therapy is used as a treatment method on its own or in conjunction with individual psychotherapy; it may be conjoint, that is, additional members of the patient's family are in the same group with him; it may consist of a family or families (at least one school uses the combined term 'conjoint family therapy' for family therapy); and though there is usually one therapist, there may be co-therapists or multiple therapists.

Group dynamics

In an introduction to group therapy such as this, we shall avoid looking in any detail at the multitude of studies that have been made to determine what goes on in groups—the dynamics of a group.

Briefly group dynamics is the study of the interplay of psychological forces which may be involved in the formation and functioning of any group, be it a treatment group or not. Group dynamics denotes the study of (a) the structure and functioning of groups, notably the psychological aspects of 'small groups' with especial reference to the changing pattern of intra-group adjustment, tension, conflict and cohesion; and (b) the shifts in relationships of one group with another (*A Dictionary of the Social Sciences*, Gould and Kolb).

Some practical considerations in group therapy

We shall begin by clarifying the meaning of a number of terms such as open, closed, heterogeneous.

An open group is a group from which improved patients are leaving and into which new members are entering during the life of the group. A closed group on the other hand signifies a group commencing with a particular number of patients and continuing with those patients for the prescribed life of the group. Some groups may be comprised of people with the same type of problem, a homogeneous diagnostic group, while in other situations the diagnostic composition of the group, and this is probably more frequent, is mixed or heterogeneous.

Whether or not there is an ideal size for a group engaged in group therapy is open to some argument, and depends to some extent on the purpose or aim of therapy. G. C. Homans defines a group as 'a number of persons who communicate with all others not at second hand through other people but face to face'. While appreciating the therapeutic value of properly conducted ward meetings with a relatively large number of patients, the general consensus of opinion would seem to indicate that 8-12 members is the most effective size for a group run as a free interaction group.

Such questions as ages of group members, the most suitable diagnostic categories for treatment, the length of each group session, and the number of sessions for which a group should run, will not be discussed here.

As a guide to conducting group therapy however, particularly in a hospital setting, the following points are given as suggestions. These will not suit all situations, but have been found to be of some value to nursing staff in an admission centre setting.

General

1. Seating is to be arranged in as circular a manner as possible, the group leader forming part of the circle.
2. Of the staff present, a nurse should sit within reasonable distance of the door but should not give the impression that she is acting as gaoler keeping people in the group.
3. The door should be kept unlocked and may be left open if the room is stuffy.
4. Should a patient wish to leave the room, he or she will be directed to make a request to the group leader. The group leader may indicate to a member of the nursing staff that she should accompany the patient outside. The nurse's function in such a situation is to try to understand why the patient has left the room and, if it seems appropriate, to encourage him to return to the group to discuss the difficulty which caused him to leave.
5. All members of the therapeutic team should feel free to make any contribution they consider relevant to the discussion in progress during the group.

Therapist's role

1. The therapist is as non-directive as possible, allowing patients to develop their own themes.
2. In open groups with rapidly changing members, some comment on what is expected of patients may be helpful. To this end, at the beginning of each group where new members are present, the therapist should introduce himself or herself, e.g. 'For those of you who do not know me, my name is Dr——— or Mr——— or Nurse———. These meetings are held primarily so we can learn together where your difficulties lie, so that you can help each other in finding solutions to them. Illness may arise out of difficulties in your relationships with other people, so you are expected to say exactly what you feel about other people in the group, including myself. In fact, to derive most benefit from the group, say whatever comes into your mind during the group session'.
3. When patients are obviously resisting personal involvement by talking about trivia, the therapist should comment on this and try to relate apparent irrelevancies to the group situation, e.g. 'It is easier to talk about the hostility in the world than about your own angry feelings in the group'. All communications made by patients should, in general, be dealt with as if representing a common group problem. It will soon become apparent if they are not, and frequently they are.
4. The therapist should examine the countertransferences that develop in himself or herself.
5. It may be necessary for the therapist to initially support some patients when they find difficulty in coping with outspoken group members, but such support should be minimal. A comment such

as, 'Do you usually withdraw like this and not stand up for yourself?' might be more helpful than taking the cudgel for such a person. As mentioned earlier, nothing is done for patients which they can reasonably be expected to do for themselves.

6. With regard to tension developing in a group, it is well to remember that this tension is the driving force of the group, and it is not always helpful for the therapist to deliberately reduce this. Groups usually find their own ways of dealing with tension and they should be allowed to do so.

After the group

After each group therapy session, which may last 1-1½ hours, all staff present should meet for say 30 minutes to discuss the particular group meeting and perhaps relate it to previous meetings. This reviewing time, which should be mandatory after every group, provides an excellent learning situation for staff who may later run groups themselves.

Areas which lend themselves to discussion are as follows:

1. THEMES
   (a) Overt—what were the main topics discussed by the group?
   (b) Latent—what does one think was the unconscious significance of the main topics, and why were they chosen?
2. LEVELS OF TENSION. A quick survey of levels of tension throughout the group session may be made. Peaks and lows of tension should be correlated with themes, and causative factors analysed.
3. INTRAGROUP RELATIONSHIPS. The development of relationships between patients and between patients and staff, including the leader, should be discussed, and the possible significance of them in terms of patients' personalities is worthy of study. Some emphasis should be placed on the role of the leader in stimulating or interpreting such relationships between groups members, and comment should be made by staff on his general handling of the group (was he directive, permissive, etc.?). In this way the leader's blind spots in his countertransference to group members may be brought to light.
4. A GENERAL APPRAISAL of the group is worthwhile even though one can be so wrong. The question is asked: 'Was it a good group?' If so, 'Why?'; or if not, 'Why not?'.

Training groups for staff

In the author's view, experience as a member of a training group is a prerequisite for any staff member to function as a group leader. In a sense the post-group staff meeting is itself a group experience, but an extremely watered-down one which does little, in comparison with a more formal group, to help the staff member look at himself and develop sensitivities and qualities essential in the group leader.

Sensitivity training

What has been said about the development of sensitivities in staff members leads one to comment on 'sensitivity training', about which there is a growing body of literature. A new language has grown up around this concept, and one hears such terms as sensitivity groups, marathon groups, confrontation, and encounter groups. In these groups, participants may meet for periods of up to 8 or 10 hours in a day for the purpose of developing sensitivity and understanding, leading to more satisfactory interpersonal relationships. Marathon groups may be held for as long as 48 hours or more, the participants taking time out for meals, rest, etc. Sensitivity training is practised in various business and professional groups, and, in expert hands, has proved beneficial. In the hands of amateurs however, the same process may have disastrous results.

PSYCHOPHARMACOLOGY

The use of drugs to calm excited mental patients dates back to the fifth century B.C. or earlier. Most drugs used until recently had many drawbacks. Many certainly would reduce agitation, anxiety and disturbed behaviour, but they frequently caused clouding of consciousness or had addictive properties. A very big advance was the introduction of the major tranquillisers in 1952; in that year the first favourable report on chlorpromazine in the treatment of disturbed psychotic patients was published. Since that time, numerous major and minor tranquillising drugs and specific antidepressant drugs have been added to the psychiatric armamentarium.

It is most unusual in these times when new drugs are rapidly and continuously appearing on the market, to find a chapter dealing with drugs that is up to date. This book will be no exception. All that can be hoped for is to touch upon certain of the more commonly used drugs. The few mentioned are not necessarily better than unmentioned ones, but receive attention because of a certain bias arising out of their satisfactory use by the author. It is worth remembering that it is often not the pill, but who gives it that counts; and that it is far better to learn to use a limited number of drugs properly and to know their actions and side effects thoroughly, than to flit in an ephemeral fashion from one drug to another, never getting to know a drug's true capabilities. It might be said that an inferior drug in practised hands is better than the most active drug in the hands of a meddler.

With this introductory apologia for the benefit of those whose favourite preparations are missing, we shall look briefly at examples of major tranquillisers, minor tranquillisers, antidepressant drugs and sedatives.

Major tranquillisers*

The major tranquillisers, also termed ataractic drugs (from 'ataraxy' meaning freedom from confusion), reduce agitation and anxiety and produce only minimal clouding of consciousness. They also diminish the intensity and duration of psychotic symptoms such as delusions and hallucinations. As far as is known today, these drugs suppress symptoms,

* The discoverer of chlorpromazine called this group of drugs 'neuroleptics', the term still used in European medicine. The name 'tranquilliser' was later coined by a sales-conscious group who were promoting a drug known as a minor tranquilliser, and the somewhat inappropriate term is found in most Anglo-American literature to describe neuroleptic drugs.

but do not eliminate the basic structure of the psychosis. They are said to act mainly in the midbrain and reticular substance, that is, at subcortical levels, but their precise mode of action has not yet been clearly elucidated.

The two main groups of major tranquillisers in use are the phenothiazines and the butyrophenones. The rauwolfia alkaloids from the root of the rauwolfia serpentia have a powerful action, but have fallen into disfavour in psychiatric practice as they have cumulative action, and in dosages required are prone to cause depression sometimes leading to suicidal attempts.

Numbered among the phenothiazines are chlorpromazine hydrochloride (Largactil), trifluoperazine (Stelazine), thioridazine (Melleril), fluphenazine (Anatensol), perphenazine (Trilafon or Fentazin), prochlorperazine (Stemetil), promazine (Sparine), pericyazine (Neulactil), and thioproperazine (Majeptil). This list could be extended to more bewildering limits.

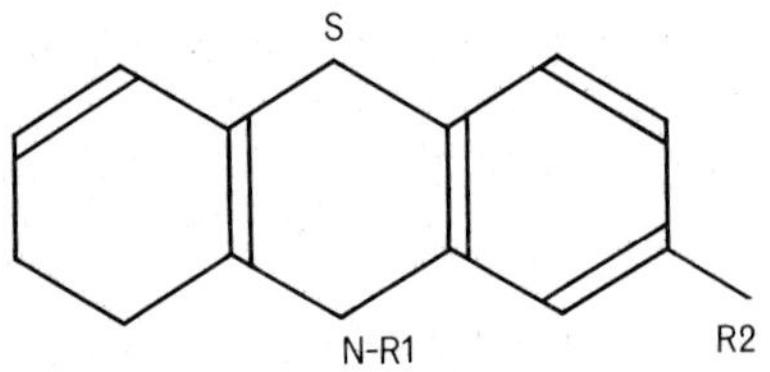

Fig. 13. **Basic phenothiazine nucleus**

The different chemicals mentioned above are derived by altering side chains R_1 and R_2 on the basic phenothiazine nucleus shown in Fig. 13.

The butyrophenones are represented by haloperidol (Serenace) and trifluoperidol (Psychoperidol).

Phenothiazines

The members of this group that will be briefly described are chlorpromazine, trifluoperazine, thioridazine, and fluphenazine.

The main indications for the phenothiazines are given below (1-4), though not all drugs are equally useful in each of the groups of disorders mentioned. For example, an agitated patient is, generally speaking, better served by giving chlorpromazine or thioridazine rather than trifluoperazine, and if the patient is withdrawn, then trifluoperazine rather than the aforementioned is indicated. In some cases it is sound practice to give mixtures of the phenothiazines. For example, the doctor who understands trifluoperazine best and knows its capabilities as a drug to counteract psychotic manifestations, may indeed prescribe it along with chlorpromazine or thioridazine for his deluded and hallucinated patients who are also agitated.

1. *Manic States.* Phenothiazine derivatives are used effectively in quieting manic states, whether of schizophrenic or manic-depressive origin. Their use in depression without the concurrent use of an antidepressant drug is in general, contra-indicated. If agitation is marked in a depressed

patient, phenothiazines alone may be used to initiate treatment followed closely by an antidepressant drug or electroplexy. Patients presenting with a mild depression and given phenothiazines alone may become more deeply depressed.

2. *Schizophrenia.* When phenothiazine derivatives were first introduced, it was the experience of some authorities that 10%-15% of schizophrenic long-stay hospital patients improved to such a degree that they could go back to the outside community and function adequately. These drugs however are most effective in patients who have not been overtly sick for a long time. They do not affect the mental symptomatology uniformly in schizophrenia, and evaluation must be made on an individual basis. Sargent (1956) stated that one's search must continue until the most suitable drug for each individual is found. The author believes however, that only in exceptional cases will the therapist have to move from a limited number of well-tried drugs. A few general points will be made on the effects of the phenothiazines in schizophrenic illnesses.

Symptoms such as anxiety and aggression are influenced effectively and reliably, delusions and hallucinations are controlled, and the drugs are able to reduce the emotional push behind delusional ideas. There is less effect on schizophrenic thinking and disorganised cognitive processes.

Paranoid and catatonic types of schizophrenia generally respond better to these drugs than do the simple and hebephrenic forms, but there are many exceptions to this.

3. *The arteriosclerotic and senile psychoses.* The phenothiazines have a beneficial effect on the patient's behaviour by controlling agitation, anxiety, delusions, hallucinations and disorderly conduct. They have no beneficial effect on dementia *per se.*

4. *States of delirium.* These drugs appear to be effective regardless of the cause of delirium and appear to work equally well whether the delirium is due to alcohol, drugs or infections. The confusion, agitation, and hallucinations subside relatively quickly. Needless to say, other treatment appropriate to the cause of the delirium, must be instituted along with the phenothiazines.

Brief notes will now be given on some of the phenothiazines in common use.

CHLORPROMAZINE HYDROCHLORIDE

Administration and dosage

The main routes of administration are oral or intramuscular. For oral medication, sugar-coated tablets in stregths of 10 mg, 25 mg, 50 mg, and 100 mg, and a mixture or syrup containing 25 mg per 5 ml are available. For parenteral use chlorpromazine in prepared in aqueous solutions—25 mg in 1 ml (2.5%), 50 mg in 2 ml (2.5%) and 50 mg in 5 ml (1%). These strengths are used intramuscularly. The intramuscular injections must be deep as the solution causes irritation and sometimes abscess and necrosis at the injection site. When used intravenously, chlorpromazine is injected slowly after dilution of the 2.5% solution to 10 times its volume with normal saline solution.

A 100 mg suppository for rectal use is also available but is rarely used. The dosage varies from 75 mg to 1,000 mg daily for psychotic manifestations, though higher doses have been used. It is customary to commence medication on a T.D.S. basis. Maintenance dosage after stabilisation is usually one half the therapeutic dose, but each case must be treated on its merits. Some patients who respond rapidly may not require long term maintenance therapy, while others will. Chlorpromazine, along with other phenothiazines, takes many weeks to be excreted from the body. This fact leads to two practical issues. Firstly, patients can be maintained on a single daily dose preferably given at night, and secondly, one should not be too sanguine that a patient does not require further medication if he remains well even for some weeks after cessation of the drug.

Complications and side-effects.

Among the minor side effects are drowsiness, dryness of the mouth, pallor of the skin, heartburn, constipation (occasionally diarrhoea), polyuria (excessive urine), tiredness, weakness, lowering of the body temperature (occasionally pyrexia), tachycardia (increase in pulse rate), photophobia (sensitivity to light) and skin rashes, dizziness and postural hypotension, sometimes headache, attacks of abdominal pain, and weight gain. In view of a severe photosensitive skin rash that may occur in some people taking or handling chlorpromazine, or even being in an atmosphere where it is present, one must never crush tablets.

Persons suffering from arteriosclerosis and cardiovascular disease are more susceptible to the hypotensive effects, and should be closely observed. Cerebral thrombosis and even coronary artery thrombosis have been attributed to the lowering of blood pressure caused by this drug. Urticaria or other skin conditions may be extremely severe. Patients who are on a high dose of chlorpromazine should not be exposed to much sunlight owing to the photosensitivity which the drug produces. Some people who have become sensitive in this way will develop quite a severe rash when exposed to sunlight even after the drug has been stopped.

Psychic complications may be seen. The patients may complain about feeling peculiar, strange, or out of contact, weak, lethargic or depressed. Others complain of being restless. Depersonalization or distortions of the body image (the sense of awareness of body outline) may occur, and some therapists will not use chlorpromazine in schizophrenics who present with depersonalization. Convulsive seizures may occur in people so predisposed, usually in the first two weeks of treatment.

Engorgement of the breasts with lactation has been observed in some patients.

Chlorpromazine prolongs and intensifies the effect of many sedatives, especially barbiturates and narcotics. Patients on high doses of chlorpromazine should not drink alcohol because the combination has a potentially strong sedative action.

A Parkinsonian syndrome and/or excitomotor effects of extra-pyramidal origin sometimes occur with continued high dosage, but it is spontaneously reversible on withdrawal of the drug. If it is desired to carry on the high dosage of chlorpromazine or other phenothiazines, the Parkinsonian-like syndrome can be treated with drugs such as procyclidine (Kemadrin) 5 mg B.D., benzhexol hydrochloride (Artane) 2-5 mg B.D., orphenadrine hydrochloride (Disipal) 50 mg T.D.S., benztropine mesylate (Cogentin) 2 mg mane, or one of the anti-histaminics e.g. promethazine hydrochloride (Phenergan) 25 mg T.D.S. Acute torticollis, torsion spasm, or a type of movement of the head and eyes similar to an oculogyric crisis occasionally occurs, and can be distressing to the patient. These side effects also respond to the above drugs, or to parenteral sedation with a barbiturate.

Oedema and thrombocytopenic purpura have also been reported, and difficulty in accommodation may be experienced.

Among the more serious side effects is jaundice occurring in 1% of people receiving chlorpromazine. It is not common in those who have received and tolerated the drug well for several months. The jaundice is due to stasis of bile in the bile canaliculi with lymphocytic infiltration. After withdrawal of the drug the jaundice usually subsides in about two weeks, but may last longer. Special treatment for jaundice may be necessary, for example a high protein and high calorie diet, and ACTH or cortisone is recommended by some physicians.

More serious than jaundice is chlorpromazine's influence on the white blood cells. Leucopenia is fairly common, and at times becomes so marked that an agranulocytosis is present. Any patient receiving chlorpromazine who develops a sore throat or fever should have an immediate white cell count. If there is a serious drop in the count, the drug should be discontinued immediately, and antibiotic treatment instituted.

With long-continued use, a slate blue discoloration of the skin may occur in areas exposed to the sun, with or without dustlike opacities of the cornea, and central lens opacities. Pigmentation of the retina may also occur with long continued use.

Treatment of side effects

In cases of a large overdose, the stomach should be emptied by emesis or gastric lavage. This is a reasonably safe procedure if the patient is still conscious. It must be remembered however, that neither of these procedures should be carried out on an unconscious patient, unless the doctor has first introduced a cuffed laryngeal tube into the trachea to prevent the inhalation of vomitus.

In the unconscious patient, an intravenous infusion of 1,000 ml of Hartmann's solution given over four hours, or less if hypotension is marked, is indicated. The management of the unconscious patient requires the specialised skills of an anaesthetist who, among other things, will ensure that adequate hydration and electrolyte balance is maintained. Noradrenaline (Levophed) may be given by intravenous drip to assist the elevation of blood pressure, and antibiotics should be given to prevent pheumonia.

The severe headache which occasionally occurs with chlorpromazine will probably respond to the intravenous injection of dihydroergotamine.

The management of jaundice has been touched upon above, as has the treatment of extrapyramidal side effects.

Contra-indications

Chlorpromazine should not be given to comatose patients who are under the influence of alcohol, barbiturates, narcotics, or other central nervous system depressants. Caution is required in giving it to patients with arteriosclerotic conditions, cardiovascular disease, or other conditions in which a sudden drop in blood pressure may be undesirable. It is best not given to patients with a history of liver dysfunction or jaundice. It should also not be given in the presence of a low leucocyte count. When given prior to anaesthesia, post operative unconsciousness may be prolonged, and it is best to omit the drug before patients receive ECT under general anaesthesia.

TRIFLUOPERAZINE

Administration and dosage

1 mg, 2 mg and 5 mg tablets, a sustained-release capsule containing 15 mg, and a syrup containing 1 mg in 5 ml are available for oral use. For intramuscular injection, ampoules of 1 ml and 2 ml, containing 1 mg of trifluoperazine in 1 ml are used. For anti-hallucinatory and anti-delusional effects (termed the ataractic effect) 10-30mg orally is given daily in divided doses, usually B.D.

Trifluoperazine is valuable in rapid tranquillisation (page 305).

Side effects

The most frequently-occurring side effects are due to the action of the drug on the extrapyramidal centres in the brain, and fall under three groups, namely, Parkinson-like symptoms, akathisia, and dystonia or dyskinesia. These may occur with any of the phenothiazines but, in doses usually used, are perhaps somewhat more common with trifluoperazine than with chlorpromazine. Gradual increase of dosage to the optimal therapeutic level is stated to minimise these side effects, which usually occur in the first week of treatment only, and rarely reappear. In practice, even with an initial dosage of 15 mg per day, drugs which are used to counteract these side effects are rarely necessary.

Parkinson-like symptoms include masklike facies, tremor, salivation, muscular rigidity, ataxia, and a shuffling gait. Akathisia is a peculiar motor restlessness which can be mistaken for anxiety. Patients may experience an initial transient period of jitteriness. They find they cannot keep still and will move their legs or tap their feet. One rather pathognomonic feature is seen in the patient who oscillates between sitting on a seat and almost standing up, only to return his buttocks to the seat in a repetitive fashion. Patients in such a state of restlessness due to phenothiazines have been known to run considerable distances without purpose.

Dystonias are bizarre neuromuscular reactions in which certain muscle groups go into spasm leading to a variety of strange postures and movements. Among the symptoms experienced are spasm of limbs, spasm in the oropharyngeal region, opisthotonos (arching of the back), torticollis, or a combination of these, difficulty in swallowing, extreme difficulty in articulation when the tongue is affected, often seeming to the patient to be too large for his mouth (it may even protrude), and oculo- gyric crises which consist in forced upward deviation of the eyes with head retraction. Convulsions have been reported. Autonomic signs such as sweating, pallor or pyrexia may occur.

Patients may be alarmed by many of the extrapyramidal effects and should be reassured of the fact that they will shortly subside. These effects are counteracted by the use of the anti-Parkinsonian drugs mentioned earlier, or the simple reduction of dosage may suffice. Among other side effects are minor ones such as nasal congestion, mild drowsiness, and sweating. An embarrassing though rare side-effect is precipitancy of micturition. As with chlorpromazine, jaundice has occurred, and blood dyscrasias such as agranulocytosis, leucopenia and thrombocytopenia (deficiency of blood platelets) have occasionally been seen.

THIORIDAZINE (MELLERIL)

This drug is more sedative in its action than trifluoperazine, and may be used instead of chlorpromazine, especially in patients who have developed a photosensitive rash.

Administration and dosage

For oral medication, tablets of 10 mg, 25 mg, 50 mg, and 100 mg or a 3% solution (30 mg per ml) may be used. Thioridazine is also prepared for I.M. injection in a solution of 25 mg per ml, available in 2 ml ampoules.

In psychosis, a useful commencing dose is 50 mg T.D.S., but for very disturbed patients an initial loading dose of 200 mg followed by 100 mg fourth or sixth hourly may well be indicated until control is obtained. Maintenance doses vary from 75 mg to 300 mg daily with 150 mg daily as the average.

Side effects

Thioridazine shares with other phenothiazines autonomic system reactions such as dry mouth, postural hypotension and drowsiness. Rarely, if ever, do jaundice, agranulocytosis and photosensitivity occur. Extrapyramidal symptoms and convulsions are seen less frequently than with most other phenothiazines. The dermo-lenticular corneal pigmentations occurring in association with long-continued large doses of chlorpromazine are said to occur less frequently with thioridazine, but one could not be dogmatic about this. Thioridazine may however, with long-continued high dosage, lead to pigmentation of the retina with some visual impairment. For this reason it is recommended that a safe upper margin for continued use is 800 mg per day.

A symptom complained of by some males taking thioridazine is an inability to ejaculate, and females may experience amenorrhoea.

FLUPHENAZINE HYDROCHLORIDE (ANATENSOL)

Administration and dosage

Fluphenazine is available in tablet form in strengths of 1 mg and 2.5 mg, and as an elixir containing 0.5 mg in 1 ml.

For intramuscular or intravenous injection, 10 ml vials containing 2.5 mg per 1 ml are available.

The clinical application of fluphenazine is the same as for other phenothiazines, and the side effects are similar and respond to reduction of the dosage or to anti-Parkinsonian drugs. Adult psychotic patients will require an initial daily dose ranging between 2.5 mg and 10 mg, given at six or eight hourly intervals.

A preparation of considerable value for psychotic patients who are unable or unwilling to take oral therapy, is fluphenazine decanoate. A 1 ml injection of fluphenazine decanoate, which contains 25 mg per ml,* provides eighteen to twenty-one days of controlled anti-psychotic activity. The term depot fluphenazine is applied to this preparation.

It is best to stabilise a patient on oral phenothiazines in hospital,† as one can more readily tailor the dose to the patient's needs when divided doses are given. After stabilisation, and while the patient is still in hospital or in full-time day hospital care, these long-acting preparations are introduced, starting with a dose of say 0.5 ml (0.25 ml for those over sixty years of age) and doubling this after five to ten days. After this second injection, the dosage is 'tailored' according to clinical response and to the length of action of the drug. Wide variations may be found in amounts required. With fluphenazine deconoate for example, the dose may range from 0.5 ml every five weeks to 1 ml every two weeks, 1 ml every four weeks being the average requirement.

Such preparations, which are given by deep intramuscular injection, are valuable to the domiciliary nurse and doctors working in community services, for patients who would otherwise fail to take medication and as a consequence relapse and return to hospital.

Obviously once such drugs have been injected they cannot be withdrawn, and special care must be taken with the elderly. These drugs are contra-indicated in patients with marked arteriosclerosis or Parkinsonism, in patients who have developed jaundice or allergic reactions (including skin rashes) to oral phenothiazines, and in patients who have a history of obstructive jaundice. As with any of the phenothiazines it is unwise to administer these long-acting drugs in the presence of phaeochromocytoma, renal or liver failure, or severe cardiac defect.

Butyrophenones

Examples of this group of major tranquillers which were discovered by Paul Janssen are haloperidol and trifluoperidol. Of these, haloperidol will be briefly described.

* A 1 ml preparation is available in ampoules or preloaded sterile disposable syringes. There are also same strength preparations in 0.5 ml and 2 ml ampoules.

† If the patient's and his family's drug histories do not reveal extrapyramidal reactions to neuroleptics many therapists commence treatment with a depot preparation. If there has been such a reaction, a test-dose of 0.1 cc (2.5 mg) is first given and the dose increased at short intervals.

HALOPERIDOL (SERENACE)

Haloperidol is available as tablets of 0.5 mg, 1.5 mg and 5 mg, and in solution of 5 mg in 1 ml for I.M. or I.V. injection. Its mode of action appears to be similar to that of the phenothiazines, and it is used to control delusions and hallucinations. Its main value however, would seem to lie in the control of manic states whether of schizophrenic or manic-depressive origin.

For rapid control of a disturbed patient, 5-10 mg given I.M. or I.V. T.D.S. is usually adequate.

Some markedly disturbed and aggressive patients may require 100 mg of haloperidol or more in twenty-four hours and this amount can safely be given to physically well patients. A method of *rapid tranquillization* or *rapid neuroleptization* has been developed wherein 10 mg (and in some instances a larger dose) is given I.V. or I.M. The dose is repeated every thirty minutes until the desired therapeutic effect is achieved. Should there be no evidence of a response after six hours of the above regime it is well to try an alternative therapy.

Regimes of rapid tranquillization have also been developed for the phenothiazines, particularly fluphenazine.

It is an interesting fact that the larger doses of haloperidol produce less extrapyrimidal side effects than smaller doses, and in rapid neuroleptization with haloperidol the prophylactic use of anti-Parkinsonian drugs is not recommended both because they are often unnecessary, and because at least some anti-Parkinsonian drugs appear to counteract the antipsychotic effect of major tranquillisers. Extrapyramidal side effects should however be watched for and treated if they appear.

After stabilization oral dosage may be substituted, and the dose for a twenty-four hour period is arrived at by doubling the parenteral dose required for a similar period. As with all drugs the dosage is tailored to suit the individual patient, one aim being to reduce it to the minimum required for a therapeutic effect.

Diphenylbulylpiperidines

A recently developed group of drugs, the diphenylbutylpiperidines, related to the butyrophenones, are, at the time of writing, undergoing extensive trials in Europe. Representatives of this group of neuroleptics are: pimozide, which is given orally once daily in doses of 2-4 mg, though a higher dosage may be required; fluspirilene, 1-3 mg given I.M. once weekly; and penfluridol given orally once weekly, the dosage being 10-40 mg.

In antipsychotic doses, so wide is the margin between the dose that is therapeutic and the dose that produces side effects, that side effects are minimal or non-existent.

If the early promise of these drugs stands the test of time, their obvious advantages will ensure their widespread use, and the maintenance of schizophrenic patients outside hospitals will be greatly facilitated.

Tardive dyskinesia

A special note is made of serious neurological side effects which may occur after high dosage long-continued use of any of the neuroleptic drugs. These side effects comprise a syndrome referred to as persistent or tardive dyskinesia, or extrapyramidal insufficiency. The syndrome is characterised by facial tics, grimacing, sucking and smacking movements of the lips, fly-catching and lateral movements of the tongue, lateral jaw movements, choreiform movements of the arms, athetoid movements of the upper extremities or fingers, ankles and toes, and tonic neck and back contractions. When the disorder develops it continues unchanged or worsens unless the causal drug is withdrawn. On such withdrawal the symptoms may be modified but there is a tendency for the state to persist, unresponsive to or even worsened by anti-Parkinsonian drugs. Tardive dyskinesia sometimes develops after a neuroleptic drug is stopped, possibly due to the side effect of muscular rigidity passing off.

Minor tranquillisers

Minor tranquillisers diminish anxiety and tension but do not have any appreciable effect on psychotic symptomatology. They can be useful adjuncts in psychotherapy for neurotic patients, tiding them over periods of otherwise disabling anxiety. Examples of minor tranquillisers are: the benzodiazepines, namely chlordiazepoxide (Librium), diazepam (Valium), oxazepam (Serepax), clorazepate (Tranxene); and meprobamate (Equanil, Miltown). Any of these may lead to drug dependence.

CHLORDIAZEPOXIDE

For oral medication, tablets of 5 mg, 10 mg, 25 mg and capsules of 10 mg are available. Ampoules containing 100 mg of dry preparation are mixed with 2 ml of solvent for I.M. injection, and with 10 ml of solvent for I.V. injection. The drug acts mainly in the limbic areas of the brain, reducing anxiety. It is only slightly hypnotic and produces muscle relaxation. The dosage range used to allay anxiety and reduce muscle spasm associated with anxiety is anything from 15 mg-40 mg daily, with much individual variation.

High doses given I.M. or I.V. have been used in the treatment of alcohol and drug withdrawal states. The indications for chlordiazepoxide are the alleviation of tension, anxiety, fear and agitation associated with anxiety neurosis, tension headaches and insomnia, the agitation associated with some depressive illnesses, and obsessive-compulsive neurosis.

There appear to be few side effects. No toxicity in the liver, bone marrow or central nervous system has been described. Water retention giving rise to ankle oedema, ataxia, drowsiness, skin rashes, nausea and constipation may occur. Chlordiazepoxide is contra-indicated in myaesthenia gravis.

DIAZEPAM

Tablets of 2 mg, 5 mg and 10 mg and a syrup containing 2 mg per 5 ml are the oral preparations in use. 2 ml ampoules of diazepam containing 10 mg in 2 ml are used for I.M. or I.V. injection.

The action of diazepam is similar to that of chlordiazepoxide but less is required mg for mg. For oral use, the average range is 10-30 mg per day. Its antispasmodic activity is superior to that of chlordiazepoxide. The indications for diazepam, apart from its value in relieving anxiety and tension, are epilepsy, and especially status epilepticus for which it is given by injection, Huntington's chorea, malignant neoplasia, motor neurone lesions, multiple or disseminated sclerosis, radiation sickness, and the so-called stiff man syndrome, a syndrome of unknown aetiology characterised by bouts of severe rigidity and spasm of somatic musculature, lasting hours or days, and often precipitated by physical or emotional stimuli. Diazepam's muscle relaxing property is the one mainly called for in the management of these conditions.

Side effects include ataxia and sedation if given in high dosage. Visual disturbance, tinnitus (ringing in the ears), incontinence, skin rashes and hypotension may also occur. Diazepam is contra-indicated in patients suffering from myaesthenia gravis or glaucoma.

MEPROBAMATE (EQUANIL, MILTOWN)

Meprobamate is supplied as scored tablets of 400 mg and is given in amounts of 1-4 tablets daily. It is used in the treatment of anxiety and tension states. Certain headaches, premenstrual tension and psychosomatic pains are among its indications. It has been used to ease the symptoms resulting from withdrawal of alcohol or other drugs, and in managing behaviour problems in children.

Side effects include drowsiness, dizziness, gastric discomfort, urticaria and angioneurotic oedema.

Antidepressant drugs

Drugs which regulate mood are known as thymoleptics. There are two main groups of these drugs used in the treatment of moderate to fairly severe depressions, namely the tricyclids and the monoamine oxidase inhibitors (MAOIs).

In general, the MAO inhibitors appear more effective in what Sargent calls 'atypical depressions', and in depressive neurosis, while the tricyclid group is more effective in those depressions in which the 'depressive syndrome' is present, namely, manic depressive psychosis, depressed type; involutional melancholia; and reactive depressive psychosis. There are however, many exceptions to this general rule, and as yet no clear-cut way has been devised of prophesying on clinical grounds which particular patient will respond to which particular group of drugs. Indeed, there is some evidence to show that response to a particular group of drugs might be more dependent on hereditary factors than on the clinical picture of the depressive illness.

If the depression suffered is a severe one, there is no doubt that electroplexy is still the most effective treatment for the attack.

Tricyclids

This group of drugs are so named because their basic chemical formula, which is similar to that of chlorpromazine, contains three rings. Members of the group include: imipramine (Tofranil), amitriptyline (Tryptanol, Saroten, Laroxyl, Elavil), nortriptyline (Allegron, Aventyl, Nortab), trimipramine (Surmontil), protriptyline (Concordin, Triptil), doxepin (Sinequan).

The precise mode of action of these drugs in the central nervous system is unknown, but they have come to replace ECT in the treatment of many mild and moderately severe depressions.

IMIPRAMINE AND AMITRIPTYLINE

Oral preparations of imipramine consist of tablets of 10 mg and 25 mg. An ampoule containing 25 mg in 2 ml is available for I.M. injection, but is rarely used. The usual therapeutic dose of imipramine, which was the first of the tricyclids to be marketed, is 50 mg T.D.S. There is however, wide individual variation in the response of patients, and 25 mg T.D.S. or 75 mg T.D.S. may be the effective dose for a particular patient. In older people, particularly if arteriosclerotic changes are suspected, initial dosage at least should be low, owing to the possibility of hypotension developing with this drug—as is the case with any of the tricyclids.

Amitriptyline may be given orally as tablets or capsules of 10 mg and 25 mg, and as a mixture containing 10 mg in 5 ml. A preparation of 2 ml containing 25 mg per ml is also available for intramuscular injection.

Amitriptyline has a more beneficial effect on agitation than does imipramine. It is more often necessary to give a small dose of a major tranquilliser or a minor tranquilliser with imipramine to settle agitation or anxiety, than it is with amitriptyline. Amitriptyline appears to be a slightly more superior antidepressant, though what has been said earlier about a drug being as good as the person who prescribes it, applies here. As well as being effective in the treatment of the psychotic depressions, amitriptyline has a place in the treatment of neurotic depression.

The usual dose of amitriptyline is 25 mg T.D.S., and if it is necessary to increase this, an extra tablet is given in the evening. The maximum dose for those depressions that are going to respond is rarely more than 50 mg T.D.S.

Improvement with both imipramine and amitriptyline is generally noticeable within one or two weeks of adequate medication. One should not be unduly concerned however, if there is not a marked response before three weeks, as improvement in the patient's clinical state has been observed as long as five or six weeks after commencement of medication.

It is an interesting fact that some patients suffering from a mild depressive illness will improve with as little as one 25 mg tablet of amitriptyline in the evening. (This also applies to other antidepressant drugs.)

Once a depressed person's mood level has returned to normal, and he is clinically well, it is important to maintain medication at the effective dosage level, usually 25 mg T.D.S. for several months, after which time medication should be reduced by 25 mg per day monthly, returning to the previous dosage level should any re-exacerbation of symptoms occur. The reason for this treatment regime is that an untreated depressive illness usually runs a course which may be anything from a few weeks to many months, or even years in rare instances. Unless guided by previous attacks, one cannot really determine how long the illness is likely to continue. If medication which has caused a raising of the mood level is stopped too soon, the patient's mood will return to a point consistent with the expected untreated level. This is shown diagramatically in Fig. 14 where the heavy line represents the patient's untreated mood level and the interrupted line the alteration caused by antidepressant medication.

If antidepressant medication is commenced at A, the mood level rises and usually flattens out at a normal level. If medication is stopped at B, mood level will fall to the untreated level. It is therefore important to continue medication at therapeutic levels, maintaining the 'artificially' induced rise in mood to a point in time at least as far ahead as the untreated depression would have lifted, as shown by dotted line. These same principles apply of course to any antidepressant therapy.

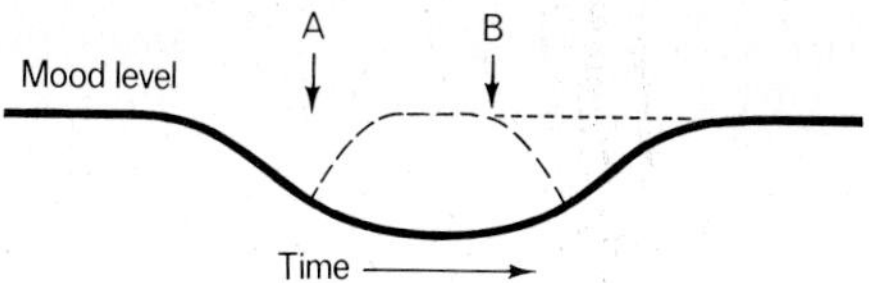

Fig. 14. **Mood level in depressive illness influenced by anti-depressant medication**

In severe depressions where it is felt that ECT is indicated early in treatment, for example, if the patient is in a stuporose state, not eating, or if he has gross depressive delusions, or in some instances if he is considered acutely suicidal, antidepressant medication may be commenced along with the ECT and continued for some months after its completion. In this way, though the medication does not significantly reduce the number of electroplexy treatments required, the relapse rate is lowered. One point to be remembered when embarking on any form of treatment for those psychotic depressive illnesses in which the patient is grossly retarded, is that a reduction in suicidal ideas may not run parallel with the activation of the patient, who becomes better able to put into effect his suicidal tendencies, because he is no longer grossly retarded in action.

Having embarked on some more general points relevant to the management of depression we shall return to the side-effects of imipramine and amitriptyline, which to a greater or lesser extent are common to all tricyclic antidepressants.

Side-effects of imipramine and amitriptyline

Side effects are usually minimal, and may be lessened by lowering the daily dose if this is feasible. The most common side-effect is dryness of the mouth due to reduction in the production of saliva. Something that may result indirectly from this if oral hygiene is poor, is infection, evidenced as a stomatitis or even as a parotitis. Drowsiness, tremulousness, agitation and palpitations may be encountered. Some patients complain of inordinate sweating, especially at night. Flushing of the skin, erythematous patches and rashes may occur. Difficulty in accommodation may lead to blurring of vision. Hypotension leading to dizziness, giddiness and even syncope, especially of the postural type, may be caused by large doses. Constipation may occur and will need to be counteracted with a mild laxative, for example, bisacodyl (Durolax) 5 mg, two tablets at night.

Difficulty in micturition may be encountered, and one should be wary of over-prescribing in older men with possible prostatic hypertrophy in case acute retention of urine is precipitated.

Impotence in males and lack of sexual urge in females may be due to treatment with the tricyclic antidepressants, and it is sometimes difficult to ascertain whether the depression itself or the drug is to blame. Dysarthria is a rare side effect, as are epileptic seizures though they may occur in people with low fit thresholds.

A few patients are difficult to maintain at a reasonable mood level as they readily swing over into a hypomanic state. Reduction in dosage, or the concurrent administration of one of the phenothiazines or haloperidol may be indicated in such cases.

Imipramine and amitriptyline should be used with extreme caution, if at all, in patients suffering from glaucoma. Mention should perhaps be made again of the value of these drugs in the management of nocturnal enuresis, their effectiveness appearing to be related to the anticholinergic effects of these drugs. Doses ranging from 20 mg-50 mg or even greater amounts of either, are given some $\frac{1}{2}$-1 hour before retiring.

NORTRIPTYLINE

This drug appears to be as equally effective as imipramine and amitriptyline, and its side effects are similar, as is its contraindication in glaucoma. It is prepared in tablet and capsule forms in strengths of 10 mg and 25 mg and also as a paediatric elixir containing 10 mg per 5 ml.

DOXEPIN

Doxepin hydrochloride is one of the latest of the tricyclic antidepressants to be approved by the Food and Drug Administration in the United States of America. Its use in Australia at this time is not widespread, but from an appraisal of clinical reports of its use in Europe and the United States, it would appear to be an effective antidepressant and anti-anxiety agent, with less intense anticholinergic side effects than are produced by the other tricyclids mentioned above. Enhanced therapeutic activity, said to be due to a seven-membered central ring instead of six as in other tricyclids, is claimed for this drug.

Doxepin is prepared in pink and red capsules in strengths of 10 mg, 25 mg, and 50 mg. For mildly to moderately depressed patients, the usual initial dosage is 25 mg T.D.S. or Q.I.D. This may be increased by increments of 25 mg per day until the effective therapeutic level for the particular patient is reached, usually 75 mg-150 mg daily. More severely depressed patients will require 150 mg-300 mg daily. Elderly patients and patients with cardiac conditions would appear to tolerate the drug very well.

The above drugs are given as examples of the many tricyclic antidepressants available. Manufacturers produce comprehensive brochures which, in general, give sound information on the other preparations with which you may come into contact. There is not much to pick between this whole group of drugs in terms of antidepressant potency. More important than erudite dissertation on finer shades of their action is the need to get to know how to use one or two of these drugs effectively, and to be able to diagnose depression satisfactorily.

Not included with the tricyclids is another antidepressant, dibenzepin hydrochloride (Noveril) which is stated by its manufacturers to be 'the first representative of the dibenzodiazepines, a new group of compounds with psychotrophic activity'. This drug would appear to be as effective as say amitriptyline. It is available in tablets of 80 mg and in ampoules containing 40 mg in 2 ml. Initial doses vary between 160 mg and 400 mg daily, which is increased to 240-480 mg daily after a few days.

Monoamine oxidase inhibitors

Drugs of this group are called monoamine oxidase inhibitors (MAOIs) because they inhibit the enzyme amine oxidase, thus preventing it from destroying 5-hydroxytryptamine or serotonin. It is believed that the antidepressant effect of the MAOIs is due to the resultant raising of the level of serotonin which is said to briefly excite cerebral neurones between its liberation and destruction.

There are two types of these enzyme inhibitors, the hydrazines represented by such drugs as iproniazid (Marsilid) and phenelzine (Nardil), and the non-hydrazines of which tranylcypromine (Parnate) is an example.

It has been stated above that tricyclic antidepressants are in general more effective in psychotic depressions, and the monoamine oxidase inhibitors more effective in the management of 'atypical depression' and neurotic depression, but there are many exceptions to this. Monoamine oxidase inhibitors are falling into disfavour, not because of their lack of effect in suitable cases, but because of serious side effects and the necessity to obviate some of these by strict dietary precautions. Iproniazid, the first widely-prescribed monoamine oxidase inhibitor may be very toxic to the liver, and fatal liver damage has been attributed to its use.

Phenelzine is available in tablets of 15 mg. The usual dose is 15 mg T.D.S. which is gradually reduced after maximum benefit is obtained. Tranylcypromine is prepared as 10 mg tablets, and the starting dose is 10 mg morning and afternoon. If no response occurs after two or three weeks this may be increased to 10 mg T.D.S.

Side effects to these drugs may occur early, or weeks or months after commencement of therapy. They appear to be more common in elderly women.

The number of medical conditions to which the monoamine oxidase inhibitors are anathema, and the large number of drugs with which they are incompatible will not be enumerated here, but anyone contemplating their use should be thoroughly cognizant with the deleterious possibilities.

Among the less serious side effects are dry mouth, headache, dizziness, postural hypotension, gastric disturbance, constipation, difficulty in initiating micturition, oedema, skin rash and mild hypomania.

Severe headache may be associated with hypertension, and there is no way of telling who will experience this cephalalgia and hypertension. Out of a clear blue sky at any time, on any dosage, a throbbing occipital headache, becoming generalised, may develop. This may be associated with nausea and vomiting, tachycardia, dizziness, sweating, muscular twitching, pallor, dilated pupils, severe chest pain, photophobia and neck stiffness. The clinical picture is similar to that occurring in subarachnoid haemorrhage or in hypertensive crises associated with a phaeochromocytoma which is a tumour of the adrenal medulla.

Subarachnoid haemorrhage may indeed occur, as seen from the following anecdote. The author some years ago examined a middle-aged woman admitted to an admission centre and suffering with typical depressive neurosis which had not responded to a monoamine oxidase inhibitor prescribed by her local doctor. She was admitted and examined in the evening and showed no abnormal physical signs but gave a history of some mild headache one or two weeks earlier, and she had a mild headache on admission. Medical undergraduates were attending a teaching session in another building at the hospital on the following morning and the patient expressed her willingness to be present. In the morning, word came back from the lecturer running the teaching session, inferring that we were utter fools for sending along a patient with a subarachnoid haemorrhage. This patient, showing no neurological signs on the evening before, had given a hand with some ward chores, and by morning had a stiff neck and a Babinski sign due to a small subarachnoid bleed. (She made a satisfactory recovery.)

Such hypertensive crises which may lead to cephalalgia or subarachnoid haemorrhage are precipitated in patients on monoamine oxidase inhibitors, by the presence of a pressor amine, tyramine, in food eaten. The main culprit is cheese, as all types of cheese, except perhaps cream cheese and cottage cheese, contain quite a high concentration of tyramine, the highest being in cheddar cheese. Among other tyramine-containing food and drink are the protein extracts such as Marmite and Bovril, and alcohol (especially Chianti). It would appear that other pressor substances are also implicated, one being the aminoacid, dihydroxyphenylalanine (DOPA) which is found in broad beans, in higher concentration in the pods than in the seeds. Sour cream, pickled herring, chicken livers and canned figs are other foods it is advisable to avoid. It has been stated that monoamine oxidase inhibitors should not be used with any of the tricyclic antidepressants as such combinations may lead to serious hyperactivity, convulsions, hyperpyrexia, and even death, but real evidence that such co-administration is unduly hazardous appears to be lacking. Such combined antidepressant therapy can be used with considerable benefit to patients who are refractory to single antidepressants and who are not considered suitable for ECT, provided that both drugs are started simultaneously and given orally in doses lower than would be used if each drug was given on its own. Also, it seems that no problems will be encountered if therapy is started with a tricyclid and an MAO inhibitor added later.

If sympathomimetic drugs such as adrenaline, ephedrine, amphetamine and methedrine are taken by patients under treatment with an MAO inhibitor, severe headache, hypertension, hyperpyrexia and subarachnoid haemorrhage may occur. On the other hand, their combination with morphine or pethidine may lead to collapse.

This is merely an introduction to possible pitfalls in the use of monoamine oxidase inhibitors. In spite of all this however, some patients appear to be able to use them under medical direction with relative impunity if they are well instructed in the hazards, and avoid dangerous combinations with certain foods, drinks and drugs.

Sedatives

Sedatives are used to decrease agitation, restlessness and excitement, and to promote sleep.

Earlier chapters dealt with misuse or abuse of a number of sedatives, and here we shall dwell briefly on clinical use only. Because a drug is potentially one that can be abused, and any drug that tranquillises or sedates can become a drug of dependence, one should not throw rational therapy with such drugs out the door.

Barbiturates are relatively cheap, and a large range is available for the management of insomnia and to control such symptoms as agitation and restlessness. It is sound practice to prescribe them for as long as is necessary in those psychiatric conditions in which insomnia is a symptom and which respond to treatment, for example, manic depressive psychosis, depressed type. Their use in chronic states of tension needs to be weighed carefully, as tolerance to them, as well as physiological dependence, is developed.

The dosage of barbiturates will depend of whether they are being used primarily as tranquillising agents or as promoters of sleep.

The choice of barbiturate for the promotion of sleep will depend on the duration of action required. Longer acting barbiturates (8-12 hours) include amylobarbitone, butobarbitone and cyclobarbitone, while pentobarbitone and quinalbarbitone are short-acting (4-6 hours). Sleep disturbance may be classified as initial insomnia, or difficulty in getting off to sleep, middle insomnia, which implies frequent waking, and delayed insomnia or early morning waking. Obviously there may be mixtures of these patterns. Knowing the length of action of these drugs one can choose the cap that fits. It would be unsatisfactory, for example, for a person suffering from early morning waking to be given a short acting barbiturate.

There are many non-barbiturates available, and the development of these is to be applauded. Ones in fairly common use include methaqualone hydrochloride, nitrazepam and methyprylone.

Though, for reasons related to limiting sensitive prescribing, combinations of drugs in the one tablet are in general eschewed by psychiatrists, an excellent sedative consists of a combination of methaqualone and the antihistamine drug, diphenhydramine hydrochloride.

More recent psychoactive drugs

Lithium

It may seem inappropriate to speak of lithium as a recent addition to the drug armamentarium, as its value in the treatment of 'psychotic excitement' was demonstrated by J. F. J. Cade as far back as 1949. Much earlier than this, in the mid 19th century, lithium had been introduced into medicine as a remedy for gout. Later, various lithium salts were prescribed for a variety of conditions, and in the 1940s lithium chloride was used rather indiscriminately as a taste-substitute for common salt in the low-sodium treatment of oedema due to congestive cardiac failure. There were a number of fatal outcomes as a result of this unbridled enthusiasm, and by 1949, the year of Cade's publication, the drug was withdrawn from medical use in the United States of America. This set back some two decades the assessment and development of lithium as a therapeutic substance. In 1970, the United States Food and Drug Administration permitted its reintroduction strictly for the treatment of mania. It is now used effectively in a variety of illnesses, and mostly as lithium carbonate.

INDICATIONS

Cade summarises the indications for lithium therapy as follows:

1. It is given for mania, both as treatment and as prophylaxis.
2. It is given for manic-depressive (bipolar) illness, both as treatment and as prophylaxis; it is less effective in depressive swings.
3. In recurrent endogenous (unipolar) depressive illness it is highly effective as prophylaxis in a number of cases, and is probably useful as treatment, especially if there is a family history of manic-depressive illness and lithium responsivity.
4. In some cases of schizo-affective illness and so-called chronic schizophrenia, it is dramatically effective. Those in the latter category who do respond have frequently had affective symptoms at some time.
5. It is used in character or personality disorders in young people with clear evidence of cyclothymia.
6. Other uses are in as yet only thinly explored areas—explosive aggressive prisoner psychopaths, childhood hyperkinesis, hyperthyroidism (as lithium iodide) and Huntington's chorea.

Lithium carbonate

Lithium should never be prescribed for a first affective swing in early adult life as the person may not have another for years, and once a decision is made to use lithium it is in Cade's words a 'life sentence'. The decision to use lithium will be influenced by the frequency of manic-depressive swings and the family history.

A usual therapeutic dose is 1,800 mg of lithium per day designed to produce a therapeutic serum level of 0.8-1.2 mEq/*l* in five to ten days. When remission has been produced in seven to fourteen days the dosage is reduced to a dose sufficient to maintain the blood level within the therapeutic range. This is usually between 600 to 1200 mg/day. It is important that patients on lithium therapy should have an adequate sodium intake.

Obviously, because lithium is a potentially toxic drug and because minimal serum levels have to be attained for it to be therapeutic, facilities for monitoring blood levels must be available. These are usually estimated at least twice weekly in the beginning of treatment, thereafter weekly for the next month, monthly for the next year, and then quarterly as a routine unless there is a recurrence of symptoms. In lithium poisoning which may lead to death, the blood level exceeds 2.0-3.0 mEq/*l*.

Side effects described are some degree of lassitude, difficulty in initiating action and a fine tremor of the fingers, none of which are disabling. Most toxic effects are attributable to the drug's action on the gastrointestinal tract and the central nervous system. These consist of anorexia, nausea, vomiting, severe abdominal discomfort and diarrhoea; lassitude, ataxia, slurred speech, marked tremor and muscle twitching; and in severe intoxication, choreoathetosis, increasing lethargy and stupor leading to coma, and sometimes generalized seizures.

Two other effects of lithium are the depression of thyroid function leading to goitre which responds to thyroid hormone medication, and a so-called diabetes insipidus syndrome where polyuria is marked. This latter paradoxically responds to chlorothiazide, a diuretic drug.

As renal tubular damage may occur with toxic doses, lithium is contra-indicated in patients with pre-existing circulatory and renal disease.

Propranolol

Propranolol is a Beta-adrenergic blocking agent first used in medicine in the 1960s for the treatment of angina pectoris and cardiac arrhythmias, and later for the management of hypertension and familial essential tremor.

It has been found to alleviate the physical symptoms associated with anxiety which are mediated via the sympathetic nervous system. Its main site of action is peripheral as opposed to the benzodiazepines and neuroleptic drugs which influence brain metabolism.

It is suggested that in a state of anxiety a vicious circle is established where anxiety gives rise to distressing physical symptoms (page 56) which in turn perpetuate feelings of anxiety. If the physical concomitants of anxiety can be ameliorated then an anxiety attack may well be cut short.

The drug propranolol (Inderal) is prepared in tablets of 10 mg and 40 mg. The effective dose range is between 80-320 mg per day, the average maintenance dose being 160 mg given in two divided doses. Side effects consist of feelings of lethargy or fatigue and sometimes nightmares which are avoided by taking the evening dose earlier. As the drug in effective doses diminishes cardiac output and slows the pulse rate, it is contra-indicated where the patient has a low cardiac reserve as in congestive cardiac failure, and in heart block. Bronchospastic airways disease (asthma) is also a contra-indication. There are enthusiastic claims for its efficacy in the treatment of anxiety, but in a review article by Whitlock and Price, the following conservative statement is made:

> The assessment of new drugs for the treatment of anxiety presents many problems. Subjective assessment is made difficult by placebo effect. Objective measurements may appear to slightly benefit but if the patient does not feel an overall sense of improvement the drug must be

deemed to have failed. Using this creterion, the performance of Beta-blocking agents in anxiety states is not impressive. Nevertheless, where autonomic symptoms are troublesome, and particularly where these are referable to the cardiovascular system, the addition of a Beta-blocking drug to conventional anxiolytic therapy, such as a benzodiazepine, would seem likely to prove useful.

Other possible uses of propanolol in psychiatry are in the amelioration of alcoholic and opiate withdrawal symptoms, and as a counter to the fine tremor produced by lithium.

It is too early to comment on its use in schizophrenia where only a limited number of trials have been carried out.

Conclusion

This section on psychopharmacology is not intended to take the place of a pharmacopoeia, but merely to indicate some general principles. Drugs favoured by many prescribers have no doubt been omitted, but adequate literature is available on this expanding area of psychiatry.

To know your drugs requires more than book learning. One must be familiar with the colour, shape, size and nature of the preparations being used, talk about them and listen to one's patients.

To some extent, drugs may have done away with the need for close contact with patients suffering from certain illnesses, but people caring for patients must never lose sight of the fact that the way they relate to them is still of inestimable value in therapy; it is often not the pill but who gives it that counts.

PHYSICAL TREATMENTS

In this section on physical treatments, we shall look briefly at electroconvulsive therapy, modified insulin therapy, prolonged (or continuous) narcosis, leucotomy and amygdalotomy.

Electroconvulsive therapy (ECT)

Electroconvulsive therapy goes under a number of names, such as electroplexy, shock treatment, and some, supposedly euphemistically, refer to it as electrocerebral therapy. The name however, is not as important as how the nurse or doctor explains the treatment to the patient who is about to receive it. Convulsive therapy was first used by a Hungarian, Dr Von Meduna, in 1935, who injected camphor-in-oil intramuscularly into patients. Later the camphor-in-oil was replaced by intravenous injections of leptazol to produce convulsions. Its use was based on the belief of another Hungarian, Dr Nyiro, that epilepsy occurred much less frequently with schizophrenia than could be accounted for by chance alone. This is now known not to be so, and it was found also that convulsive therapy was of marked value only in sufferers from schizophrenia who experienced mood changes such as depression, and in schizophrenic patients who were stuporose (catatonic stupor). It later became apparent that this form of treatment was much more effective in depressive illnesses, than in schizophrenia generally. It is an empirical treatment, which means that there was no scientific rationale worked out before it was applied. The use of electricity to produce convulsions was introduced by two Italians, Cerletti and Bini, in 1938, replacing the previous pharmacological methods which were disagreeable to patients. ECT was first given unmodified or 'straight', but nowadays it is preceded by the injection of a general anaesthetic and a muscle relaxant which minimises the actual convulsions produced when the cerebral neurones discharge upon the passing of an electric current through the brain—a procedure which is known as Modified Electro Convulsive Therapy.

The technique essentially consists of giving a general anaesthetic, usually I.V. thiopentone sodium (pentothal) up to 0.25 G (usually less) in a 2½% solution, and following it with an intravenous injection of a muscle relaxant, for example suxamethonium bromide (Brevidil-E) or suxamethonium chloride (Scoline) 50-100 mg. The muscle relaxant is injected through the same needle as the general anaesthetic, the needle being left in the vein between injections.

When the muscle relaxant has caused complete relaxation by its blocking action at the neuromuscular junction (this relaxation is preceded by muscle fasciculation or fibrillation), and the patient has been adequately oxygenated by means of face mask and bag connected to a cylinder of oxygen, an electric current of 90-160 volts is passed for 0.1-1 second between padded electrodes moistened with a saline solution and placed over both temples (bilateral) or over one temple and a point on the scalp on the same side of the head (unilateral).

There is fairly conclusive evidence that unilateral placement over the nondominant hemisphere leads to less post ECT confusion and memory impairment, the latter usually being short lived in any case.

The passage of the electric current causes discharges in the cerebral neurones, and if no muscle relaxant were used this electrical activity would cause a generalised convulsion with tonic, clonic and flaccid paralysis stages. The general anaesthetic and muscle relaxant having been used however, little movement results. It may be as slight as a flickering of the eyelids and fanning of the toes. If too well modified, no movement is observable, and in order to tell if the cerebral neurones have fired, it is worthwhile checking the pupils within seconds of passing the current. The pupils will not react to light but remain dilated for a time if generalised neuronal discharge has occurred. If the pupils still react to light it is worthwhile checking the electrodes and their application and passing the current a second time.

Indications for ECT

1. *Manic depressive psychosis, depressed type; reactive depressive psychosis; involutional melancholia*: In these conditions the average number of treatments is six to eight, usually given two or three times weekly. It is sound practice to give two further treatments after clinical improvement, as this lessens the relapse rate.

2. *Manic depressive psychosis, manic type*: One or two treatments are given daily until the patient has received eight and sometimes more treatments.

3. *Depressive neurosis*: Four to six treatments are usually adequate.

This condition is a doubtful indication, and patients may become depersonalised and feel worse than they did before treatment.

4. *Schizophrenia*: In these days with our improved drug armamentarium there is little or no place for ECT in the management of schizophrenia, save when affective symptoms, gross retardation, or catatonic symptoms (stupor or excitement) are in evidence. Catatonic stupors respond dramatically. In catatonic excitement the giving of up to three treatments in 24 hours may be life saving. Acute paranoid states respond, but sufferers from hebephrenia or simple schizophrenia, or people with an insidiously developing paranoid schizophrenia generally do poorly.

5. *Epilepsy*: An artificially induced fit may cut short the irritability and depression that precedes a seizure in some sufferers.

6. *Other*: Electrotherapy has been used to treat the affective component present in certain organic cerebral conditions, some acute organic states and, rarely, psychosomatic disorders such as asthma and neurodermatitis.

Contra-indications

Advanced age is not a contra-indication in the absence of cardiovascular degeneration. In fact, first attacks of depression occurring at any age over fifty respond very well unless some organic cerebral factor is complicating the picture.

Acute pulmonary infection is a contra-indication from an anaesthetic point of view but pulmonary tuberculosis is not.

Simple hypertension is not a contra-indication; in fact, the blood pressure in agitated patients may subside after treatment.

Recent coronary thrombosis requires expert anaesthetic care but fatalities are not common.

Bone complications, particularly recent fractures will require adequate relaxation.

Probably, the only absolute contra-indication to electrotherapy is the presence of a cerebral tumour.

Complications of treatment

With the advent of modified ECT, fractures and dislocations have become extremely rare. The risk of anaesthetic complications is the same as for any short general anaesthetic, and the nurse should remain with patients after each treatment until they are fully conscious, and should report any abnormality in breathing or colour to the doctor after ensuring that the airway is clear.

Some degree of post-treatment memory impairment may occur, especially for little details such as names, particularly with bilateral ECT, though this generally clears up within two weeks. In older patients with organic brain syndromes, confusion may be aggravated, but wider spacing of treatments will do much to obviate this.

Fatalities are said to occur in 1 in every 1,000 cases treated.

As a result of massive treatments with ECT carried out over a period of years, necessary in schizophrenia before the advent of suitable drugs, and probably related to anoxia of parts of the brain associated with unmodified ECT, a number of long-hospitalised patients have developed irritable foci of electrical activity in the brain and are prone to suffer epileptic seizures. Whether this state of affairs would follow massive treatment with modified ECT in which patients are adequately oxygenated before each treatment is still an open question.

Modified insulin therapy

Modified insulin therapy consists in giving soluble insulin in doses of 10-30 units or more some 3 hours before giving the patient food in the mornings. The procedure lowers the level of blood sugar, reduces emotional tension, produces drowsiness and relaxation and increases appetite. The commencing dose is 10 units of soluble insulin which is increased by 5-10 units daily, so long as the patient can still take his meal at the end of three hours without needing to be roused. Sweating may be profuse. Threatened coma is averted by sitting the patient up and giving sweetened tea. Intravenous glucose may be required in rare cases of insulin sensitivity. Treatment is omitted on one day per week. The procedure has been used in the treatment of drug addicts suffering from withdrawal symptoms, and to increase appetite and produce relaxation in many forms of psychiatric illness. Nowadays it has largely been replaced by other pharmacological means.

Modified insulin therapy should not be confused with Insulin Coma Therapy or 'Deep Insulin Therapy' which until a decade or more ago was used extensively in the treatment of schizophrenia (page 191ff).

Prolonged (or continuous) narcosis

Continuous narcosis has few advocates today, its place being largely taken by other forms of treatment. The object of the treatment is to keep the patient asleep for about 20 out of 24 hours a day for a period ranging from 5 to 14 days, the patient being roused for meals and other nursing procedures.

Indications for this treatment are:

1. Depression with much agitation and anxiety;
2. Obsessional illness with agitation.
3. Mania.
4. Drug withdrawal symptoms.

A special darkened quiet room and skilled nursing care are necessary.

Among sedatives used are amylobarbitone, chlorpromazine, paraldehyde.

10-15 units of soluble insulin followed by one ounce of glucose given twice daily seems to combat toxic effects due to accumulation of barbiturates in the body.

Charts and records of temperature, blood pressure, respiration, urinalysis, and fluid balance must be kept.

Diet must be adequate and the body warm. Breathing exercises and regular turning of the patient will help to prevent the development of hypostatic pneumonia; and bowels, bladder and skin require close attention.

The procedure may be dangerous in elderly or infirm patients or in presence of organic disease.

Complications include:

1. Toxic effects.
2. Hypostatic pneumonia.
3. Cardiovascular collapse.
4. Venous thrombosis in calf.
5. Abscess formation at site of injections. This may particularly occur with paraldehyde which, with age, breaks down chemically to form acetic acid.
6. Withdrawal fits.

Leucotomy

Leucotomy is a surgical operation on the intact brain for the relief of mental symptoms, and particularly for the reduction of emotional tension. Tracts of white matter between the thalamus (dorsomedial nucleus) and the frontal cortex are severed. This operation should not be undertaken until emotional stress has failed to respond to all other reasonable treatment measures. It was conceived by Moniz of Lisbon, in 1933, and first carried out under his direction by Lima, in 1935.

The original standard prefrontal leucotomy carried out in the plane of the coronal suture led, in many instances, to personality changes (page 178) and it has been modified in various ways, among which are included:

1. Transorbital leucotomy (Freeman and Watts).
2. Selective cortical undercutting (Scoville).
3. Topectomy consisting of excision of portions of the frontal cortex (Pool).
4. Thalamotomy—electrocoagulation of the dorsomedial thalamic nuclei (Grantham).
5. Rostral leucotomy, in which a brain needle is directed from trephine holes anterior to the coronal suture towards the midpoint of the supraorbital plate (first performed by Wylie McKissock in London, 1948).

J. Pippard (1955) compared personality changes after rostral and standard prefrontal leucotomies. He found negligible personality deficit after 95% of rostral leucotomies which gave good symptomatic relief, compared with only 44% after standard leucotomies.

Indications for leucotomy

Pippard states that, where all other physical and psychological methods of treatment have failed, leucotomy may be considered in the treatment of the following conditions:

1. Obsessive tension states.
2. Phobic states.
3. Obsessive-compulsive neuroses.
4. Persistent depressive states in older patients, especially those with obsessional personality.
5. Some schizophrenic syndromes, particularly the paranoid and (so-called) pseudoneurotic.

6. Cases where serious emotional distress has failed to respond to other reasonable treatment measures.
7. Some cases of intractable pain.

Complications of leucotomy

Surgical mortality is 1-3%. The incidence of epilepsy as a complication of leucotomy varies with the type of operation and averages about 10% of cases. Seizures may appear shortly after or up to ten years post operatively. Gain in weight is usual. Personality changes occur if the incision is too extensive (see frontal lobe syndrome).

Surgical convalescence after operation is a matter of days but social convalescence may take months or years. If psychosurgery has been extensive, doctors, nurses and the patient's family have the job of helping the patient to grow up from his surgically induced childhood.

Amygdalotomy

Amygdalotomy is an operation wherein the amygdaloid nuclei which are part of the visceral brain and situated medial to the uncinate cortex are destroyed at operation. This is a recent and still a relatively uncommon procedure and its main indication is the control of aggression in some patients when other methods of treatment have failed.

The part played by nursing staff both before, during and after physical treatments is of major importance. The emotional and physical preparation of patients for ECT and post treatment observations cannot be stressed too much. Prolonged narcosis can bring in its train many physical complications if nursing care is not of a high standard. Following leucotomy and amygdalotaomy, surgical convalescence is relatively short, but social convalescence may take months or even years, and nursing staff can play a major part in such convalescence or rehabilitation.

SOCIAL AND MILIEU THERAPY

Faulty interpersonal relationships in some instances contribute towards psychiatric disorder. Also, whatever the factors in the genesis of such disorders, sufferers frequently show a marked lack of confidence and find it difficult to mix with others and to apply themselves to their occupations and to those activities that form part of the normal person's day-to-day existence.

Social therapy is therapy designed to correct faulty interpersonal relationships, to increase a person's self awareness and self assurance and to enlarge his scope of activities, especially in as much as they involve interpersonal relationships. Various activities, such as occupational therapy, industrial therapy, homemaking and beauty courses, ward socials, dances, sport, music and painting conducted in group situations, all serve as media for social therapy.

Milieu therapy consists of the production in a treatment situation of an environment or atmosphere which is helpful or therapeutic. The French term 'milieu' means literally, environment or social surroundings.

We have already discussed the change from a custodial to a more permissive regime in hospitals which develop as therapeutic communities. In such hospitals, the whole atmosphere becomes more hopeful and patients are seen as individuals who have potential and who, in fact, may play a part in planning their own management. This represents a helpful change in a hospital milieu and any change in such direction constitutes milieu therapy.

It is really somewhat artificial to separate these two forms of therapy as it is obvious that, if social therapy is undertaken, the treatment milieu is changed for the better, and any steps to improve a ward or hospital milieu will involve improvements in social relationships. For this reason, it is more practical to speak of social and milieu therapy as a single entity.

Within the general framework of this approach, many other forms of treatment may be undertaken such as drug and physical therapies; and the application of principles of social and milieu therapy may add much to any psychiatric, medical and surgical treatment programme. The development of a therapeutic community in a treatment setting described in Chapter 2 is an aspect of social and milieu therapy.

SPECIAL TECHNIQUES

In this section we shall somewhat arbitrarily deal with the following: behaviour therapy, cognitive therapy, abreactive techniques and hypnosis.

Behaviour therapy

Behaviour therapy consists in the application of principles of learning (and of experimental psychology) to the treatment of disorders of behaviour that may be subsumed under a number of different diagnostic labels. The therapist looks objectively at both environmental events and the patient's behaviour, and analyses the maladaptive responses of the patient, or more specifically, those behavioural patterns which in response to environmental events are distressful to a person, or limit his satisfactions or effectiveness.

On the basis of this analysis, a programme that may be modified in the light of individual response to treatment, is worked out.

Systematic desensitisation

A common procedure used by behaviour therapists is known as systematic desensitisation. Three steps are described. Firstly, the patient is taught to produce muscle relaxation in a progressive fashion in himself. This may be done by teaching him to tense groups of muscles then relax them in turn until muscle relaxation has spread throughout the body and extremities. Some therapists use hypnotic techniques to produce this muscle relaxation.

Next, the patient and therapist determine all the situations that give rise to inappropriate anxiety in the patient and these are grouped in themes and graded in terms of anxiety produced. This grading of stimuli that produce anxiety or ineffectual behaviour is referred to as *hierarchy construction.*

In the third step, the patient imagines an anxiety-producing scene while in a relaxed state, commencing with the one he finds least anxiety-producing; and when this can be imagined without distress, the patient, again in a state of muscular relaxation, progresses to the next scene in the heirarchy, and so on until he can imagine the most anxiety-producing scene with equanimity. Between sessions the patient is encouraged to enter the particular situations he has coped with in imagination in therapy, and approval of the therapist for undertaking such activity acts as reinforcement to the patient's efforts.

Work done in therapy may well be undone by actions of others in the patient's day-to-day world. For example, relatives who show over-solicitous concern and even undertake on behalf of a patient, functions that he wishes to avoid, may well be rewarding maladaptive functioning. This could happen, for example, if washing clothes is anathema to a patient on the basis of a phobia that she will contaminate them, and relatives show over-concern and undertake this chore for her. It is important for relatives to be made aware of the possible effects of such action.

On page 224, mention is made of the therapist or other person accompanying the patient, aided initially by an anxiolytic drug, into a phobic situation. This act of the patient entering actual anxiety-producing situations with support, be they heights, open spaces or proximity to phobic objects, is known as *in vivo desensitisation* or reinforced practice. Systematic desensitisation may be seen as an application of Pavlovian or classical conditioning (page 324), the unadaptive activity having previously been conditioned to certain environmental cues.

Positive reinforcement

If a behavioural response to a situation is followed by a rewarding experience, for example the receipt of praise or food, or the avoidance of pain, the particular behavioural response is strengthened and will occur later with greater frequency in the same situation. The obtaining of a reward following a particular behavioural response to a situation is termed positive reinforcement. Positive reinforcement procedures have been used in a variety of clinical settings, for example to foster acceptable social habits in long-stay hospital patients, in speech training, in teaching and other management of mentally retarded children, in the management of specific neurotic and habit disturbances, and in the treatment of sexual deviations.

Some treatment and training situations lend themselves to the development of what is termed a *token economy*. In addition to reinforcing acceptable behaviour or performance by giving praise, it may also be reinforced by rewarding patients with tokens which may be used as a means of exchange by them to procure additional comforts and privileges.

One must be aware that positive reinforcement may be given unwittingly by hospital staff to inappropriate or undesirable behaviour. This can occur when a patient's unacceptable behaviour engenders more interest in, and involvement of staff with him than is usually the case. Why change behaviour that produces a greater degree of attention from, and social intercourse with staff?

Extinction and aversion

When a particular form of behaviour is followed by no stimulus at all, that is, when no reinforcement is given, it may well lead to weakening or extinction of that behaviour; and actual punishment of behaviour (an aversive stimulus), or the use of what is termed negative reinforcement, will also lead to a weakening of a behaviour and its less frequent occurrence.

These concepts of positive reinforcement, extinction and aversive stimulus are applications of instrumental or operant conditioning (see below).

Aversive stimuli are said to be less effective in modifying behaviour than are positive or rewarding stimuli, and the current trend in behaviour therapy favours positive reinforcement or non-aversive techniques. This is not to say that the giving of an aversive stimulus (a form of aversion therapy) is not of value in certain clinical situations, including the treatment of homosexuality.

A note on conditioning

Brief comment will be made on animal experimentation out of which have developed behaviour therapy procedures. It will be left largely to the student to make his own comparisons with human behaviour.

Ivan Pavlov (1849-1936), a Russian physiologist, noted that not only food placed in a dog's mouth produced salivation, but this response ocurred also at the sight of food. He made the assumption that salivation at the sight of food must have been learned. The flow of saliva produced by food he termed an unlearned or unconditioned response, while salivation at the sight of food he called a learned or conditioned response. Pavlov experimented to find out how conditioned responses are formed, and taught the dog to salivate in response to various signals or stimuli, proving that a stimulus-response association could be developed in the laboratory.

In the experimental situation, if a light (the conditioned stimulus) is switched on, initially the dog will make an irrelevant response or none at all and will not salivate. Giving meat powder (the unconditioned stimulus) a few seconds after giving the light signal, the dog eats and salivates. If this procedure is repeated a number of times, in the order, showing the light first (conditioned stimulus) and then the food (unconditioned stimulus) which produces salivation (the response), a process known as reinforcement, in time the dog will salivate when the light is turned on even though food does not follow. When this occurs, a conditioned response has been established. This method of conditioning is referred to as classical (or Pavlovian) conditioning. It is quite possible that certain human behaviour may be conditioned to certain environmental cues.

A second form of conditioning also occurs, this being instrumental or operant conditioning. This differs from classical conditioning in that in the experimental situation the animal is not harnessed but is freely moving and it has some choice in the action it takes. If an approved form of behaviour occurs and this is rewarded, the animal is more likely to repeat the approved form of behaviour. Operant conditioning is used in animal training. If one wishes to train a dog to bring the paper in each morning, one would probably say, 'Paper', hold the paper in his mouth and lead him to where the paper had to be deposited. After giving a reward and strong approval following this action on a number of occasions, the dog may learn to bring in the paper himself when one says 'Paper', in order to receive the reward or approval.

Rats and monkeys may learn to press bars or pull levers in order to obtain food. The bar-pressing and lever-pulling may be chance happenings initially, but if they lead to the appearance of food, the food acts as a reinforcer to the activity that produced it and it will be repeated to obtain more food. Should no food appear, bar-pressing and lever-pulling activities diminish in frequency, or, in other words, non-reinforcement of an action (or operant response) will lead to extinction of that response. There seems little doubt that operant or instrumental conditioning occurs continuously in our daily lives.

Aversive techniques

As well as the aversion techniques which utilise negative reinforcement or punishment in treatment procedures based on operant or instrumental conditioning theories, aversion to noxious habits may also be conditioned. This is seen when intramuscular injections of apomorphine, a powerful emetic, are given at the same time as alcohol is taken by mouth. The nausea and vomiting induced by apomorphine becomes associated with the drinking of alcohol; and it is hoped that the patient will develop a distaste or disgust for alcohol.

Assertive training

Assertive training covers a range of methods of promoting change of behaviour. There are many who suffer from anxiety in interpersonal situations with a subsequent inhibition of appropriate action and the inability to express basic feelings.

Techniques which fall under the rubric of behaviour therapy have been devised to help such individuals overcome these limitations and so come closer to achieving their desires and goals in life.

At the simplest level a graded list of assignments is worked through starting at the easiest and progressing to things that are more difficult. The task may be to stand up to friends or acquaintances who are exploiting one, or not to submit to the crippling domination of a spouse, or to modify an over-deferential attitude to authority figures. Appropriate motor acts of assertion usually provide rewarding consequences such as diminution of anxiety and greater control in interpersonal situations.

Relationship to psychotherapy

In recent years there has been much discussion on those elements in the practice of behaviour therapy which appear in essence to be psychotherapeutic techniques, and vice versa. Looking at one side only of this, there seems little doubt that long-term psychotherapy contains elements of a conditioning process. Emotions felt and expressed, or actions performed by patients in the past may have produced expected punishment of an unreasonable nature from parents. The thought or behaviour comes to be associated with anxiety that punishment will follow. If, in treatment, a person can express feelings to an accepting therapist who does not judge or criticise in the same unreasonable way as did parents, then the expressions of such feelings are no longer related to punishment, and having or expressing them may come to produce less anxiety in the person concerned.

Cognitive therapy

Classical conditioning takes cognisance essentially of what is observable. In other words one is interested in the response to a particular stimulus without postulating whether anything happens between the stimulus and the response.

In psychoanalysis or analytical psychotherapy, the therapist postulates that something happens between a stimulus and a response namely an unconscious process which may be an impulse, wish, memory or thought. This unconscious process (called an intervening variable) is considered to give rise to the response (or emotion). In psychoanalysis or analytical psychotherapy an aspect of therapy is to bring these unconscious processes into consciousness.

A more recent development is that of cognitive* therapy which like psychoanalysis postulates an intervening variable which consists of the meaning attached to a particular sitmulus or situation by a person.

It is hypothesised that it is the particular meaning attached to a situation that determines what emotional response occurs. Different people may attach different meanings to the same stimulus; that is, their conceptions of a situation or stimulus may differ. For some the experience of being in an aeroplane may be exhilarating and enjoyable, but for the person who equates being off the ground with a high risk of dying in a crash, the emotional response is the opposite and he may develop anxiety or phobic symptoms (his response) when he is about to board an aeroplane (the stimulus). Quite obviously there may be some risk attached to being 30,000 feet above the ground and this may not be the best example, but what of the woman who has a phobia of pigeons and won't walk across the street if there is one of these birds on the opposite footpath? It is hardly conceivable that a pigeon can harm one, so for this woman there is a particular meaning attached to pigeons (the stimulus), something that causes her anxiety and makes her avoid them (her response). Whatever has led to her phobia, it may be assumed her thinking is aberrant when it comes to pigeons.

Cognitive therapists recognise that common psychological disorders centre around certain aberrations in thinking leading to different meanings being attached to stimuli. These aberrations may be direct distortions of reality—for example, the paranoid person who believes everyone is against him—or they may arise from illogical thinking which includes drawing wrong conclusions from observations. How many people, after discovering a few minor faults in a newly-purchased car, jump to the wrong conclusion that the whole vehicle must be a 'bomb' and even the make of car terrible, when in fact everything else is in excellent condition.

* Cognition (L. *cognoscere*, to know) is that activity of the mind by which one 'knows' things, i.e. the means by which one is aware of the processing of thinking and perceiving. The faculties of understanding and reasoning are also entailed in cognition.

This type of thinking may lead to aberrant meanings being attached to objects or situations, and these aberrant meanings are important in determining faulty emotional and behavioural responses to otherwise neutral or even pleasurable situations.

While for example, loss, danger or attack may indeed be real in some situations, it is possible, due to incorrect judgements, to erroneously perceive loss, danger or attack in inappropriate situations; or, in other words, to attach inappropriate meanings (or cognitions) to situations where they are not warranted. In this way inappropriate emotions of sadness, anxiety and anger may arise. The inappropriate or aberrant attachment of meanings to objects or situations may be an ingrained habit of which the person is not consciously aware.

In cognitive therapy, attention is directed towards these faulty cognitions. Firstly, the patient must become aware of the meaning he attaches to an object or situation. Secondly, he must recognise that his thoughts in this area are illogical or inaccurate. He must then substitute accurate judgements on the object or situation for inaccurate ones, and finally, test out the validity of his substituted judgements in a practical way.

Cognitive therapy requires a close collaborative effort between patient and therapist, the patient in a sense learning to become the master of his own fate as early in therapy as possible. Techniques drawn from the field of behaviour therapy, for example 'assertive therapy', are used in conjunction with cognitive therapy. It is beyond the scope of this book to try to delineate the techniques used, and the interested student is referred to specialised texts (see Bibliography, Beck, A. T.)

Commented on above is the relationship between psychotherapy and behaviour therapy. Cognitive therapy bears an even closer relationship to behaviour therapy, even apart from its use of some behavioural techniques.

Abreactive techniques

Abreactive techniques are used to assist the patient to remember and talk about painful emotional experiences. The procedures involve the very slow intravenous injection of drugs such as methylphenidate (a stimulant) and/or amylobarbitone or thiopentone (sedatives). An example of the use of this technique in the exploration and management of hysterical paralysis is mentioned on page 221. It is important that 'recovered' memories resulting from these procedures be 'worked through' in psychotherapy.

Hypnosis

Hypnosis has been known for centuries, and still the process leading to the state of hypnosis and the nature of the hypnotic state remain a mystery. The term 'hypnosis' refers both to the process and the state produced. It is known however, that hypnosis is not the same as sleep and that under hypnosis a person becomes highly suggestible. The increased suggestibility under hypnosis is used in attempts, frequently successful, to correct distressing or harmful habits, to increase concentration, to increase a feeling of confidence, to relieve pain and so forth. Such effects however, are unfortunately not necessarily long-lasting. Deep trance subjects may be regressed to an earlier age under hypnosis and may recall events hitherto lost from consciousness. The uncovering of such events still needs to be 'worked through' in psychotherapy. The true deep trance subject has no recollection of the events occurring in the trance state, including memories revived, when he is 'wakened' from it. Symptoms may be removed by suggestion under hypnosis, but the removal of a symptom does nothing towards alleviating its cause and the symptom may recur or others take its place if the basic underlying conflict is not adequately dealt with, for example by psychotherapy.

From all the evidence available it may be categorically stated that hypnosis is not a therapy in itself but an adjunct to therapy. As Marceuse quotes in his book *Hypnosis, Fact and Fiction*: 'Just as surgical conditions are treated not by anaesthesia but under anaesthesia, so psychiatric or psychological matters are treated not by hypnosis, but the process is aided and facilitated by hypnosis'.

THE NURSING APPROACH

At this stage little will be said save that differing behaviour in patients, and patients with differing psychiatric disorders, will require the utilisation of a variety of management techniques on the part of the nursing staff. Some of these points have been touched upon earlier in sections dealing with specific conditions. There is no substitute for actual experience with patients and discussion with senior colleagues if one is to learn the finer points of patient management.

REHABILITATION TECHNIQUES

Just as rehabilitation is an essential aspect of the treatment of patients who have suffered physical disabilities, so the hospitalised psychiatric patient requires rehabilitation to fit him for his place in society. A person who breaks his leg may have perfect union of bone and the leg may be capable of withstanding all the normal strains likely to be imposed upon it. The muscles of the leg may have become less efficient or even wasted through disease, and specially designed exercises are performed to bring them to a state of normal functioning. Even when bone and muscle are normal the patient may be fearful of using the leg, and encouragement and practise must be given until such fears are dispelled and the patient can approach the business of using his leg as if nothing had ever happened to it. Of course, in modern physical rehabilitation techniques, the patient is helped to maintain the image of his leg as a useful limb and as extensive movement as possible is encouraged from the outset to enable the patient to maintain a normal body image.

The principles applying in physical medicine apply also to psychiatric patients who must be encouraged to see from the outset of their illness, the possibility of a normal future existence. To be realistic, in some psychiatric conditions we meet, as in some physical disabilities, a fully and permanently productive future may be difficult to guarantee, but the maximum of functional ability must be the aim and the patient must be encouraged to maintain his self-image as a useful citizen. There is always the possibility of some improvement. Rehabilitation techniques in psychiatric patients involve such things as:

1. The development of sustained periods of concentration in work situations—here the utilisation of occupational and industrial therapy plays an important part.
2. The development of more satisfactory social relationships in patients through the medium of such measures as socials and sporting activities.

The nurse, who is with the patient for a longer time in the day than any other discipline, must learn to work with the occupational therapist, the recreational officer and others who may be playing a specific role in patient rehabilitation.

The patient is not fully rehabilitated until he is once again functioning satisfactorily in the community. This later stage involves the specialised skills of social workers and welfare officers, and the nurse who functions as a domiciliary nurse may play a very active role in helping the patient take this final step from in-patient care.

Some hospitals have specialised designated positions as Work Advisors or Rehabilitation Officers whose particular role concerns itself with this final step in a psychiatric patient's return to the community.

Mention should be made of those patients suffering from concomitant psychiatric and physical disabilities. Such patients constitute an immense challenge in rehabilitation programmes, involving a team of experts including doctors, social workers, physiotherapists, occupational therapists and nursing staff. The concept of 'total care' in handling such diverse handicaps has been developed wherein physical, mental, domestic and social factors are all seen as requiring concurrent attention.

COMMUNITY MEASURES

A review of factors in the causation of psychiatric illness (Chapter 10) will show that there is no single cause for a person's behaviour, and that there are many factors apparent in the community relevant to the development of psychiatric illness.

Even though little can be done to combat adverse hereditary and constitutional factors *per se,* the adverse environmental factors which may aggravate the effect of heredity or constitution are open to modification. The effects of early or remote environment on the developing child may be modified through education and psychological treatment of adults, and by the application of medical treatments. But even in this area, as in most of the other stress areas mentioned, including the critical periods of normal life, socioeconomic and sociocultural factors intertwine, leaving the individual therapist of whatever discipline feeling like a stunned mullet enmeshed in an intricate net which he cannot on his own unravel.

With such an expanding knowledge of factors relevant to the development of psychiatric disorders, and following the contributions of the social scientists, something more than just the clinical approach to psychiatric illness had to be developed. Community psychiatry is evolving to cater for this need.

Community mental health services

It is probably better, at this stage of development, to reserve the phrase 'therapeutic community' for those activities occurring within the hospital or unit as described in Chapter 2, and to employ the term 'community psychiatry' for those activities occurring outside the unit or hospital setting. These will include activities such as liaison with local doctors and outside organisations, the setting up of therapeutic facilities outside the hospital and the development of mental health consultation programmes, with all their ramifications.

When mental health services are provided for a community, a number of basic services are necessary, and these include inpatient services, out-patient services, facilities for part time care such as day or night hospitals, 24-hour a day emergency services, consultation and educational services available to community agencies and professional personnel. In addition to these basic or essential services, a comprehensive community service would also include diagnostic services, pre-hospital care and after-care services, the latter including such facilities as hostels, half-way houses, rehabilitation services, vocational and educational services, foster home placements and home visits. In addition, the machinery should be set up to undertake research, both into areas of need where preventive measures can be undertaken and into the results of one's community endeavours.

This becomes an enormous undertaking requiring the cooperation of a large number of different services. Liaison with them must be sound and regularly maintained if this complex treatment network is to remain workable. Whether the headquarters for such a comprehensive service is the regional psychiatric hospital or some other place in the community will depend on factors relevant to a particular area. In the state of New South Wales, the large psychiatric hospitals are, in the main, providing the impetus for community psychiatric endeavours, and so have become the organisational centres for developing work in the community. This does not mean that potential patients necessarily visit or are admitted to the hospital, for in many instances assessment centres in the community screen people in need of help, and deal appropriately with the problems presenting. It may well be that the citizen can receive help while remaining in the community by virtue of utilising one of the services there, by attendance at an outpatient clinic or day hospital centre in the community, or by dint of members of a domiciliary team helping him through a crisis.

In providing a mental health service the importance of making known what facilities are available to people in key positions, for example, doctors, teachers, clergy, lawyers, is of paramount importance. In fact, anyone in a position to detect emotional disturbance in people whom they serve should be made aware of the avenues of help into which they may steer their troubled fellow citizens.

Regionalisation

It becomes apparent that community psychiatry must be developed on a regional basis in order that the multiplicity of essential communications does not become unmanageable. In practice, in many parts of the world, this means that a particular geographical area is allotted to a particular hospital for the oversight of the community psychiatric programme. The hospitals themselves may contain units each of which is made responsible for a particular sub-region of what is uneuphemistically termed the 'catchment area' of the hospital. This limits the number of general practitioners, community services personnel and other key figures with whom personal liaison must be maintained by the staff of a particular hospital unit, thus improving the quality of communication.

Mental health consultation

A brief comment will be made on mental health consultation which differs from the traditional idea of consultation carried out by specialists in various fields of medicine. Restricting ourselves for the moment to a traditional medical consultation, the usual pattern is for the doctor who, either at his own or his patient's instigation, desiring a second opinion from a colleague or specialist in a particular field, requests a second doctor to see his patient. This second doctor who is called actually examines the patient in the appropriate fashion, then confers with the patient's doctor, giving his opinion as to diagnosis and appropriate management.

Mental health consultation differs from this and has been defined by Milton Greenblatt as 'an interaction between a consultant and a consultee on behalf of a client. The consultant is a person with a specialised knowledge in the mental health field; his consultee requests help in increasing his skills in handling a disturbance, crisis or troublesome situation, or in raising the mental health of a person or group for whom he is responsible. The client may be an individual, a group, an agency, or an institution.'

In this way the mental health consultant does not come into contact with the client (our patient in the traditional medical model above), but helps the consultee, who alone remains in contact with the client, to deal with the situation. Such a consultee may be a school teacher, domiciliary or public health nurse, social worker, clergyman, general practitioner, guidance counsellor, or any other professional community health worker.

Mental health consultation allows the mental health consultant with his high degree of expertise to have a wider field of helpful influence in the community, and provides a learning experience for the consultee whose degree of expertise increases with such 'supervised' experience. On the other hand, the consultant learns much from such a relationship with a consultee.

Prevention in psychiatry; domiciliary nursing

Many nursing staff will spend at least portion of their working life as specialised domiciliary, public health or community nurses, who are involved more in the care of patients in the community than in the care of those in hospital.

These nurses will be involved in learning about and cooperating with helping agencies that are outside the psychiatric hospital, and collaborating with these agencies to maintain the patient in the outside community. Community psychiatry involves techniques designed to prevent both long-continued psychiatric disability and the return of patients to inpatient care following discharge from hospital (*Tertiary prevention*). Adequate follow-up of patients to ensure that medication prescribed is being continued, the provision of support at stressful periods and the utilisation of ex-patients' clubs are three ways of preventing such readmissions.

The detection of psychiatric disorders in people at an early stage enabling early management to be initiated thus preventing a severe degree of break down, and the utilisation of more effective treatment measures constitute *Secondary prevention.* Adequate outpatient facilities, the detection of early signs of illness through aid societies and a variety of other social agencies, adequate education of the general practitioner to 'home-in' on early indications of psychiatric disorders all constitute part of a secondary prevention programme.

Primary prevention consists in dealing with situations that are known to have deleterious effects on personality development or to lead to breakdown before such unsatisfactory changes occur. It is known for example, that widows recently bereaved are prone to develop psychiatric disturbances. If some planned steps can be taken to help women who have experienced loss in this way, the incidence of ensuing depressive illness may well be lowered. Intervention at the time of such a crisis has come to be known as 'crisis intervention'.

The man responsible for developing the above concepts in psychiatry is Gerald Caplan, who acknowledges that the idea of primary prevention emanates largely from the work of Erick Lindemann (1944). Lindemann studied the effects of personal loss on American citizens whose relatives died in a large night club fire in 1943 and formulated what is termed *Crisis theory.*

CONCLUSION

We have looked in a general way at the various treatment methods utilised in the practice of psychiatry, namely psychotherapy, group techniques, drug therapy, physical treatments, social and milieu therapy, special techniques, the nursing approach, rehabilitation techniques, community measures. In actual practice many of these will be seen to overlap. The purists who consider that treatment involves only the management of the patient with a developed illness may object to the inclusion of the preventive techniques mentioned under community measures, but until we can change our focus and see such preventive measures as an essential part of treatment, we are likely to perpetuate the situation where psychiatric hospitals, with the deleterious effects of long term hospitalisation, remain as the first line of defence against mental illness. In truth, they should at most be places of brief haven providing highly specialised care where this is indicated and frequently the last line of defence in the battle against mental illness.

It is obvious however that in some instances the psychiatric hospital must provide the first line of defence, for example, where families are under inordinate stress due to current behavioural disturbances in close relatives.

ANTIPSYCHIATRY

When but at this point, following an outline of treatment, should one draw attention to a movement which goes so far as to deny the existence of functional psychiatric disorders which, if true, would invalidate much of what has been said above. It is well for students who observe rumblings against and denigration of psychiatry to know something about the antipsychiatry movement, and a little space will now be given to this topic.

Professor Wallace Ironside, in an editorial annotation appearing in the Australian and New Zealand Journal of Psychiatry, has delineated three dominant features of the early medical antipsychiatry stereotype. Firstly, psychological aetiology was denied by patients. Secondly, if denial by patients failed, there was rejection of this concept of aetiology. Thirdly, obloquy (abuse or being generally ill-spoken of) not only by patients but by one's family and friends and medical colleagues reinforced this denial and rejection. With the value of psychiatry now more accepted by medical practitioners, this medical antipsychiatry stereotype is disappearing to a large extent except in the thinking of some entrenched rigid practitioners of medicine.

There are, however, other manifestations of what is now known as the antipsychiatry movement spearheaded by psychiatrists themselves and spreading to some non-medical groups. This movement began in the early 1960s, though long before this, some psychoanalysts had been loud in their declamation of psychiatric institutions. Of the early well-known antipsychiatrists, Szasz and Laing are psychiatrists, and Goffman a sociologist.

In essence, the antipsychiatry movement commenced by championing the cause of people given the diagnosis of schizophrenia. The aim was to re-define schizophrenia as a social-interpersonal situation rather than as a mental disorder or disease. Szasz claimed that 'to classify a person psychiatrically . . . is to rob him of his humanity', claiming also that non-organic mental illness is a myth nurtured by the vested interests of psychiatrists. Laing goes as far as envisaging a schizophrenic episode as being maybe the welcome liberation from the shackles of a destructive family or a sick society. Antipsychiatry affirms that to make a diagnosis of schizophrenia gives a non-illness the status of an illness and places a difficult-to-remove stigma on the person so labelled. In claiming that schizophrenia is not a mental disorder, the movement avers that it should not be treated in accordance with the medical model by the medical profession, including psychiatrists.

Other objections raised by antipsychiatrists to the medical model management of schizophrenia include the detention of people in large inhumane psychiatric hospitals. They see mental hospitals as places where people who deviate from the behavioural norms of society are incarcerated and attempts are made to have them conform. ECT is seen as an amnesia producer and neuroleptic drugs as chemical straitjackets.

There is a rooted objection to the search for somatic agents to reverse what they see as a non-existent disease process. They also point the finger at the doctor-patient relationship which they claim is a distant one, and fraught with difficulties as the psychiatrist in a hospital setting has to act as father-confessor and gaoler rolled into one.

One can accept that there are elements of truth is some antipsychiatry affirmations, and if one cuts through the highly emotive and sometimes misrepresentative statements, they serve to emphasise points and stances taken by psychiatrists over a long period of time. Who but psychiatrists have, over past decades, tried to influence medical colleagues in other disciplines as to the importance of psychological factors and interpersonal relationships? Many successful attempts have been made by psychiatrists to minimise the institutionalising effects of large hospitals and to take the patient out of the hospital into the community setting. Endeavours of psychiatrists and other workers in the mental health field to mitigate the very things the antipsychiatrists are disparaging are far too great to enumerate, and in practically all instances have pre-dated the rumblings of this group.

There are elements of truth in the stance of most movements and if antipsychiatry serves to hasten socio-political initiatives, these aspects are to be welcomed. However, people working in psychiatry owe it to a worthwhile helping profession to conceptualise their own stance in their calling and back this stance with knowledge in order to deflect those emotionally-charged half-truths that are found on the fringe of any movement, no matter how valid and pure are its central aims.

21

ADMISSION WARD PSYCHIATRY

Most larger psychiatric hospitals have special wards set aside as admission wards where admitting procedures are carried out, patients are initially assessed, and management programmes are instituted. The implementation of management programmes makes these wards more than assessment centres, the majority of patients being treated successfully and discharged home after a relatively short stay in hospital. An effectively run admission ward obviates to a large extent the necessity for intermediate and long-stay wards, thus militating against the process of institutionalisation.

Admission wards are best organised on a regional basis, each taking responsibility for given segments of a hospital's catchment area. This enables closer links to be made with community agencies and general medical practitioners, and leads to less dissipation of effort and skills of those ward personnel who undertake community follow-up.

The nature of referrals to an admission ward will depend to a large extent on other special facilities existing in a particular region, and on the ability of these facilities to cope with presenting problems.

In the author's experience in admission wards up until the late 1960s, it was necessary to deal with the problems of alcoholic patients, both in withdrawal states and on Inebriate Orders for transfer to other treatment centres. In a six-month survey carried out in the mid 1960s, these patients comprised over 20% of admissions. In addition to this population which would better be managed in a setting other than an admission ward, were some 10% of admissions diagnosed as suffering from dementia, the majority being geriatric patients with no psychotic or behavioural manifestations necessitating the specialised skills of psychiatric staff. The development of units to deal with the special problems of geriatric patients is a heartening move. Whilst speaking of diagnostic categories, one finds from experience that the presence of more than two antisocial personalities at any one time in an admission ward of say forty beds can effectively wreck a ward programme, and one has to carefully weigh up whether it is prudent to attempt inpatient treatment of these people or to discharge them for the welfare of the rest of one's patients.

Some patients enter admission wards on a voluntary basis and some on a non-statutory basis, and others are admitted on legal restraining orders for a variety of reasons. There will therefore be wide variations in the motivation of admission ward patients to enter treatment programmes, and attitudes will range from full co-operation to open hostility to treatment endeavours. This variation in patients' attitudes to hospitalisation requires the development of particular skills by the therapeutic team to deal with the variety of attitudes expressed and acted upon by patients. More important than this factor of motivation influencing patients' behaviour is the nature of the patient's illness itself, and more so in an admission ward than in any other treatment situation does one find a diversity of diagnostic categories and behavioural manifestations.

As well as behaviour resulting essentially from psychiatric disorders, it is in the admission ward that one is most likely to encounter patients' symptoms and mental state abnormalities associated with a variety of physical illnesses. For this reason the person working in admission ward psychiatry must be the one par excellence to view the total person, not just looking above the neck but being attuned to the possibility of pathology in any bodily system. This calls for accurate observation and an ability to sense the presence of organicity based on sound clinical experience. Some behavioural manifestations that create problems in management are found in any psychiatric setting and in the community. There is, however, a concentration of these in admission wards and we shall look briefly at some of them before overviewing admission ward organisation.

Management problems

Involuntary admissions

Mention has been made above that some patients may be admitted under a legal restraining order for observation and treatment. This occurrence would normally arise out of a situation where a person is considered to be a danger to himself or others, and he does not agree to inpatient care. Quite obviously such a patient can fall under a variety of diagnostic categories some of which will receive mention later in this chapter.

In general, unless the patient is violently overactive and psychotic, it is possible to establish some degree of rapport with him if one maintains a calm objectivity showing confidence and an expectation of co-operation from the patient. How often has one seen a reluctant and even hostile patient brought struggling to the reception area of an admission ward by some custodians of the law, probably anxious themselves, settle down in the presence of a diminutive admitting nurse who makes the patient feel less threatened by her attitude?

The suicidal patient

The most common psychiatric disorders leading to suicide are psychotic depressive illnesses which show features of the depressive syndrome. Not all patients with these symptoms have thoughts of suicide, but when feelings of hopelessness become marked, and particularly when the patient entertains delusions of worthlessness or sin, observation must be of the strictest nature and appropriate treatment instituted as soon as possible. Initial treatment will frequently consist of modified electroconvulsive therapy, or the giving of tricyclic anti-depressants, or both, but whatever regimen of treatment is embarked upon, at no stage should a seriously depressed patient be out of sight until one is certain that a suicidal risk no longer exists.

A crucial risk period in which suicide is likely to be attempted is in the early hours of the morning when the patient, suffering from delayed insomnia is plagued with thoughts consistent with feelings of hopelessness and despair. Two examples of early morning suicide known to the author will be cited. The first was a middle aged man who made his way to a gas oven in the kitchen of a somewhat ancient hospital and sucessfully gassed himself sometime between 2.00 a.m. and 4.00 a.m. The second was a female patient whom the relatives wished to take back home for treatment in another part of the country. This patient at the last interview with the author was loathe to leave the interview situation, lingering somewhat imploringly at the door, an action that should add to one's alertness of the possibility of suicide. Immediate medical supervision was available in the form of a relative living in the house in which the patient was to sleep prior to making the trip the next day, and the risk of suicide was thoroughly aired and understood by all.

This woman did not make the trip—a tragedy for the relatives who had assumed responsibility for her. Before daybreak her body was found on nearby railway tracks.

The use of siderooms, where observation of potentially suicidal risk patients may be intermittent only, should be avoided at all costs. It is a simple matter for a desperate patient to rig up bed sheets and attempt hanging.

Staff should not be distracted from the observation of suicidal risk patients at change of shift. Things can happen quickly. In five minutes, a psychotically depressed patient in an admission ward made her way to the bathroom, unscrewed the wire hook from a coat hanger, placed one end in her mouth, and presumably fell upon it, as one end penetrated the oropharynx and protruded subcutaneously in the posterolateral aspect of the neck, the broken end being jammed behind her upper teeth. Fortunately no really serious damage was done and the patient later responded to modified ECT and took up the business of living again.

These cases are mentioned, not in any macabre spirit, but to warn against the complacency that may develop when things have been running smoothly in an admission ward for some time.

There are a number of principles to follow in the management of a patient who has been assessed to be highly lethal or acutely self-destructive. Practical issues concerning observation have already been touched upon, and in terms of the attitude to adopt towards severely depressed patients, it is a good rule of thumb to see these people as having suffered a severe loss. This will determine to a large extent the way one, as a professional helper, behaves towards these patients. One offers them friendship and genuine care as a replacement for the loss they have sustained. One shows preparedness to accept any communication the patient may make especially ones pertaining to feelings of hopelessness and despair, as this indicates to the patient that someone is prepared to share his misery. Having accepted the misery, it can realistically be pointed out that he will not always feel as he currently does. Severely depressed patients should not be exhorted to do things beyond their current capabilities. One may be asked by the patient about current environmental difficulties and every effort should be made to resolve these. The social worker and community resources may well need to be involved in the management of the patient.

Other aspects of management of the suicidal patient include at least a daily lethality rating, assessment of the domestic environment, and if indicated, involvement in the treatment situation of significant persons in the patient's life.

These principles will apply to the severely depressed patient, no matter what the diagnostic label.

The recent suicide attemptor

Most suicide attemptors are probably seen initially in a general hospital casualty department and psychiatrically assessed there or in the general hospital ward. Some will present in a psychiatric admission ward. Firstly, it is important to assess the suicide potential or lethality of the patient, and to this end one must appraise whether or not a psychotic depression or other psychotic illness is present. There are probably eight suicide attemptors to every one actual suicide and some authorities believe that those who attempt suicide represent a different population from those who commit suicide. Be that as it may, there are many reasons why, apart from really wishing to die, a person will, for example, take an overdose or cut his wrists; and there is frequently the element of a gamble in the act. It often seems to be the case that the goal of attempted suicide is to alter one's life or to produce changes in attitudes or behaviour of those people significant to the attemptor.

One does not need to be psychotic to commit suicide, and areas to be assessed include: the strength of the intention to suicide, whether the circumstances of the act involved the probability of rescue, existing precipitants including the necessity to alter other people's behaviour, and whether the precipitants are modifiable.

On the answers to the above questions one can formulate a management programme which will initially involve friendly support for the patient who has been in a state of crisis.

The violent patient

The potentially violent patient feels threatened by what is going on inside himself. He is often engaged in a desperate struggle to prevent his imagined annihilation, and if his panic is added to by incompetent handling or unnecessary strictures, then naturally he will respond by attacking something or someone. In a non-authoritarian ward atmosphere, outwardly-directed violence is relatively uncommon because strictures on patients are the minimal necessary for their welfare and that of the staff.

A lesson was there to be learned when the open-door policy was first introduced in large hospitals. Phenothiazines had already been introduced and served to control violent behaviour to some degree, but it still persisted, only to diminish in an extraordinary fashion when doors were unlocked by day.

Having made this broad generalisation that a relatively permissive atmosphere will minimise violent behaviour in patients, it should be pointed out to the inexperienced worker that unpredictable behaviour does occur in admission wards, emanating as it does from a patient's inner delusional and hallucinatory world. This underscores the necessity for differentiating between the psychotic violent patient and the non-psychotic violent patient. The former is largely governed by forces within himself, is less responsive to environmental change, and less amenable to reasoned argument. Nevertheless there is a core of rational ego function in most psychotic patients, and if one can, in a quiet respectful manner, convey reassurances to a disturbed patient, getting it across that one is interested in his welfare, violent activity may be averted. It is sometimes evident from the outset in undertaking such an approach that it will be ineffective, and one rapidly has to resort to other means to avoid damage to property or person.

Examples of conditions in which behaviour may be irrational and destructive include schizophrenic catatonic excitement, paranoid schizophrenia, manic depressive psychosis (manic type), states of delirium, alcoholic intoxication, and psychomotor seizures. The management of these disorders is outlined in the relevant sections of this volume.

It is mandatory that the psychiatrist team leader or medical officer should anticipate destructive behaviour in patients and initiate adequate treatment regimes, both for the welfare of patients and of staff faced with the task of nursing them.

Many potentially violent patients are frightened of their destructive potential, and at least one patient in the author's experience, at a time when protective rooms were still in use, expressed great relief that a padded room was available as a refuge for him when he could no longer control his aggression.

As it is the nursing staff who are mostly confronted with the possibility of violence from patients, a few general points will be made with the nurse in mind.

It is essential to differentiate other unexpected or unpredictable behaviour from violent behaviour. An example of a failure in discernment comes from a ward where a female patient was reported on two successive days to be violent. She was mute and was given to touching staff on the shoulder or putting her arm around staff members' necks and dragging them towards her. At times she lay on the floor and rolled about. As it turned out this patient was merely drawing attention to the fact that she was in considerable pain resulting from acute pyelonephritis which was subsequently diagnosed and treated, leading to cessation of the supposedly violent behaviour.

We have already noted that potentially violent patients are afraid, and may resort to acts of violence because of this fear and insecurity. If a nurse is tentative and afraid this will make the patient more insecure and may precipitate destructive behaviour. Therefore, she must never try to cope with a potentially agressive patient on her own. There is safety and less fear in a nurse if she has the moral support of numbers. So one should obtain assistance before attempting to control an explosive situation. A show of strength gained from numbers may indeed be settling to the patient. A corollary to this is that the nurse should never be isolated on her own with patients in the ward, especially as the chances for unpredictable patient behaviour are high in the mixed population of an admission ward.

While in an earlier discussion on the therapeutic community the statement was made that the worker there is as permissive as the patient's mental state will allow, in terms of some potentially violent patients in the admission ward, which may obviously be run on therapeutic community lines, one would be wise to look at the other end of the authoritarian-permissiveness continuum and emphasise the point that the degree of stricture exercised should be sufficient to control behaviour which can be damaging to the patient, to materials and to staff.

Admission Ward organisation

Only broad principles will be touched upon as staffing, architectural considerations, and facilities available will to a large extent determine how a particular ward may be developed.

It is important to have a separate reception area manned by a doctor and nursing staff where the legal and domestic admitting procedures can be carried out and an initial history taken, and where relatives may be interviewed and given requisite support and the opportunity to ask questions about the patient and the hospital. The admission of a patient constitutes the culmination of a crisis situation for relatives and appropriate cognizance must be taken of information volunteered by and requested from them, and friendly realistic support should be offered. It is self-evident that relatives can be important factors both in the genesis of a disorder and in its ultimate resolution, and their active support is to be sought at all times. To be less starry-eyed about them, some relatives can be an utter nuisance and quite unhelpful, but this first encounter in the reception area is an important one when their potential for co-operation can be initially assessed, and psychiatric first aid can be given.

Bathing of patients occurs at a convenient time before they are settled in the ward. This provides an opportunity for nursing staff to establish communication with patients and to note any physical abnormalities that may require attention.

Efforts should be made to orientate the newly-admitted patient in the ward. Fears are allayed even by the simple expediency of showing the patient around a ward and its facilities.

If an admission ward is equipped with single rooms, extreme care should be exercised in the selection of patients to occupy these, and it may be a good general principle for new admissions initially to be placed in a bed bay along with those patients known to require strict observation and care within view of the nursing station, which must at all times be manned.

Decisions will need to be taken on the degree of freedom that can be allowed each individual patient, with the emphasis on early ambulation in the patient's own clothes, and involvement in ward programmes. The therapeutic team in the ward must be flexible enough to do things for the patient when they are necessary and to withdraw support at the optimal time in the interests of the patient developing an independent stance and heightened self-esteem. This latter can be fostered by involving the patient in programme-planning and encouraging him in the variety of occupational and social activities that should be built into the daily life of an admission ward.

Probably the most importaint elements to develop in an admission ward where relatively rapid change both in the patient population and in an individual's mental state may occur, is sound communication. This can be achieved in a number of ways, namely through the therapeutic team's daily meetings where new patients are discussed and older ones reviewed, through total ward meetings and other group meetings and activities, through written reports, and nursing staff meetings held at change of shift.

In some instances it is important to involve patients' relatives in the treatment situation. This may be achieved by holding group discussions in the evenings. Where marital discord exists, special therapy groups may be held for dissident couples by a member of the therapeutic team who has appropriate skills. If a number of geriatric patients emerge and they do no benefit from the ward meeting, some separate group activity may be planned for them. The types of therapeutic activity obviously can vary greatly, depending on the present needs and on the skills of the staff.

As stated earlier in this chapter, many patients are discharged home from admission wards and the responsibility of these wards does not cease at discharge. Letters must be written to referring doctors and agencies. The patient may be discharged to the care of his local general practitioner, it may be appropriate for him to attend for follow up at some community clinic, domiciliary ward personnel may visit him in his home at intervals, or the patient may attend an out-patient section of the hospital, just to mention a number of the possibilities open if further surveillance is necessary.

Working in an admission ward can be, as in any area of psychiatry, a rewarding experience, and the satisfactions gained by both patients and staff are proportionate to the effort expended in developing realistic management programmes which can run the gamut of all treatment modalities.

The migrant patient

Not as an afterthought but for emphasis, a separate section is set aside to comment on the fact that, with movement of world populations in recent decades on a scale greater than ever before, one is being confronted more and more in the admission ward by patients who stem from a variety of cultural backgrounds.

Apart from a language barrier, broken down to some extent by the provision of official interpreters or by the use of indoor or outdoor hospital staff who speak the same language, migrant patients may prove difficult to help on a number of counts. They may have culturally-determined ways of coping with emotional stress and pain, different value systems and beliefs, different family structures and different attitudes to the sick family member, and other variables including differing interpretations of non-verbal communication cues which may hamper our understanding and render some aspects of our management ineffectual.

Ellard, in an article entitled 'The problems of the migrant', has highlighted some of the difficulties that may be encountered. In some parts of the world a vital interest is now being taken in what has come to be termed transcultural psychiatry which, among other things, studies the ethnic differences mentioned above.

Psychiatric staff have a responsibility to acquaint themselves with this developing subspecialty which, in essence, means learning about customs, attitudes, values and beliefs in other cultures, in order to understand and so be more effective in the management of patients from other cultural backgrounds.

22

GENERAL HOSPITAL PSYCHIATRY

Psychiatric and psychological principles have their application in any hospital ward, or for that matter in any treatment setting, and to undertake an extensive coverage of general hospital psychiatry would constitute a marathon endeavour when one considers the great variety of patients, investigation and management situations in a modern general hospital.

Apart from a psychiatric unit or services in a general hospital, mentioned first so not forgotten, one finds medical wards and surgical wards with their various subspecialty sections, numbered among which could be gastroenterology, endocrinology, neurology, gynaecology, urology, and ear nose and throat, to mention but a few. There may exist a renal transplant unit, special clinics dealing with diabetes, asthma or arthritis. The neurologist will have beds. Neurosurgical problems may be dealt with. Patients may require admission for certain skin conditions. There will probably exist a coronary care unit and/or an intensive care unit. Those hospitals interested in oncology, or the science of new growths, will have special cancer wards, and there may be a special section for treatment by deep ray therapy. Behind all the treatment modalities conducted by the various specialties, and the above is by no means an exhaustive list, there exist the diagnostic services of pathology, bacteriology, haematology, diagnostic radiology, electrocardiography, electroencephalography and radioisotope units, again by no means an exhaustive list, as newer and more refined techniques of investigation are rapidly emerging.

Feeding into this enormous complex of investigatory and treatment modalities are the Casualty and Outpatients' Departments, plus the wheels and wings of ambulance transport.

What a potentially frightening patchwork quilt is the patient going to harbour under when he is forced to assume the sick role and enter a general hospital! He is apprehensive unless he is thoroughly aware of what is facing him, that he knows he can cope adequately with it, and that the ultimate outcome will see him restored to full health; and probably nobody entering hospital knows these facts.

Unless they occasionally make a conscious effort to look at things through patients' eyes, staff working every day in the atmosphere of a general hospital may, through familiarity with the environment, become somewhat oblivious to the strangeness and even fear felt by newcomers to the surroundings.

The importance of human contact in unfamiliar surroundings should need no emphasis. This can be achieved by the simple act of hospital staff speaking with patients, answering their queries when they can, and offering information about the hospital and ward.

Effects of hospitalisation

We shall now look more closely at what the act of hospitalisation means to the adult patient. Apart from the general apprehension felt by him arising out of unknown or only partly understood facts about his illness and the procedures he will undergo, which could be allayed to a large extent by proper management by the referring agency whether this be the general practitioner, the outpatient specialist or someone else, there are three areas of adaptation to be faced by the patient. The first of these concerns his *family* which is disrupted because of the separation entailed in hospitalisation. Depending to a large extent on relationships existing within the family prior to hospitalisation will be the reaction of the patient, ranging from a sense of loss and despair through to feelings of hostility for imagined rejection by the family. The patient may feel he is letting them down, or he may, on the basis of earlier separations, see his entry to hospital as a punishment.

The second area of adjustment involves the cessation of the patient's *work*. Working effectively involves satisfaction and a sense of achievement. It is concerned with financial security and a host of other possible fulfilments. To be separated from work can therefore produce an enormous sense of loss, or a feeling of under-achievement. There are also anxieties associated with the possibility that the patient may not be as efficient or capable following hospitalisation.

The third major area of adjustment is to separation from *society* or the community. If a person has depended to a great extent on social relationships and community activities to produce in himself a feeling of achievement or of being a needed and useful citizen, hospitalisation cuts these supports from under him.

On the other side of the coin, providing hospitalisation is not seen as a life-endangering experience by the patient beset with the daily problems in these three spheres, he may be relieved to be away from family, work and society for a time.

Being sensitive to these possibilites, hospital staff will be able to empathise with the patient and help him to come to terms with the reality of his situation, as well as substituting to some extent for his losses, even at the simple yet important level of offering friendship, albeit temporary.

Psychological reactions to physical illness

Psychological reactions to acute physical illness in adults are well described by Peterson in a requested article of similar name mentioned in the bibliography, and the interested reader is referred to this. In summary, it is pointed out that there are three goups of factors which influence the patient's psychological reaction to illness, these being: (i) factors in the illness itself; (ii) factors in the patient; and (iii) situational factors.

Among *factors in the illness* must be considered: the severity of symptoms such as pain, the degree of disability and the perceived threat to life; the duration of the illness and its rate of progression which will have a bearing on the patient's adaptation to it; the organ or system involved and the degree to which the patient places importance on the predominant site of illness.

Factors in the patient include age, sex, body image and premorbid personality. The body image is made up of a person's perceptions, thoughts and feelings about his own body. The head, heart and sexual organs are of particular importance to most people both from a functional point of view and in respect of what they symbolise. For example the head is concerned with intellectual capacity and control, the heart with life itself, and sexual organs with masculinity or femininity. Arising out of the patient's personality which determines his fairly consistent habitual responses to stress of any sort, a variety of reactions is possible. The paranoid person tends to be suspicious and jealous of other patients; the schizoid personality may find the closeness of being cared for and nursed somewhat threatening; the explosive personality incapacitated by illness may react with hostility; the anankastic (obsessive-compulsive) personality, perfectionistic and needing to remain in control of situations, may feel particularly anxious and find it difficult to allow things to be done for him even when this is essential, and the hysterical personality may react to illness in an attention-seeking, exhibitionistic fashion. Reactions seen are often responses arising out of ways that different personalities have of coping with stress rather than directly implicating those caring for these patients; and staff will be more comfortable if they do not accept at too personal a level the hostile or scapegoating manoeuvres of some when these arise essentially out of patients' reactions to the stress of illness.

Situational factors include aspects of family, work and social environment which have already received mention. Added to these are the very fact of hospitalisation and the necessary adoption of the sick role, and very importantly, relationships with doctors, nurses and others in the therapeutic team.

Coping strategies of patients

Strategies to cope with the stress of illness and hospitalisation are to a great extent peculiar to a given person and they follow the pattern the person has developed to cope with previous stresses in life. Peterson quotes Verwoerdt, who classifies three categories of coping strategy. The first is aimed at a retreat from the threat and the conservation of energy, and involves the defence mechanism of repression. Defences aimed at excluding the threat or its significance from awareness include suppression, denial, rationalisation, projection, and the mechanism of depersonalization.

Intellectualisation is a defence aimed at the coping strategy of mastery and control.

To quote Peterson:

> Acceptance of the illness, coupled with a realistic redirection of anxiety, using it to energise the body-mind fight against the noxious threat by all available

means, are healthy, ideal reactions to the stress of sickness. As the patient recovers, he becomes less dependent and egocentric. He gradually relinquishes the sick role as he turns his attention more and more to the needs of others, and regains his interest in work, recreation and everyday affairs. After it is all over, the patient may sometimes come to realise that the illness was a beneficial experience, even if some scars are left.

Stresses on staff

It is necessary to dissect out reactions to the stress of illness and hospitalisation, and the coping mechanisms of patients in order to try to understand their behaviour, but what of the stresses placed upon hospital staff? Do they cope, and if not what can be done to help them? One must remember that hospital staff of all disciplines are average citizens who have their own private lives and who live in much the same society as their patients. They find themselves for a part of most days away from normal family and society in a working situation where they are confronted with the management of a high concentration of sick people, and if working in a renal unit for example, could well be inclined to overestimate the amount of kidney trouble in the community and become somewhat sensitive about their own renal function. Similarly, if working in a special unit concentrating on the problems of malignant melanoma, one could well become mildly apprehensive about the state of one's own benign melanomatous skin lesions.

The greatest concentration of dying people, at least in civilisations with a stable political climate, are to be found in hospitals, and hospital staff, especially nurses who are more consistently in contact with patients, have had little previous exposure to dying and death, due to advances in preventive medicine and treatment. Under-exposed as they are, they have had little opportunity to come to terms with these realities and frequently feel the need for guidance and support when faced with the dying patient. Perhaps it is this very thing, this lack of exposure to death and dying, that has lead to an explosive interest in these subjects over the past decade, and the development of thanatology (Gk. *thanatos*, death) which concerns itself with the study of death, dying, bereavement, and life-threatening behaviour.

Be this as it may, rather than philosophise about illness and the inevitable lot of us all, we shall look at an example of a functioning ward in order to gain some insight into the questions that have been raised. The particular ward to be described is a surgical ward and cannot be said to be representative of all general hospital wards, especially as it deals largely with serious surgical problems many of which, up to this time, have defied the endeavours of medicine to provide a cure, and one is here speaking of various forms of cancer which not infrequently lead to death. Nevertheless, death is not the prerogative of a predominantly cancer ward, and all staff in health professions must at one time or another be faced with the care of dying patients. As it is the nurse who is with the patients more than any other discipline, in the interest of conciseness what follows will concern itself mainly with nursing.

The ward in question has three surgical teams utilising its thirty-eight beds; one general surgical team having fifteen beds, an ear nose and throat team eight beds, and a third team having fifteen beds, ten of which are utilised for patients suffering from malignant melanoma.

A method of *team nursing* is used in which two or three nurses under a more senior person attend to the complete nursing management of a number of patients. In favour of this technique is the fact that nurses can develop a more helpful relationship to the whole patient, not just to his back or bowels. If a nurse is responsible for the whole person her nursing techniques will be of the highest order, for she feels accountable to someone she knows, not just to a series of backs. One outcome of this closer relationship is that the nurse is more exposed to the emotional difficulties of her patients, many of whom have a Damoclean sword of death poised over their heads.

Looking specifically at patients with malignant melanoma, of the first forty interviewed by the psychiatrist on the Melanoma Clinic team, and this was but a fraction of those treated, eighteen had died within twelve months of the first patient having been seen. This proportion of deaths in less than one year is high because the majority of patients seen already had complications. Five of these patients died in the surgical ward and most were treated and nursed there in paraterminal stages prior to discharge home or to a nursing home. If we add patients treated on the ward by the other two surgical teams an idea can be grasped of the burden of nursing patients both in extremis and following major surgical procedures.

In order both to assist nurses in handling a difficult nursing job and to determine areas of concern to them, weekly discussion groups were commenced for nurses working on the surgical ward, and the topics raised spontaneously in the first thirty of these open-ended groups were analysed.

Considering the nature of the nursing involved, it is not surprising that questions dealing with the care of dying patients came to the fore in the majority of discussions: in fact, in the first thirty meetings questions relating to the management of dying patients arose on twenty-seven occasions.

Queries raised included:

How does one talk to a dying patient?
How does one keep a patient occupied so he won't think of death?
How does one manage a terminal patient afraid of death who keeps on talking of death to other patients thus casting gloom?
What does one do when a patient says, 'Let me die, Nurse'?
Should one agree with a dying patient that he is dying and possibly destroy his last hope?
What does one do when a patient wants to die and doctors put tubes in and prolong his life?
Should a nurse show her emotions, for example depression, on the ward or bottle them up and let them out later?
How does one speak to a patient readmitted with extending cancer?
Why not euthanasia?

Other topics falling within this category included:

emotional distress caused by seeing patients suffer, vis à vis dying;

the possibility that seeing death frequently would lead to either callousness or emotional breakdown in a nurse;
denial by other patients for a time of the death of one of their number;
feelings of futility and uselessness which develop in some who nurse dying patients, their feelings being related to lack of therapeutic returns at the physical level as opposed to satisfactions derived from the caring aspects of nursing;
the development of emotional involvement with dying patients with consequent increase in disturbance in nursing staff when death comes;
attitudes of different nurses to death, ranging from unconcern to depression and hostility;
feelings of frustration and a sense of inadequacy when a dying patient does not respond to the nurse's ministering overtures.

Other topics raised by nurses fitted into six other broad categories, namely, nursing generally; discussion of specific patients; communication; relatives and visitors; disfiguring operations; and miscellaneous topics. No breakdown will be made of these areas, save to point out two things. Firstly, lack of communication by some doctors to the nursing staff on what has been told to patients about their condition puts the nurse in an untenable position when discussing some matters raised by patients. Secondly, dealing with relatives and visitors is frequently found more difficult than coping with patients in bed. What, for example, does one say when an agitated relative shakes a patient who is in extremis demanding that he speak? How does one tactfully deal with a husband who is forcing a ham sandwich on to his emaciated dying wife asserting that it will build her up? Is it right for the nurse to crave moderaion from a visiting man of religion who is praying loudly over a dying patient upsetting many other patients in the ward?

In addition to a breakdown of topics in group discussion, a questionnaire was prepared and answered by Melanoma Clinic staff of a number of disciplines and was returned by sixteen nurses with varying levels of experience. The same questionnaire with minor modifications was distributed to first and second year resident doctors working throughout the general hospital. Responses by the sixteen nurses and the first sixteen medical staff questionnaires were analysed. Pertinent to earlier comments on nursing group discussions, an item on questions posed by patients and found most difficult to answer showed that 68% of nurses and 56% of doctors experienced difficulties in answering questions related to the prognosis of terminal illness. Again, on questions posed by relatives, 70% of nursing staff and 44% of the resident doctors found discussions with relatives about bad prognosis and death the most difficult to handle. Much could be said about the heavy load of nursing procedures allowing less time to talk with patients, about staff personality clashes producing tension in a whole ward, about the difficulty of avoiding emotional involvements with patients, about difficulties arising out of being rostered in a ward where patients ask nurses questions on procedures and conditions before the nurses have learned about them in training, and about the junior nurse's uncertainty as to the expectation of sisters in respect of her work. Emphasis however, has been given to dealing with patients at the end of life, with ages ranging from the late teens to old age, the majority falling in middle life. The age, incidentally, bears a relationship to the degree of identification of the nurse with a patient, most finding it more difficult to come to terms with the inevitable demise of a younger patient in the same age group as the nurse.

It is customary for the psychiatrist to discuss with melanoma patients the areas of difficulty produced by the illness and its management. Such areas include: physical incapacity or lack of physical mobility and movement, physical pain, nausea and vomiting from chemotherapy, having to give up previous sporting or recreational activities, consciousness of scarring; the effects on the family which range from extra work for the spouse to whether a mother should tell her ten-year-old son of the seriousness of her condition; the financial burden of travelling to the clinic from afar plus the separation from the family that is entailed; loss of libido, irritability, emotional lability and frank depression. The general nurse must be in a position to allow her patients to ventilate on these and other areas of concern.

To allude to questions raised earlier in this section, the stresses of physical nursing and the emotional stresses on the nurse are heavy especially in a ward situation where dying and death are not infrequent attenders, and this can be so in any ward. Whether nurses cope can be gauged to some extent from the types of questions raised in group discussions, but that they do assist greatly in seeing patients through hospitalisation, illness, and impending death may be gauged from the following facts.

When patients with secondary melanoma or on surveillance following their first operation were asked routinely at initial interview by the psychiatrist what had helped them most in coping with their illness, 38% said the Clinic and/or Ward staff and 28% said the surgeons and their Melanoma Clinic team, while the spouse and/or family was most helpful in 18% of cases.

Teaching about death and dying

Many nursing and medical curricula still do not encompass formal teaching in the area of death and dying. Indeed the effectiveness of formal teaching is a moot point. Milton (1972) said, 'Lectures on the subject of dying are all very well, but nothing brings home to the student (nurse or doctor) the real emotional stress of dying so well as contact with and a share of the management of patients'. This is a sound view providing of course that time is set aside for staff to discuss experiences with a professional worker who understands something of the functioning of the human mind and emotions.

Sandford and Deloughery (1973) described a study using nine items from Scheidman's 57-item questionnaire, 'You and death', 'in order to involve their students in death as much as possible without actually dying, so as to create an environment for self-appropriated learning'. Two weeks after the presentation of the questionnaire, a class discussion was held based on a 'Discussion Guide on Death'. Of this teaching experience, these writers reported that the response to questionnaire items was not as important as the later discussion which provided opportunities for changes in attitude, the questionnaire merely providing a stimulus for discussion.

One possible means of helping hospital staff to acclimatise to aspects of the type of management involved in the care of dying patients is for them to attend discussion groups prior to commencing work in this area. Perhaps discussion could be based initially on Dr Kubler-Ross's book *On Death and Dying.* Work situations will very often determine what is possible logistically, and the discussion groups held with staff on the ward described seem to fill some need judging by requests from staff for more of them plus a deeper understanding of 'psychology'. Probably the best method of helping students to face the problems of caring for dying patients is for an experienced person to interview terminally-ill patients in their presence, with the students being free to ask relevant questions. After all, the dying patient is the expert in the field and many are pleased to offer what help they can in this difficult area.

BEREAVEMENT

As hospital staff indicate that they often have difficulties in coping with relatives, mention will be made of what constitutes a distressing yet normal process for these survivors of patients who die.

Whilst the patient is ill in hospital, relatives use all the coping mechanisms that patients use, often to the discomfort of hospital staff, particularly when they displace feelings such as guilt and hostility on to staff criticising their management, and virtually laying the blame for the patient's condition on them. When denial of serious illness in a loved one gives way to the realisation that death is likely if not inevitable, the relative experiences bereavement which 'refers to the process by which a person suffers, sustains and then recovers from the wound inflicted by the loss of someone essential to his reality' (Weisman).

A number of stages of bereavement are described and only the initial stages will be observed in the hospital setting. Firstly, when the possibility of death of a patient is grasped by the relative he passes through a stage of *anticipatory grief.* This is a period of anxiety for relatives who virtually become mourners preparatory to the death of their loved ones. In protracted deaths, one may see relatives display all the stages that Kubler-Ross (1969) uses to describe the experiences of the dying patient during this period of awaiting the death of a loved one, namely, denial, anger, bargaining, depression and acceptance, though the last-mentioned rarely occurs before ultimate death.

After death comes *mourning* for the survivor. This mourning may commence with acute anxiety followed by denial of the event and the bereaved may feel and appear numb and shut off for a period. This is followed either by copious weeping or severe self control of emotions, both extremes being said to represent a craving and searching for the lost one.

Depression and grief follow the acute mourning period and feelings that the lost one still survives are not uncommon. For many months after this the bereaved frequently experiences great *loneliness* and feelings of isolation. This is followed in the normal course of events by *relief* and *resolution.*

This same sort of sequence of events may be seen after any form of severe loss for example, after marital breakdown. In this latter situation the distress often appears worse, for there is no finality such as death, and the one who has been abandoned has difficulty in adjusting if thoughts of the possibility of restitution are difficult to erase.

Staff can be most helpful in the early stages of the bereavement process by simply accepting and sharing the grief of the bereaved, a difficult task if it rekindles painful emotions of separations experienced by staff. The important thing to appreciate is that the bereaved person, in a state of distress and displaying a variety of emotions and behaviour is grappling virtually with loss of a part of himself and one can do little at this stage except show the empathy one feels and accept and share his emotions.

Not all people who suffer loss pass normally through the process of bereavement, and more specific psychiatric intervention may become necessary if abnormal bereavement supervenes. The criteria for making this diagnosis according to Weisman are as follows: (i) arrest of the process, in which afflicted patients show typical symptoms for long periods without evidence of relief, recovery, or restitution; (ii) exaggeration of symptoms during the course, such as absolute denial that death has occurred, the belief in a full hallucination about the dead or communication with the dead; and (iii) deviant behaviour that violates conventional expectations or jeopardises physical health or safety.

Bereavement, a crisis for the survivor, lends itself to the application of crisis intervention techniques. Raphael, in the *Australian and New Zealand Journal of Psychiatry* has dealt with theoretical and methodological considerations of crisis intervention, and the interested student is referred to this article listed in the bibliography. She quotes Bellak and Hurvich, who state that the functions of the ego that have to be considered for support are: affective, defensive, cognitive, reality aspects, and object relations. There is a growing literature on the fields of bereavement and crisis intervention, and it is beyond the scope of this text to do any more than state that much work is being undertaken to evaluate the worth of preventive intervention in this area.

Comment

It is hoped that dealing with aspects of hospitalisation, illness, dying and bereavement using a busy surgical ward of a general hospital as a base from which to look at these areas has not painted too grim a picture of general hospitals, which in the main are places where hope is generated, where cures are effected and from where the vast majority of patients return to normal living. However, dying and death are facts of life in any hospital setting and need to be looked at, and through a better understanding of them we may come a little closer to providing what some say is unattainable for our patients, namely 'death with dignity'.

23

ASPECTS OF CHILD PSYCHIATRY

The sub-speciality of child psychiatry has until recent years been a much neglected field, a fact which must appear surprising in view of the importance of this stage of life, when patterns of behaviour having a great influence on adult functioning are being laid down. Indeed, the satisfactory resolution of problems arising in childhood would appear to be the best form of preventive psychiatry, though there is insufficient factual evidence to date to state dogmatically that such early intervention reduces the incidence of adult psychiatric disorders.

The child is an individual in the process of development, still very flexible, and more easily modified by environmental factors than is the adult. So intertwined in the general matrix of the family is he, and so important is the whole family in the genesis of patterns of behaviour and attitudes in the child, that there are those working in child psychiatry who would delete the concept of child psychiatry with its traditional overtones of treating an individual, and instead use a term something like 'child and family psychiatry'.

Standard classifications of disorders, though satifactory for adults, have been found wanting when applied to children and adolescents. This is because the child is developing, and at each stage of development, a variety of factors relevant to the formation of attitudes and behaviour patterns impinge upon the child, with differing degrees of influence at each level and in each area of development.

To remedy this deficiency, the American Group for the Advancement in Psychiatry (G.A.P.) in 1966 produced a classification of Psychopathological Disorders of Childhood which has many adherents. In addition to this the American Psychiatric Association has produced a third edition of its *Diagnostic and Statistical Manual* (D.S.M. III) which is currently being tested.

We shall adhere to our policy of following the I.C.D.-9, and perusal of Appendix I will show that conditions specific to childhood fall under a number of different rubrics, namely, Psychoses with origin specific to childhood, Disturbance of emotions specific to childhood and adolescence, Hyperkinetic syndrome of childhood, and Specific delays in development. In addition to this, diagnoses appearing in other categories of disorders in the I.C.D. may be applied to children, for example, schizophrenic psychoses, manic-depressive psychoses, personality disorders, special symptoms and syndromes, disturbances of conduct etc.

As certain stages of development will be mentioned later in the text, it should be stated at this point that such stages are designated as follows:

Infancy—covers the period from birth to two years.

Pre-school period—ranges from two to five years.

School age period—is from six years to the onset of puberty (approximately 11-13 years of age for girls and 13-15 years of age for boys).

Adolescence—is the period from the onset of puberty until the completion of biological maturity, and is divided into early, middle and late phases.

To do even minimal justice to the subspeciality of child and adolescent psychiatry would require another tome written by an expert in the field. Within the confines of this volume one can provide but a descriptive introduction, and that largely borrowed from I.C.D.-9. The student working in the subspeciality is referred to more comprehensive texts.

Psychoses with origin specific to childhood

This category of disorders is limited to those psychoses which always begin before puberty.

Infantile autism

The I.C.D. describes infantile autism as

> a syndrome present from birth or beginning almost invariably in the first 30 months. Responses to auditory and sometimes to visual stimuli are abnormal and there are usually severe problems in the understanding of spoken language. Speech is delayed and, if it develops, is characterized by echolalia, the reversal of pronouns, immature grammatical structure and inability to use abstract terms. There is generally an impairment in the social use of both verbal and gestural language. Problems in social relationships are most severe before the age of five years and include an impairment in the development of eye-to-eye gaze, social attachments, and cooperative play. Ritualistic behaviour is usual and may include abnormal routines, resistance to change, attachment to odd objects and stereotyped patterns of play. The capacity for abstract or symbolic thought and for imaginative play is diminished. Intelligence ranges from severely subnormal to normal or above. Performance is usually better on tasks involving rote memory or visuospatial skills than on those requiring symbolic or linguistic skills.

Childhood autism, infantile psychoses and Kanner's syndrome are other names for this condition.

Disintegrative psychosis

Disintegrative psychosis, or Heller's syndrome, is

> a disorder in which normal or near-normal development for the first few years is followed by a loss of social skills and of speech, together with a severe disorder of emotions, behaviour and relationships. Usually this loss of speech and of social competence takes place over a period of a few months and is accompanied by the emergence of overactivity and of stereotypies. In most cases there is intellectual impairment, but this is not a necessary part of the disorder. The condition may follow overt brain disease—such as measles encephalitis—but it may also occur in the absence of any known organic brain disease or damage.

There may also occur a variety of atypical infantile psychoses showing some, but not all, the features of infantile autism. The description of these disorders, also referred to as Atypical childhood psychosis, appears in Appendix I.

Disturbance of emotions specific to childhood and adolescence

These are less-well-differentiated emotional disorders characteristic of the childhood period that are classifiable neither as neurotic disorders nor as acute reaction to stress. Glossary definitions of the descriptive titles appear in Appendix I. Titles included are: with anxiety and fearfulness, with misery and unhappiness, with sensitivity, shyness and social withdrawal, relationship problems, and other or mixed.

Hyperkinetic syndrome of childhood

The I.C.D. includes

> disorders in which the essential features are short attention-span and distractibility. In early childhood the most striking symptom is disinhibited, poorly organised and poorly regulated extreme overactivity but in adolescence this may be replaced by under-activity. Impulsiveness, marked mood fluctuations and aggression are also common symptoms. Delays in the development of specific skills are often present and disturbed, poor relationships are common . . .

A number of subcategories are described. These include *simple disturbance of activity and attention, hyperkinesis with developmental delay*, and *hyperkinetic conduct disorder* (see Appendix I).

Specific delays in development

These are a group of disorders in which a delay in development in one or more specific skills is the main feature. The delays are related to biological maturation but may be accentuated by other nonbiological factors.

Specific reading retardation

Developmental dyslexia and specific spelling difficulty are other terms applying to these

> disorders in which the main feature is a serious impairment in the development of reading or spelling skills which is not explicable in terms of general intellectual retardation or of inadequate schooling. Speech or language difficulties, impaired right-left differentiation, perceptuo-motor problems, and coding difficulties are frequently associated. Similar problems are often present in other members of the family. Adverse psychosocial factors may be present.

Specific arithmetical retardation

Also called dyscalculia, this refers to

> disorders in which the main feature is a serious impairment in the development of arithmetical skills which is not explicable in terms of general intellectual retardation or of inadequate schooling.

'Other specific learning difficulties' applies to

disorders in which the main feature is a serious impairment in the development of other learning skills which are not explicable in terms of general intellectual retardation or of inadequate schooling.

Developmental speech or language disorder

These are

disorders in which the main feature is a serious impairment in the development of speech or language (syntax or semantics) which is not explicable in terms of general intellectual retardation. Most commonly there is a delay in the development of normal word-sound production resulting in defects of articulation. Omissions or substitutions of consonants are most frequent. There may also be a delay in the production of spoken language. Rarely, there is also a developmental delay in the comprehension of sounds. Includes cases in which delay is largely due to environmental privation.

Developmental aphasia and dyslalia fall within this category of disorder.

Specific motor retardation

The term includes

disorders in which the main feature is a serious impairment in the development of motor coordination which is not explicable in terms of general intellectual retardation. The clumsiness is commonly associated with perceptual difficulties.

Clumsiness syndrome or dyspraxia syndrome are synonyms.

Mixed development disorder is the final named specific delay in development. The diagnosis is made only where the mixture of delayed skills is such that no one skill is preponderantly affected.

Treatment in child psychiatry

As with any rational therapy, the management of the child is undertaken after a thorough appraisal of the factors implicated in the illness.

We have seen how important the child's immediate environment is to his normal development, and how an unsatisfactory environment is a large factor in the genesis or aggravation of psychiatric disorders.

The most influential factors in the child's environment are his parents, and for this reason parents are involved in child management programmes to a greater extent than they are in the psychiatric treatment of adults. As the child is still flexible and modifiable by parental attitudes, it becomes important to help parents understand their part in his development, and where necessary to help them modify their attitudes. Parents will frequently need help to accept and cope with a sick child. Many will feel an unnecessary sense of responsibility and guilt for their child's illness. It is for these reasons that contact with parents of a sick child by at least one member of the psychiatric team becomes of paramount importance.

At its simplest level, treatment may comprise explanations or advice to parents. At the other end of the scale however, the management of a disturbed child will require all the facilities and skills of a variety of specialist staff available in an in-patient centre.

The principles of primary, secondary and tertiary prevention as outlined in our next chapter, Mental Retardation, can be applied here, and the student would do well to organise his thinking on these lines. Principles only will be covered, some being possible to apply at consulting room or outpatient level, others requiring day hospital or inpatient facilities:

1. Psychotherapy in childhood requires rather special training and experience as children differ from adults in several ways. Their motivation for treatment is frequently not high as, in general, they have not chosen to undergo treatment, some adult in their environment having made this choice for them. The adult can often accept the fact that internal changes may result in solutions to their problems, but the child barely recognises internal conflicts, tending to relate difficulties to environmental factors, as most children have a limited capacity for self observation. Experts in this field can list many more problems inherent in this form of treatment, nevertheless psychotherapy on an individual or group basis remains a firm plank in the management of suitable cases. Play therapy, including drawing, is important, and in essence it is a substitute for the verbalised free associations of adults.
2. Physical treatments such as electroconvulsive therapy and certain neurosurgical operations aimed at modifying behaviour may be indicated, the latter, in the present state of knowledge, being last-resort measures when all else has failed. Any physical defect which has an influence on the child's psyche should be corrected.
3. Drug therapy has become an important adjunct in the treatment of disturbed children. The child's reaction to a drug however, does not always parallel that seen in the adult. Stimulant drugs such as amphetamine, and a wide range of major and minor tranquillisers have their place in management.
4. Under the treatment heading 'social and milieu therapy' has to be considered the child's psychological environment, and the obtaining of co-operation from parents and other significant people, for example school teachers. The most satisfactory placement of a child to overcome environmental difficulties requires careful consideration. If the home situation appears untenable, would the child be better off with a relative, in a foster home, in a hostel, or in an inpatient treatment facility? The pros and cons of such projected moves must be weighed carefully.
5. While under treatment, it is important that a child's education continues. This can range from programmes of training designed to foster socially acceptable behaviour and to teach simple procedures such as eating and dressing, to attendance at more formal educational facilities.
6. The nurse may function in two major ways in the child psychiatry setting. As a member of the domiciliary team, she will find herself dealing primarily with parents in supportive and advisory roles. In the hospital setting, her role becomes largely that of parent substitute, and it is important that a consistent relationship with particular children be allowed to develop.

Child Health Clinics

We have mentioned that treatment may be carried out at consulting room or outpatient level and also in day hospital or inpatient facilities. Special mention should be made of the child-guidance movement which developed in the United States of America under the pioneering drive of William Healy who, with his associates, established the Institute for Juvenile Research in 1909. Healy became the director of the Judge Baker Foundation in 1917 and work was directed towards evaluation and diagnosis of children referred to the Boston Juvenile Court. The name of the Foundation was changed to the Judge Baker Child Guidance Centre, and the method of its operations in the 1920s and 1930s was the forerunner or model for present day child health centres. People from other parts of the United States of America and from overseas studied Healy's writings and many studied under him, later to leave and set up similar centres in many parts of the world. The emphasis on suitable clientele moved from the management of delinquent children only to that of a broad spectrum of unhappy and emotionally disturbed children, in the belief that such unhappiness and disturbance if adequately managed would prevent the later development of delinquent behaviour.

There currently is some confusion in the designation of child clinics as they are in a state of evolution and cut horizontally across the whole spectrum of children with problems—in the general community, in schools, in paediatric hospital settings, and in juvenile and divorce courts, to name but a few areas where services for children are established.

The name 'child health clinic', or simply 'health clinic' is customarily used for clinics established in the community. These are frequently under the general oversight of a community paediatrician. Not infrequently within this complex will be the child psychiatry group (or the erstwhile child guidance clinic) whose basic personnel would comprise, for example, a child psychiatrist, a psychologist, two social workers, and two community nurses. Other components of a child health clinic are a speech therapy group and a hearing assessment team. The child health clinic liaises with the school medical teams, whose essential role is seen as case detection, whether the child has a physical or psychological disorder, and with other health professionals in the community.

A child-psychiatry group situated in a paediatric hospital setting would obviously concentrate more on paediatric liaison. There would also exist a close relationship with school medical officers and school councillors. All child health centres are geared to evaluate physical abnormalities, particularly those of the special senses, to evaluate and manage emotional difficulties in children, and to modify unhealthy family influences through working with parents.

It might be mentioned also that Alfred Adler greatly influenced the decision to organise child guidance clinics in Vienna at the beginning of this century. His methods consisted of a diagnostic exploration of the child's familial and educational situation, using questionnaire methods, family interviews and family treatment, and the combined efforts of a 'therapeutic team' which included a counsellor, parents, teachers, truant officers where indicated, and others.

Adler's approach has similarities to the American model, with the essential difference that the latter, since the 1940s and 1950s, has concentrated on individual long term psychotherapy with children and their parents.

24

MENTAL RETARDATION

Mental retardation refers to 'a condition of arrested or incomplete development of mind which is especially characterised by subnormality of intelligence'. The student, if not familiar with earlier comments on mental retardation and intelligence, should at this point refer back to the brief reference made to these topics in Chapter 8.

The I.C.D. divides mental retardation into four grades:

Mild mental retardation (IQ 50-70)
Moderate mental retardation (IQ 35-49)
Severe mental retardation (IQ 20-34)
Profound mental retardation (IQ under 20)

Synonyms for these states are provided in Appendix I (page 388). The grading of mental retardation is made on the basis of an individual's current level of functioning irrespective of its nature or causation be it psychosis, cultural deprivation, Down's syndrome etc.

Such grading is a guide to the capabilities of people falling within each range, in terms of possible social adjustment, ability to learn, and the acquisition of skills. More precisely, it has been worked out for each level of intelligence what maturation and development can be expected at pre-school age, what training and education is possible and likely to be achieved at school age, and what social and vocational adequacy can be expected of the adult. One should consult larger text books for more precise details of such findings.

To give one set of examples pertaining to adults however, it is found that an adult with profound mental retardation needs nursing care and may achieve only very limited self-care, the moderately retarded adult may achieve self-maintenance in unskilled or semi-skilled work under sheltered conditions, and the mildly retarded adult can usually achieve social and vocational skills adequate to minimum self-support.

Incidence

It is estimated that 3% of the population of the United States of America are mentally retarded. This is an approximate figure as such data is difficult to gather. In the state of New South Wales, figures were prepared by the Division of Health Services, Research and Planning, in September, 1970.

Extracted from this report entitled, New South Wales Mental Retardation Survey 1970 are the following facts:

Omitting those stated to be mildly retarded, a figure that could not be gauged in the general population though it could be in institutions, it was found that in the 0-19 year age group the rate of mental retardation was 1.01/1,000 population. Omitting people 60 years and over, as well as the mildly mentally retarded, it was found that the ratio of mentally retarded people 0-19 years of age to those 20-59 years of age in institutions was approximately 1:2. This suggests that there are approximately 3/1,000 of the population of NSW in the age range 0-59 years who are more than mildly retarded. When it is considered that mild mental retardation comprises 75-85% of the total instances of retardation, it becomes likely that a little over 1% of the population of New South Wales suffers from mental retardation of one degree or another, a figure which is widely accepted as the prevalence rate.

Probably another 1% of any average population, while not falling within the ranges delineated as mentally retarded, will be of borderline or dull-normal intelligence requiring special educational facilities. So it can be seen that the problem of educating this population to a stage where capabilities of self-support and of adequate socialisation are possible, is a large one.

Aetiology

1. *Genetic Factors.* There are at least three ways in which genetic factors can lead to mental retardation. In the first of these, the defect in intelligence is less severe and is unassociated with organic pathology. These are people who fall within the lower end of the normal distribution curve. IQs are generally 50 plus, and the level of intelligence is believed to be due to polygenic inheritance.

In the second group, the defect, mostly severe, arises from pathological conditions due, in the main, to the effects of single mutant genes. Some rare conditions due to dominant mutant genes are tuberous sclerosis (epiloia), a number of conditions grouped under the term craniostenosis* in which there occurs premature closure of cranial sutures, and skull deformities. Members of this group include acrocephaly (pointed skull), and hypertelorism, in which, among other features, the eyes are set widely apart.

Recessive mutant genes are responsible for a large number of metabolic disorders, as newer techniques of analysis of the chemical constituents of the body are demonstrating. Among such disorders are phenylketonuria and homocystinuria (disorders of amino acid metabolism). Tay-Sachs disease, Niemann-Pick disease and Gaucher's disease (disorders of fat metabolism), galactosemia and glycogen storage disease (disorders of carbohydrate metabolism), and hepato-lenticular degeneration or Wilson's disease (disorder of copper metabolism). Certain varieties of sporadic cretinism occurring in individuals with adequate iodine intake are also determined by autosomal recessive genes. In these instances, defects in metabolism lead to an inadequate production of thyroxine. Most cases of gargoylism (Hurler's disease) are transmitted by an autosomal recessive gene.

The third group of disorders associated with mental retardation is due to aberrations in chromosomal number or shape. Examples of such

* In some forms of craniostenosis, recessive genes have also been implicated.

disorders are Mongolism, cat-cry (cri du chat) and Klinefelter's syndrome. Many people with Klinefelter's syndrome have normal or even superior intelligence, and some people presenting with only a few of the stigmata of mongolism, may also be of normal or superior intelligence.

2. *Factors in utero.* There is some evidence that severe dietary deficiency in the pregnant mother may give rise to foetal damage. Deficient iodine in the mother's diet occurring in certain regions gives rise to endemic goitrous cretinism. Virus infections, especially rubella (German measles) contracted by the mother during the first trimester may lead to deaf mutism, cataract, and possibly to mental retardation in the infant. Infection before birth by the protozoan Toxoplasma gondii causes toxoplasmosis, and those newborn infants who survive this have mental and neurological deficits. Congenital syphilis produces mental retardation in about 40% of cases, and the stigmata of congenital syphilis are present in approximately 75%. These stigmata consist of Hutchinson's teeth (which are notched along the cutting edge), interstitial keratitis, and nerve deafness.

Irradiation by X-rays or from radioactive fall out may damage the foetus, producing congenital abnormalities and mental retardation.

Certain chemical substances taken early in pregnancy, or large doses of insulin given to the expectant mother and producing profound hypoglycaemia, may lead to foetal damage and mental defect. Rhesus factor incompatibility of a severe nature may be associated with mental retardation.

3. *Factors during birth.* Abnormal labour giving rise to prolonged asphyxia and brain trauma during birth may lead to mental defect. Epilepsy may also follow these insults. It would appear that prematurity may also result in intellectual deficits.

4. *Factors after birth.* With severe trauma sufficient to cause paralysis, there may be associated mental defect as well as epilepsy. Infections such as meningitis, viral meningoencephalitis caused by the poliomyelitis virus, ECHO virus, Coxsackie virus, herpes simplex, and central nervous system effects of the viruses of mumps, measles, pertussis etc., may be implicated.

Lead poisoning frequently leads to chronic encephalopathy and mental retardation.

There is a group of disabilities which may affect learning ability through their isolating effect on the individual. This group includes defective vision or hearing, reading disabilities, motor handicaps, emotional disturbances or mental illnesses, petit mal and other forms of epilepsy. Unless special education and training is given, and defects are treated where possible, the intellectual development of these children will be hampered.

Apart from such disabilities which tend to isolate the individual from the normal stimuli essential for proper development, early segregation and institutionalisation or inadequate homes in poor social circumstances may also lead to inadequate stimuli and lack of educational opportunity.

These cases are referred to as 'mental retardation with psycho-social (environmental) deprivation'.

The above-mentioned disabilities affecting learning ability, and other factors leading to lack of educational opportunity are of particular importance in the so-called borderline group.

There remains a rather large group of disorders associated with mental retardation, the causes of which are multiple or unknown. Included here are congenital porencephaly (cystic formations in the cerebral hemispheres), congenital hydrocephalus, and microcephaly which covers a variety of disorders of variable aetiology in which the head is small and of peculiar shape.

Comment will now be made on a number of the better known clinical conditions associated with mental retardation, remembering that, apart from mongolism, these conditions are relatively rare.

Mongolism (Down's syndrome)

First described by an English physician, Langdon Down, in 1866, there is still controversy regarding the causes of the chromosome abnormalities associated with mongolism.

Advanced maternal and perhaps paternal age, and X-radiation are seen as likely predisposing factors. It is thought that ova which are present in germinal form from the time of conception have more opportunity to be affected by noxious factors, for example X-radiation, the older the mother is at the time of conception.

The problem of aetiology has been further complicated by the recent recognition of three distinct chromosomal abnormalities occurring in Down's syndrome:

1. Patients with trisomy 21 (3 of chromosome 21 instead of 2), have a total of 47 chromosomes instead of the normal 46. This is the most common form.
2. In mosaic mongols both normal and trisomic cells are found in various tissues.
3. Translocation, usually affecting chromosomes 15* and 21, is the mechanism operating in the inherited form of the condition known as familial mongolism.

The incidence of mongolism is stated to be 1 in 700 births. In a middle-aged mother (over 32 years) the risk of giving birth to a mongoloid child with trisomy 21 is about 1 in 100, but if translocation is present the risk is about 1 in 3.

Clinical picture

Over 100 stigmata or signs have been described in Down's syndrome, but they are rarely all found in the one individual.

The skull is rounded, face and occiput are flattened. The palpebral fissures are narrowed and slope downwards and inwards. The ears are usually small and have a simple convolutional pattern. The hair is wiry, and the tongue, being too large for the mouth, becomes coarse, cracked and fissured, due to continued sucking. The hands are broad and thick,

* Chromosomes 13, 14 or 15 may be involved.

with a single palmar transverse crease (Simian fissures), and thumbs and fingers are shorter than normal, the little fingers also being curved inwards. A large cleft may separate the great toes from the others. Laxity of ligaments and muscular hypotonicity are frequently described, but mongols who are given adequate opportunity for physical exercise do not show this.

Neuropathology

The hemispheres tend to be small with underdeveloped convolutional patterns, and the cerebellum and brain stem are also small. Abnormalities of the pituitary gland occur.

Mental state

Mental retardation is the outstanding feature. Most patients are moderately or severely retarded and very few have IQs of more than 50. Patients with very few stigmata may have normal or even superior intelligence.

People with Down's syndrome are usually good tempered, cheerful, co-operative and quite lively, in contrast to cretins.

Treatment and prognosis

No specific treatment has proved effective. Every effort should be made to develop the patient's full educational and social potential within the limits of his handicap. Nowadays, a normal or near normal life expectancy can be contemplated.

Cretinism

As well as iodine deficiency in the diet giving rise to endemic goitrous cretinism, and metabolic defects determined by autosomal recessive genes, cretinism is due not uncommonly to the congenital absence of the thyroid gland (sporadic athyreosis).

Clinical picture

Goitre, or enlargement of the thyroid, is present (except in athyreosis). If the condition is not recognised early and treatment given, the infant ceases to grow. Skin becomes coarse and dry, the voice hoarse and low pitched, and the abdomen protruberant. There are disturbances in ossification, and weakness of spinal muscles may lead to dorsal kyphosis. Limbs are stunted, ligaments lax and the patients are sluggish in their movements. The general appearance becomes podgy owing to broad coarse features, protruding tongue, tumid abdomen, and supraclavicular masses.

Mental state

Any degree of mental retardation may occur. The cretin is usually placid and lacking in animation, providing minimal nursing management problems.

Treatment

Treatment with thyroid extract usually averts most of the symptoms and signs if instituted early in infancy, hence the importance of recognizing this condition as soon after birth as possible and not confusing it with mongolism. Up to the age of three months, a daily dose of 15 mg of thyroid extract is given, and increased so long as there are no signs of overdose such as a rise in temperature, tachycardia or diarrhoea.

Thyroid extract is not effective in adult cretins. In cases of endemic goitrous cretinism the condition responds to the ingestion of small amounts of iodine.

Hydrocephalus

The central nervous system is bathed in cerebrospinal fluid (CSF) which, for the most part, takes its origin from the choroid plexuses within the ventricles of the brain. The CSF is reabsorbed into the blood stream mainly via the capillary bed of the pia and arachnoid over the cerebral hemispheres. Any obstruction to the passage of this fluid will lead to its accumulation, with subsequent enlargement of the fluid compartments between the source of CSF and the obstruction.

Common sites for such obstruction are the foramen of Munro, the third ventricle, aqueduct of Sylvius, the foramina of Majendie and Luschka, and the basilar cisternae. There may also be failure of normal CSF absorption due to obliteration of the pathways over the surface of the brain resulting from diffuse inflammation and the development of fibrous tissue.

The causes of obstruction may be:

1. Neoplasm.
2. Congenital malformations, particularly atresia of the aqueduct of Sylvius which may be inherited as the result of a sex-linked recessive gene.
3. Acute purulent infection or post infective adhesions.
4. Post haemorrhagic or post operative adhesions of the arachnoid mater.

Distension of the proximal fluid compartments leads to pressure atrophy of the cortex. In the foetus, or the infant before closure of the cranial sutures, the cranial bones become separated and greatly thinned, appearing at times almost translucent. Marked hydrocephalus occurring before birth gives rise to obstetric difficulties, and such infants are rarely born alive.

Clinical picture

The abnormality is seldom noted before the second or third month of life, when the rapid enlargement of the circumference of the head becomes apparent. The fontanelles become tense and the cranial sutures widen. Signs and symptoms resulting from the increase in intracranial pressure follow the enlarging of the head in all directions. These may include vomiting, papilloedema, muscular weakness and spasticity particularly of the legs, blindness, deafness, and convulsions. Complete mental and physical deterioration may ensue. Some cases run a more chronic course, and in others the condition may become spontaneously arrested, leaving the children only mildly mentally retarded. A degree of hydrocephalus is not incompatible with normal or even superior intelligence.

The distinctive features of the hydrocephalic skull are its general enlargement, and the finding that the greatest circumference is at the level of the temples. In average cases the circumference is about 64 cm, the normal being 56 cm, but in some instances it may be as much as 92 cm, with the excessive weight making it impossible for the infant to hold his head erect.

Treatment

In suitable cases, a variety of surgical procedures have been developed to by-pass obstructions.

Tuberous sclerosis (epiloia)

This condition due to an abnormal dominant gene possibly influenced by so-called modifying genes manifests itself with considerable variability. The clinical features of the complete form are:

1. Mental retardation which is usually severe and which increases with advancing age.
2. Adenoma sebaceum, typically distributed as a 'butterfly rash' in the skin of the cheeks and nose, though present on the rest of the body, due to an overgrowth of sebaceous glands.
3. Epilepsy, usually of the grand mal type.
4. Cutaneous fibromata usually developing in late childhood and adolescence.
5. Intracranial calcifications, usually periventricular, which may be detected on X-Ray.
6. Small yellowish tumours of the retina (phacomata), and benign tumours of the brain, kidney, heart and liver, which may become malignant.

The pathological lesions in the central nervous system consist of circumscribed, hard whitish nodules from a few millimetres to 2-3 centimetres in diameter scattered throughout the cerebral cortex.

The prognosis varies with the degree and location of the multiple lesions associated with this condition.

Specific treatment is limited to anticonvulsant medication.

Phenylketonuria

Phenylketonuria, an inborn error of metabolism, is transmitted as a simple recessive autosomal Mendelian trait, and occurs in 1 in 10,000 to 1 in 20,000 births.

The basic metabolic defect is the inability to convert the essential aminoacid phenylalanine into tyrosine due to deficiency of a specific enzyme, phenylalanine hydroxylase. This in turn leads to a number of other biochemical abnormalities. There occurs a raised phenylalanine level in the serum.

Phenylpyruvic acid, an abnormal metabolite, is excreted in the urine, where it can be tested for by adding a few drops of ferric chloride solution. In the presence of phenylpyruvic acid a vivid green colour develops. The use of Phenystix provides a simple method of testing for the condition. Unfortunately, these tests may not show a positive reaction until the infant is several weeks old, and may show false positives due to other amino acidurias. The more sensitive Guthrie test which determines the raised level of phenylalanine in the blood is therefore commonly employed.

The Guthrie test consists of making up an agar plate (culture medium) containing spores of Bacillus subtilis and a specific phenylalanine antagonist, and placing on the plate, discs of filter paper impregnated with blood to be tested. This preparation is then incubated. Bacillus subtilis requires phenylalanine for growth, and since the antagonist to phenylalanine is incorporated in the culture medium the bacterial spores receive no phenylalanine from the culture medium and will not grow unless there is a level of phenylalanine in the blood specimen being tested sufficient to counteract the effect of the antagonist. The growth of spores (a positive Guthrie test) indicates the presence of a higher than normal level of phenylalanine in the blood, and the presence of phenylketonuria.

Currently in New South Wales* a spot of blood, usually from the heel of each infant in obstetric hospitals, is collected on special filter paper, preferably on the last day of hospitalisation and certainly not before the third day. This blood is subjected to the Guthrie test.

At six weeks of age, a further Guthrie test on blood is carried out. At the same time, paper chromatography testing of urine absorbed into a 2.5 cm × 10 cm strip of blotting paper retrieved from the folds of the baby's napkin and dried at Baby Health Centres, is carried out. The one way paper chromotography method developed by Dr Brian Turner while working with the N.S.W. Department of Health has the advantage of being able to detect other amino acidurias as well as phenylketonuria. This early and later testing provides greater opportunity to cover the whole infant population, and throws up the occasional false negative Guthrie test results that may occur if carried out too early.

The organizational detail and technical skills necessary to conduct such surveys is obvious.

The importance of early detection is paramount, since the giving of a diet low in phenylalanine and commenced in the first six months of life results in improvement in developmental progress and behaviour.

Such dietary management requires the combined efforts of a team of specialists.

Clinical picture

The majority of untreated patients are severely mentally retarded, but some may go undetected throughout life with borderline or normal intelligence, as evidenced by a number of people who have been detected as late as the sixth decade and who have led useful lives.

Eczema and convulsions are present in about one third of cases.

* Personal communication from the late Dr Brian Turner.

Electroencephalograms are abnormal in 80%, even in patients who do not have convulsions.

Untreated phenylpyruvic children are hyperactive and unpredictable, and indulge in bizarre movements of trunk, upper limbs and hands. They are a management problem for nursing staff owing to these characteristics, and because verbal and non-verbal communication is poor.

The early classical descriptions of these children were of blond, blue-eyed children showing the above features, but the relative deficiency of melanin giving rise to fair complexion and hair is not present in all.

Sturge-Weber syndrome (encephalo-facial angiomatosis)

This condition, due to an irregularly dominant gene, is manifest by the presence of a facial naevus in the distribution of the fifth cranial nerve (trigeminal) which is associated with a large tortuous angiomatous formation overlying the cerebral cortex mainly in the occipital region, but extending forward from there. In the atrophic layers of cortex beneath the angiomatous formation, calcification occurs, and this appears on X-Ray looking something like a mass of worms.

The cortical damage produces contra lateral neurological signs, usually a degree of spastic paralysis. Epileptic seizures and mental retardation complete the main picture. Mental retardation is not an inevitable outcome. One patient known to the author and now aged 50 years coped very well for some years doing clerical work with minimal spasticity of the right arm and leg, but finally lost her job following a number of convulsive episodes.

Neurological procedures on the angiomatous malformations appear to have had limited success in the past.

Galactosemia

This is a metabolic defect, transmitted by an autosomal recessive gene, causing an inability to convert galactose to glucose. Clinical manifestations beginning a few days after the commencement of milk feeding, include jaundice, vomiting, failure to gain weight, and hepatomegaly.

If untreated, the condition may be fatal in a short time or may lead to progressive mental retardation, cataracts and liver insufficiency. Hypoglycaemic convulsions may be added to this picture.

Treatment consists in giving a galactose-free diet which, if instituted early, allows normal physical and mental development. Moderate amounts of milk may be taken from about school age.

Pyridoxine deficiency

Pyridoxine deficiency is another of the many recessive genetic disorders, and untreated is associated with mental deficiency and spasticity. Affected infants have abnormally high pyridoxine (Vitamin B_6) requirements. During the first week of life convulsions occur, and the administration of 100 mg pyridoxine I.V. will cause cessation of these and improvement in the E.E.G. picture. Thereafter, the addition of 10 mg of pyridoxine daily will keep the patient symptom free.

Management of the mentally retarded

It is useful to look at the management of mental retardation using the concepts of primary, secondary and tertiary prevention as developed by Gerald Caplan.

Primary prevention

Primary prevention of mental retardation will involve public education, improvement of socioeconomic standards, preventive medical measures, and genetic counselling.

PUBLIC EDUCATION

The first chapter of this book deals with some attitudes to mental illness during the ages. Superstitious attitudes with respect to mental retardation still persist in large areas of our community. Public education, which will help oust uphelpful attitudes and spell out such facts as are known, becomes important in terms of gaining supprt for acceptance of programmes aimed at limiting and treating mental retardation. It should be made clear that mentally retarded folk are individuals, essentially feeling normal emotions, having needs for love, affection and companionship and a sense of belonging, and that they are entitled to develop their full potential as is the next citizen.

Knowledge of such aetiological factors as are known will more readily enable people to take part in such preventive measures as mass screenings of blood and urine shortly after birth, vaccinations, and perhaps more importantly, the provision of a stimulating and emotionally stable environment for the infant and growing child.

IMPROVEMENT IN SOCIOECONOMIC STANDARDS

There is little point in education unless it is possible to put into practice the preventive measures indicated. Some educationally deprived individuals may be unable to grasp the facts presented, and gross poverty will prevent the production of a suitable material and emotional environment for infants and children. Poverty tends to breed nihilistic attitudes, and where a fatalistic nihilism supervenes, there exists no motivation for undertaking preventive measures.

The worse the socioeconomic standard of a community, the higher in general is the birth rate, and in such situations adolescent pregnancies and pregnancies occurring in middle life are more common, the latter giving rise to added obstetric problems and increasing the possible incidence of chromosomal abnormalities.

Socioeconomic standards are largely outside the province of workers in psychiatry, and are part of the total matrix of a community determined by the country's economy, social agencies, community leaders, educators, politicians, etc. A concerted sustained effort is required by all those in a position to create healthy change in order to produce worthwhile improvement in socioeconomic standards.

PREVENTIVE MEDICAL MEASURES

The highest standard of prenatal care of the pregnant mother is the most important factor in the prevention of mental retardation in offspring. One has but to look through our earlier section on aetiological factors to see the areas where preventive measures can be applied (Chapter 10). These are divided into genetic factors and factors occurring in utero, during birth and after birth.

Chromosomal abnormalities will be reduced by limiting the number of children born to mothers over the age of 40 years.

The prevention of prematurity, adequate nourishment for the pregnant mother, detection of rhesus factor and other blood incompatibility, adequate control of maternal diabetes, the prompt treatment of maternal infection etc. are all of importance.

Sound obstetric practice throughout pregnancy and labour, and paediatric measures to deal with both acute neonatal problems and the diseases of early childhood that can lead to mental retardation will do much to reduce the incidence of mental retardation.

GENETIC COUNSELLING

Parents who have given birth to an abnormal child, or who have close relatives affected, are naturally anxious about the possibility of defects in future offspring.

We know that the chances of affected offspring arising out of a marriage in which one parent carries an abnormal dominant gene is 1 in 2. In cases of autosomal recessive genetic disorders the parents of one child with such a disorder have a 1 in 4 chance of having a second affected child.

This is at the simplest level of genetic counselling. Many conditions are much more complicated than this and require the efforts of experts in this field working in situations equipped with a cytogenetic and biochemical laboratory where specialised tests can be carried out.

All that can be given to a parent is statistical data indicating probabilities. Given a 1 in 4 chance of producing affected offspring could mean that the next 2 or 3 or 4 children could be affected, or the parents could indeed produce a number of phenotypically normal children, either genotypically normal or carriers.

Secondary prevention

Early identification and treatment of hereditary disorders such as phenylketonuria, galactosaemia and pyridoxine deficiency, and the early identification and management of cretinism as indicated above, will forestall the gross degrees of mental retardation that usually develop in these conditions. Prompt diagnosis and treatment of conditions such as central nervous system infections, epilepsy, and lead poisoning, are important.

Surgical treatment of subdural haematomata, craniostenosis, and hydrocephalus, and the excision of epileptogenic foci may well abort the development of mental retardation.

Secondary prevention also concerns itself with the early recognition and handling of children with isolating handicaps, and with the early identification and treatment of the culturally deprived child who requires more sensory, verbal and emotional stimulation than is present in his environment, in order to widen his intellectual horizons.

Tertiary prevention

This aspect of management involves techniques designed to prevent both long-continued disability and the subsequent failure to maintain initial improvement.

After thorough assessment, a decision needs to be made as to whether the mentally retarded person is best managed at home or in an institutional setting. This decision is frequently difficult for parents to make, and the family's ability to cope with the myriad problems associated with caring for a mentally retarded child at home require assessment.

The general trend nowadays, at least in the early formative years, is for services to be provided to help the family keep the child at home. Parents who undertake to do this will usually require counselling and support, help in arranging training, and in some instances, day care in community centres for their child.

Education and training are best provided in special schools where classes are small and where teaching is directed towards personal development and social adjustment. The mother should be afforded some relief from the continuous and often demanding situation she faces when caring for her child at home. Such relief may be obtained in areas where hostel accommodation or training centres are provided.

It is obvious that very special skills will be required to manage the severely retarded, and children with certain isolated handicaps. Should neither special schools nor other facilities be available in a particular community, then institutional or residential care becomes a must in most instances if the child is to develop its full potentialities.

When residential care is mandatory, such care should not primarily be custodial, and every effort should be made to keep families in touch with their children. In keeping with the tenets of therapeutic community care, the orientation should be towards the needs of the children, adolescents or adults receiving help.

Initially of course, the staff of such hospitals may need to provide a great deal of support to patients, and particularly with infants and young children, will need to adopt the role of parent substitute, providing warmth and stability leading to emotional security and the possibility of identification with a consistent figure.

Staff must learn to appreciate the need to reduce such mothering or fathering at a suitable stage, so that patients may develop as much independence and individuality as possible.

All daily activities occurring in a residential or hospital setting should be structured as closely as possible to activities occurring at home, and the training of patients should be directed towards this end. The term applied to this aim and process is 'normalisation'. It involves such things as getting up at the normal time, getting into one's own clothes and eating under normal circumstances. It will be necessary, in many instances, to actually train the mentally handicapped so they can undertake these everyday activities. As well as residential care being developed along these homely lines, other aspects of normalisation consist in going from the 'home' to school which is usually sited in another part of the hospital, and to other places in the community, all such activities having educational and training components to maximise social potential. The more formal schooling conducted by specially trained teachers of the Education Department has an important part to play in helping the mentally retarded child to gain his full intellectual potential.

Nursing staff play the key role in the normalisation process, and the endeavours of other specialty groups should largely be directed towards helping the nurse develop further her true role of 'Nurse therapist' in these residential care programmes for mentally retarded patients.

The need for vocational or occupational training, especially for the adolescent group has been recognised, and programmes of training tailored to the individual's capabilities are now in use in many residential institutions. Though such programmes are not yet widespread, a number of ex-hospital patients have shown themselves able to hold down certain selected jobs on the competitive market. Others, more severely handicapped, are able to function in sheltered workshops, finding satisfaction in assembly work of varying types that many intellectually brighter people would find tedious.

Conclusion

A diagnosis of mental retardation should not sound the death knell on hopes of leading a reasonably productive and satisfying life. To be realistic, there are those who will never be able to cope with life outside residential care, an unfortunate fact that has to be faced, but with the application of such preventive measures as are understood today, the number of severely handicapped people can be greatly reduced, but for those who must carry the load of mental handicap, the present day approach encompassing training, education, treatment and rehabilitation, will ensure that maximum educational and social potential is attained.

APPENDIX

INTERNATIONAL CLASSIFICATION OF DISEASES

NOTE: I.C.D. Glossary descriptions of disorders which are quoted in the text do not appear in this appendix. Where they do not appear in the text, they are quoted in full below.

MENTAL DISORDERS

Psychoses (290-299)

Organic Psychotic Conditions (290-294)
includes: psychotic organic brain syndrome

290 SENILE AND PRESENILE ORGANIC PSYCHOTIC CONDITIONS

- 290.0 Senile dementia, simple type
- 290.1 Presenile dementia
  - Brain syndrome with presenile brain disease
  - Circumscribed atrophy of the brain
  - Dementia in:
    - Alzheimer's disease
    - Pick's disease of the brain
- 290.2 Senile dementia, depressed or paranoid type
  - Senile psychosis NOS*
- 290.3 Senile dementia with acute confusional state
  - Senile dementia with a superimposed reversible episode of acute confusional state
- 290.4 Arteriosclerotic dementia
- 290.8 Other
- 290.9 Unspecified

291 ALCOHOLIC PHYCHOSES

- 291.0 Delirium tremens
  - Acute or subacute organic psychotic states in alcoholics, characterized by clouded consciousness, disorientation, fear, illusions, delusions, hallucinations of any kind, notably visual and tactile, and restlessness, tremor and sometimes fever

* NOS = not otherwise specified

Alcoholic delirium

291.1 Korsakov's psychosis, alcoholic
Alcoholic polyneuritic psychosis

291.2 Other alcoholic dementia
Alcoholic dementia NOS
Chronic alcoholic brain syndrome

291.3 Other alcoholic hallucinosis

291.4 Pathological drunkenness

291.5 Alcoholic jealousy
Alcoholic paranoia

291.8 Other

291.9 Unspecified
Alcoholic:
Mania NOS
Psychosis NOS
Alcoholism (chronic) with psychosis

292 DRUG PSYCHOSES

292.0 Drug withdrawal syndrome

292.1 Paranoid and/or hallucinatory states induced by drugs

292.2 Pathological drug intoxication

292.8 Other

292.9 Unspecified

293 TRANSIENT ORGANIC PSYCHOTIC CONDITIONS

293.0 Acute confusional state
Short-lived states, lasting hours or days, of the above type:

Acute:
delirium
infective psychosis
organic reaction
post-traumatic organic psychosis
psycho-organic syndrome
psychosis associated with endocrine, metabolic or cerebrovascular disorder

Epileptic:
confusional state
twilight state

293.1 Subacute confusional state
Subacute:
delirium
infective psychosis
organic reaction
post-traumatic organic psychosis
psycho-organic syndrome

psychosis associated with endocrine or metabolic disorder

293.8 Others

293.9 Unspecified

294 OTHER ORGANIC PSYCHOTIC CONDITIONS (CHRONIC)

294.0 Korsakov's psychosis or syndrome (nonalcoholic)

294.1 Dementia in conditions classified elsewhere
Dementia in:
cerebral lipidoses
epilepsy
general paralysis of the insane
hepatolenticular degeneration
Huntington's chorea
multiple sclerosis
polyarteritis nodosa

294.8 Other
States that fulfil the criteria of an organic psychosis but do not take the form of a confusional state (293.-), a non-alcoholic Korsakov's psychosis (294.0) or a dementia (294.1)
Epileptic psychosis NOS (code also 345.-)
Mixed paranoid and affective organic psychotic states

294.9 Unspecified

Other Psychoses (295-299)

295 schizophrenic psychoses
includes: schizophrenia of the types described in 295.0-295.9 occurring in children.

295.0 Simple type
Schizophrenia simplex

295.1 Hebephrenic type
Hebephrenia

295.2 Catatonic type
Catatonic:
agitation
excitation
stupor
Schizophrenic:
catalepsy
catatonia
flexibilitas cerea

295.3 Paranoid type
Paraphrenic schizophrenia

295.4 Acute schizophrenic episode
Oneirophrenia

Schizophreniform:
  attack
  psychosis, confusional type

295.5 Latent schizophrenia
Latent schizophrenic reaction
Schizophrenia:
  borderline
  prepsychotic
  prodromal
  pseudoneurotic
  pseudopsychopathic
Excludes: schizoid personality (301.2)

295.6 Residual schizophrenia
Chronic undifferentiated schizophrenia
Restzustand (schizophrenic)
Schizophrenic residual state

295.7 Schizoaffective type
Cyclic schizophrenia
Mixed schizophrenic and affective psychosis
Schizoaffective psychosis
Schizophreniform psychosis, affective type

295.8 Other
Schizophrenia of specified type not classifiable under 295.0-295.7
Acute (undifferentiated) schizophrenia
Atypical schizophrenia
Coenesthopathic schizophrenia

295.9 Unspecified
To be used only as a last resort
Schizophrenia NOS
Schizophrenic reaction NOS
Schizophreniform psychosis NOS

296 AFFECTIVE PSYCHOSES

296.0 Manic-depressive psychosis, manic type
Hypomania NOS
Hypomanic psychosis
Mania (monopolar) NOS
Manic disorder
Manic psychosis
Manic-depressive psychosis or reaction:
  hypomanic
  manic

296.1 Manic-depressive psychosis, depressed type
Depressive psychosis
Endogenous depressive
Involutinal melancholia
Manic-depressive reaction, depressed

Monopolar depression
Psychotic depression

296.2 Manic-depressive psychosis, circular type but currently manic

Bipolar disorder, now manic

296.3 Manic-depressive psychosis, circular type but currently depressed

Bipolar disorder, now depressed

296.4 Manic-depressive psychosis, circular type, mixed

296.5 Manic-depressive psychosis, circular type, current condition not specified

Circular type (see 296.2) in which the current condition is not specified as either manic or depressive.

296.6 Manic-depressive psychosis, other and unspecified.

Use this code for cases where no other information is available, except the unspecified term, manic-depressive psychosis, or for syndromes corresponding to the descriptions of depressed (296.1) or manic (296.0) types but which for other reasons cannot be classified under 296.0-296.5.

Manic-depressive psychosis:
NOS
mixed type

Manic-depressive:
reaction NOS
syndrome NOS

296.8 Other

296.9 Unspecified
Affective psychosis NOS
Melancholia NOS

297 PARANOID STATES

297.0 Paranoid state, simple

297.1 Paranoia

297.2 Paraphrenia
Involutional paranoid state
Late paraphrenia

297.3 Induced psychosis
Folie à deux
Induced paranoid disorder

297.8 Other

Paranoid states which, though in many ways akin to schizophrenic or affective states, cannot readily be classified under any of the preceding rubrics, nor under 298.4.

Paranoid querulans
Sensitiver Beziehungswahn

297.9 Unspecified
Paranoid:
psychosis NOS
reaction NOS
state NOS

298 OTHER NONORGANIC PSYCHOSES

298.0 Depressive type
Reactive depressive psychosis
Psychogenic depressive psychosis

298.1 Excitative type

298.2 Reactive confusion
Psychogenic confusion
Psychogenic twilight state

298.3 Acute paranoid reaction
Bouffée délirante

298.4 Psychogenic paranoid psychosis
Protracted reactive paranoid psychosis

298.8 Other and unspecified reactive psychosis
Hysterical psychosis
Psychogenic psychosis NOS
Psychogenic stupor

298.9 Unspecified psychosis
To be used only as a last resort, when no other term can be used.
Psychosis NOS

299 PSYCHOSES WITH ORIGIN SPECIFIC TO CHILDHOOD

299.0 Infantile autism
Childhood autism
Infantile psychosis
Kanner's syndrome

299.1 Disintegrative psychosis
Heller's syndrome

299.8 Other
A variety of atypical infantile psychoses which may show some, but not all, of the features of infantile autism. Symptoms may include stereotyped repetitive movements, hyperkinesis, self-injury, retarded speech development, echolalia and impaired social relationships. Such disorders may occur in children of any level of intelligence but are particularly common in those with mental retardation.
Atypical childhood psychosis

299.9 Unspecified
Child psychosis NOS
Schizophrenia, childhood type NOS
Schizophrenic syndrome of childhood NOS

300 NEUROTIC DISORDERS

300.0 Anxiety states
Anxiety:
neurosis
reaction
state (neurotic)
Panic:
attack
disorder
state

300.1 Hysteria
Astasia-abasia, hysterical
Compensation neurosis
Conversion hysteria
Conversion reaction
Dissociative reaction or state
Ganser's syndrome, hysterical
Hysteria NOS
Multiple personality

300.2 Phobic state
Agoraphobia
Animal phobias
Anxiety-hysteria
Claustrophobia
Phobia NOS

300.3 Obsessive-compulsive disorders
Anankastic neurosis
Compulsive neurosis

300.4 Neurotic depression
Anxiety depression
Depressive reaction
Neurotic depressive state
Reactive depression

300.5 Neurasthenia
Nervous debility

300.6 Depersonalization syndrome
Derealization (neurotic)

300.7 Hypochondriasis

300.8 Other neurotic disorders
Neurotic disorders not classified elsewhere, e.g. occupational neurosis. Patients with mixed neuroses should not be classified in this category but according to the most prominent symptoms they display.
Briquet's disorder
Occupational neurosis, including writer's cramp
Psychasthenia
Psychasthenic neurosis

300.9 Unspecified
To be used only as a last resort.

Neurosis NOS
Psychoneurosis NOS

301 PERSONALITY DISORDERS
Character neurosis

301.0 Paranoid personality disorder
Fanatic personality
Paranoid traits
Paranoid personality (disorder)

301.1 Affective personality disorder
Cycloid personality
Cyclothymic personality
Depressive personality

301.2 Schizoid personality disorder

301.3 Explosive personality disorder
Aggressive:
personality
reaction
Aggressiveness
Emotional instability (excessive)
Pathological emotionality
Quarrelsomeness

301.4 Anankastic personality disorder
Compulsive personality
Obsessional personality

301.5 Hysterical personality disorder
Histrionic personality
Psychoinfantile personality

301.6 Asthenic personality disorder
Dependent personality
Inadequate personality
Passive personality

301.7 Personality disorder with predominantly sociopathic or asocial manifestation
Amoral personality
Antisocial personality
Asocial personality

301.8 Other personality disorders
Personality:
eccentric
'haltlose' type
immature
passive-aggressive
psychoneurotic

301.9 Unspecified
Pathological personality NOS
Personality disorder NOS
Psychopathic:

constitutional state
personality (disorder)

302 SEXUAL DEVIATIONS AND DISORDERS

302.0 Homosexuality
Lesbianism

302.1 Bestiality

302.2 Paedophilia

302.3 Transvestism

302.4 Exhibitionism

302.5 Trans-sexualism

302.6 Disorders of psychosexual identity
Gender-role disorder

302.7 Frigidity and impotence
Dysparenunia, psychogenic

302.8 Other
Fetishism
Masochism
Sadism

302.9 Unspecified

303 ALCOHOL DEPENDENCE SYNDROME

Acute drunkenness in alcoholism
Chronic alcoholism
Dipsomania

304 DRUG DEPENDENCE

304.0 Morphine type
Heroin
Methadone
Opium
Opium alkaloids and their derivatives
Synthetics with morphine-like effects

304.1 Barbiturate type
Barbiturates
Nonbarbiturate sedatives and tranquillisers with a similar effect:
chlordiazepoxide
diazepam
glutethimide
meprobamate

304.2 Cocaine
Coca leaves and derivatives

304.3 Cannabis
Hemp
Hashish
Marijuana

304.4 Amphetamine type and other psychostimulants
Phenmetrazine   Methylphenidate

304.5 Hallucinogens
L.S.D. and derivatives
Mescaline
Psilocybin

304.6 Other
Absinthe addiction
Glue sniffing

304.7 Combinations of morphine type drug with any other

304.8 Combinations excluding morphine type drug

304.9 Unspecified
Drug addiction NOS
Drug dependence NOS

305 NONDEPENDENT ABUSE OF DRUGS

305.0 Alcohol
Cases of acute intoxication or 'hangover' effects
Drunkenness NOS
Excessive drinking of alcohol NOS
'Hangover' (alcohol)
Inebriety NOS

305.1 Tobacco
Cases in which tobacco is used to the detriment of a person's health or social functioning or in which there is tobacco dependence. Dependence is included here rather than under 304.- because tobacco differs from other drugs of dependence in its psychotoxic effects.
Tobacco dependence

305.2 Cannabis

305.3 Hallucinogens
Cases of acute intoxication or 'bad trips'
L.S.D. reaction

305.4 Barbiturates and tranquillisers
Cases where a person has taken the drug to the detriment of his health or social functioning, in doses above or for periods beyond those normally regarded as therapeutic.

305.5 Morphine type

305.6 Cocaine type

305.7 Amphetamine type

305.8 Antidepressants

305.9 Other, mixed or unspecified
'Laxative habit'
Misuse of drugs NOS
Nonprescribed use of drugs or patent medicinals

306 PHYSIOLOGICAL MALFUNCTION ARISING FROM MENTAL FACTORS
A variety of physical symptoms or types of physiological malfunction of mental origin, not involving tissue damage

and usually mediated through the autonomic nervous system. The disorders are grouped according to body system. Codes 306.0-306.9 should not be used if the physical symptom is secondary to a psychiatric disorder classifiable elsewhere. If tissue damage is involved, code under 316.

306.0 Musculoskeletal
Psychogenic torticollis

306.1 Respiratory
Air hunger
Hiccough (psychogenic)
Hyperventilation
Psychogenic cough
Yawning

306.2 Cardiovascular
Cardiac neurosis
Cardiovascular neurosis
Neurocirculatory asthenia
Psychogenic cardiovascular disorder

306.3 Skin
Psychogenic pruritus

306.4 Gastrointestinal
Aerophagy
Cyclical vomiting, psychogenic

306.5 Genitourinary
Psychogenic dysmenorrhoea

306.6 Endocrine

306.7 Organs of special sense

306.8 Other
Teeth-grinding

306.9 Unspecified
Psychophysiologic disorder NOS
Psychosomatic disorder NOS

307 SPECIAL SYMPTOMS OR SYNDROMES NOT ELSEWHERE CLASSIFIED

307.0 Stammering and stuttering

307.1 Anorexia nervosa

A disorder in which the main features are persistent active refusal to eat and marked loss of weight. The level of activity and alertness is characteristically high in relation to the degree of emaciation. Typically the disorder begins in teenage girls but it may sometimes begin before puberty and rarely it occurs in males. Amenorrhoea is usual and there may be a variety of other physiological changes including slow pulse and respiration, low body temperature and dependent oedema. Unusual eating habits and attitudes toward food are typical and sometimes starvation follows or alternates with periods of overeating. The accompanying psychiatric symptoms are diverse.

307.2 Tics

307.3 Stereotyped repetitive movements
Stereotypes NOS

307.4 Specific disorders of sleep
This category should only be used when a more precise mental or psychiatric diagnosis cannot be made
Hypersomnia
Insomnia
Inversion of sleep rhythm
Nightmares
Night terrors
Sleepwalking
} of nonorganic origin

307.5 Other and unspecified disorders of eating
This category should only be used when a more precise medical or psychiatric diagnosis cannot be made
Infantile feeding disturbances
Loss of appetite
Overeating
Pica
Psychogenic vomiting
} of nonorganic origin

307.6 Enuresis
A disorder in which the main manifestation is a persistent involuntary voiding of urine by day or night which is considered abnormal for the age of the individual. Sometimes the child will have failed to gain bladder control and in other cases he will have gained control and then lost it. Episodic or fluctuating enuresis should be included. The disorder would not usually be diagnosed under the age of four years. Enuresis (primary) (secondary) of nonorganic origin.

307.7 Encopresis
Encopresis (continuous) (discontinuous) of nonorganic origin

307.8 Psychalgia
Psychogenic backache
Tension headache

307.9 Other and unspecified
The use of this category should be discouraged. Most of the items listed in the inclusion terms are not indicative of psychiatric disorder and are included only because such terms may sometimes still appear as diagnoses.
Hairplucking
Lalling
Lisping
Masturbation

Nail-biting
Thumb-sucking

308 ACUTE REACTION TO STRESS
Catastrophic stress
Combat fatigue
Exhaustion delirium

308.0 Predominant disturbance of emotions

308.1 Predominant disturbance of consciousness

308.2 Predominant psychomotor disturbance

308.3 Other
Acute situational disturbance

308.4 Mixed

308.9 Unspecified

309 ADJUSTMENT REACTION

309.0 Brief depressive reaction
Grief reaction

309.1 Prolonged depressive reaction

309.2 With predominant disturbance of other emotions
Abnormal separation anxiety
Culture shock

309.3 With predominant disturbance of conduct

309.4 With mixed disturbance of emotions and conduct

309.8 Other
Adjustment reaction with elective mutism
Hospitalism in children NOS

309.9 Unspecified
Adaptation reaction NOS
Adjustment reaction NOS

310 SPECIFIC NONPSYCHOTIC MENTAL DISORDERS FOLLOWING ORGANIC BRAIN DAMAGE

Note: This category should be used only for conditions where the *form* of the disorder is determined by the brain pathology

310.0 Frontal lobe syndrome
Lobotomy syndrome
Postleucotomy syndrome (state)

310.1 Cognitive or personality change of other type
Chronic, mild states of memory disturbance and intellectual deterioration, often accompanied by increased irritability, querulousness, lassitude and complaints of physical weakness. These states are often associated with old age, and may precede more severe states due to brain damage classifiable under dementia of any type (290.-, and 294.-) or any condition in 293.- (Transient organic psychotic conditions).

Mild memory disturbance
Organic Psychosyndrome of nonpsychotic severity

310.2 Postconcussional syndrome
Postcontusional syndrome (encephalopathy)
Status post commotio cerebri
Post-traumatic brain syndrome, nonpsychotic

310.8 Other
Include here disorders resembling the postcontusional syndrome (310.2), associated with infective or other diseases of the brain or surrounding tissues
Other focal (partial) organic psychosyndromes

310.9 Unspecified

311 DEPRESSIVE DISORDER, NOT ELSEWHERE CLASSIFIED

States of depression, usually of moderate but occasionally of marked intensity, which have no specifically manic-depressive or other psychotic depressive features and which do not appear to be associated with stressful events or other features specified under neurotic depression.

Depression NOS
Depressive disorder NOS
Depressive state NOS

312 DISTURBANCE OF CONDUCT NOT ELSEWHERE CLASSIFIED

312.0 Unsocialized disturbance of conduct
Unsocialized aggressive disorder

312.1 Socialized disturbance of conduct
Group delinquency

312.2 Compulsive conduct disorder
Kleptomania

312.3 Mixed disturbance of conduct and emotions
Neurotic delinquency

312.8 Other

312.9 Unspecified

313 DISTURBANCE OF EMOTIONS SPECIFIC TO CHILDHOOD AND ADOLESCENCE

Less well differentiated emotional disorders characteristic of the childhood period. Where the emotional disorder takes the form of a neurotic disorder described under 300.-, the appropriate 300.- coding should be made. This category differs from category 308.- in terms of longer duration and by the lack of close relationship in time and content to some stress.

313.0 With anxiety and fearfulness
Ill-defined emotional disorders characteristic of childhood in

which the main symptoms involve anxiety and fearfulness. Many cases of school refusal or elective mutism might be included here.

Overanxious reaction of childhood or adolescence

313.1 With misery and unhappiness

Emotional disorders characteristic of childhood in which the main symptoms involve misery and unhappiness. There may also be eating and sleep disturbances.

313.2 With sensitivity, shyness and social withdrawal

Emotional disorders characteristic of childhood in which the main symptoms involve sensitivity, shyness, or social withdrawal. Some cases of elective mutism might be included here

Withdrawing reaction of childhood or adolescence

313.3 Relationship problems

Emotional disorders characteristic of childhood in which the main symptoms involve relationship problems

Sibling jealousy

313.8 Other or mixed

Many emotional disorders of childhood include several elements but whenever possible a specific coding under .0, .1, .2, or .3 should be made according to the *preponderant* type of disturbance. The category of mixed disorders should only be used when there is such an admixture that this cannot be done.

313.9 Unspecified

314 HYPERKINETIC SYNDROME OF CHILDHOOD

314.0 Simple disturbance of activity and attention

Cases in which short attention span, distractibility, and overactivity are the main manifestations without significant disturbance of conduct or delay in specific skills.

Overactivity NOS

314.1 Hyperkinesis with developmental delay

Cases in which the hyperkinetic syndrome is associated with speech delay, clumsiness, reading difficulties or other delays in specific skills

Development disorder of hyperkinesis

Use additional code to identify any associated neurological disorder

314.2 Hyperkinetic conduct disorder

Cases in which the hyperkinetic syndrome is associated with marked conduct disturbance but not development delay

Hyperkinetic conduct disorder

314.8 Other

314.9 Unspecified

Hyperkinetic reaction of childhood or adolescence NOS

Hyperkinetic syndrome NOS

315 SPECIFIC DELAYS IN DEVELOPMENT

315.0 Specific reading retardation
Developmental dyslexia
Specific spelling difficulty

315.1 Specific arithmetical retardation
Dyscalculia

315.2 Other specific learning difficulties

315.3 Development speech or language disorder
Developmental aphasia
Dyslalia

315.4 Specific motor retardation
Clumsiness syndrome
Dyspraxia syndrome

315.5 Mixed development disorder

315.8 Other

315.9 Unspecified
Developmental disorder NOS

316 PSYCHIC FACTORS ASSOCIATED WITH DISEASES CLASSIFIED ELSEWHERE

Mental disturbances or psychic factors of any type thought to have played a major part in the aetiology of physical conditions, usually involving tissue damage, classified elsewhere. The mental disturbance is usually mild and nonspecific and psychic factors (worry, fear, conflict, etc.) may be present without any overt psychiatric disorder. Use an additional code to identify the physical condition. In the rare instance that an overt psychiatric disorder is thought to have caused a physical condition, use a second additional code to record the psychiatric diagnosis.

Examples of the use of this category are:

Psychogenic:
Asthma
Dermatitis
Eczema
Gastric ulcer
Mucous colitis
Urticaria

Psychosocial dwarfism

Mental Retardation (317-319)

317 MILD MENTAL RETARDATION (IQ 50-70)

Feeble-minded
High-grade defect
Mild mental subnormality
Moron

318 OTHER SPECIFIED MENTAL RETARDATION

318.0 Moderate mental retardation (IQ 35-49)
Imbecile
Moderate mental subnormality

318.1 Severe mental retardation (IQ 20-34)
Severe mental subnormality

318.2 Profound mental retardation (IQ under 20)
Idiocy
Profound mental subnormality

319 UNSPECIFIED MENTAL RETARDATION
Mental deficiency NOS
Mental subnormality NOS

BIBLIOGRAPHY

This bibliography contains both source material and suggestions for further reading.

The larger standard textbooks of psychiatry, and particularly *Comprehensive Textbook of Psychiatry* and *American Handbook of Psychiatry*, contain material relevant to most areas listed in this bibliography. They will be mentioned only under 'Psychiatry, general' but acknowledgement is given of material derived from these sources and used under other topics listed.

Psychiatry, general

ARIETI S. *American Handbook of Psychiatry*, Vols. I-III. Basic Books Inc., New York/London.

DAWSON & ANDERSON. *Aids to Psychiatry*. Baillière, Tindal and Cox, London.

FREEDMAN, A. M., KAPLAN, H. I. & SADOCK, B. J. *Comprehensive Textbook of Psychiatry*. 2nd edn., vols. I and II. Williams and Wilkins, Baltimore.

IRONSIDE, W. 'Anti-Psychiatry, Psychiatry and Medicine.' *Aust. N.Z. J. Psychiatry* 1975, 9:69.

KING, A. 'Primary and Secondary Anorexia Nervosa Syndromes.' *Brit. J. Psychiat.* 1963, 109:470-479.

MAYER-GROSS, W., SLATER, E. & ROTH, M. *Textbook of Psychiatry*. Cassell and Company Limited, London.

PARE, C. M. B., REES, W. LINFORD & SAINSBURY, M. J. 'Differentiation of Two Genetically Specific Types of Depression by the Response to Anti-depressants.' *The Lancet*, December 1962, 1340-1343.

PETERSON, B. H. 'Psychological Reactions to Acute Physical Illness in Adults.' *Med. J. Aust.* 1974, 11:311-316.

SAINSBURY, M. J. *Psychiatry for Students*, vol. I. Shakespeare Head Press (Distributed by ANZ Book Co. Pty. Ltd.).

SAINSBURY, M. J. & YOUNG , E. 'Physiotherapy and Psychiatry.' *The Australian Journal of Physiotherapy*. August 1966, 54-58.

THOMA, H. *Anorexia Nervosa*. International Universities Press Inc., New York, 1967.

PILOWSKY, I. 'Dimensions of Abnormal Illness Behaviour.' *Aust. N.Z. J. Psychiatry* 1975, 9:141.

Treatment in Psychiatry

AYD, F. J. 'The Depot Flephenazines: A Reappraisal after 10 Years' Clinical Experience.' *Am. J. Psychiat.* 1975, 132:5.

BECK, A. T. *Cognitive therapy and the emotional disorders*. New York International Universities Press, 1976.

BELLAK, L. & SMALL, L. *Emergency Psychotherapy and Brief Psychotherapy*. Grune & Stratton, New York, London, 1965.

CRISP, A. H. 'A Treatment Regime for Anorexia Nervosa.' *B. J. Psychiat.* 1966, 112:505-512.

CADE, J. F. J. 'Lithium—When, Why and How?' *Med. J. Aust.* 1975, 1:684-686.

EDITORIAL COMMENTS, 'Lithium—Futility, Disaster and Triumph.' *Med. J. Aust.* 1975, 1:669.

MARCEUSE, F. L. *Hypnosis, Fact and Fiction.* A Pelican Original, 1959, 1966.

PIPPARD, J. 'Personality Changes After Rostral Leucotomy: A Comparison with Standard Prefrontal Leucotomy.' *J. Ment. Sc.* 1955, 101:774.

PIPPARD, J. 'Leucotomy in Britain Today.' *J. Ment. Sc.* 1962, 108:249.

RAPHAEL, B. 'Crisis Intervention—Theoretical and Methodological Considerations.' *Aust. N.Z. J. Psychiatry* 1971.

WHITLOCK, F. A. & PRICE, J. 'Use of Beta-Adrenergic Receptor Blocking Drugs in Psychiatry.' October 1974, *Current Therapeutics*, Review Article.

Mental Retardation

SAX, S. *New South Wales Mental Retardation Survey, 1970.* Division of Health Services, Research and Planning, Department of Health, New South Wales.

Drug Dependence

CURRENT AFFAIRS BULLETIN. 'Drugs and Addiction.' Department of Adult Education, University of Sydney, Vol. 41, no. 7, 26 February 1968.

PATTERSON, M. A. 'Acupuncture and Neuroelectric Therapy in the Treatment of Drug and Alcohol Addictions.' *A.J.A.D.D.* vol. 2, no. 3, August 1975.

SAINSBURY, M.J. 'The Management of Delirium Tremens.' Supplement to the Bulletin of the Post-Graduate Committee in Medicine, University of Sydney, vol. 25, no. 1, April 1969.

SAINSBURY, M.J. 'Acupuncture in Heroin Withdrawal.' *Med. J. Aust.* 1974, 2:102-105.

WEN, H. L. & CHEUNG, S. Y. C. 'Treatment of Drug Addiction by Acupuncture and Electrical Stimulation.' *Asian J. of Med.* 1973, 9:138-140.

WEN, H. L. 'Fast detoxification of Heroin Addicts, by Acupuncture and Electrical Stimulation (A.E.S.) in Combination with Naloxone.' *Comparatitive Medicine East and West* 1977, V, 3-4: 257-263.

Sexual Deviation

BALL, J. R. B. 'Transsexualism and Transvestitism.' *Aust. N.Z. J. Psychiatry* 1967, 1:188 and 2:24.

BUHRICH, N. 'The Discrete Syndromes of Transvestism and Transsexualism.' *Archives of Sexual Behaviour* 6, 6, 1977.

——'Motivation for cross-dressing in heterosexual transvestism.' *Acta psychiat. scand.* 1978, 57:145-152.

ELLIS, A. & ABARBANEL, A. *The Encyclopaedia of Sexual Behaviour.* William Heinemann, London.

STORR, A. *Sexual Deviation.* William Heinemann Limited, London, 1964.

Genetics

CARTER, C. O. *Human Heredity.* A Pelican Original, 1962.

Human Dynamics

BOWLBY, JOHN. *Child Care and the Growth of Love.* A Pelican Book, 1953.

COLE, R. *Erik Erikson, the Growth of His Work.* 1975.

EIDELBERG, L. *Encyclopaedia of Psychoanalysis.* Collier-Macmillan Limited, London, 1968.

Freud, S. *New Introductory Lectures on Psychoanalysis*. Penguin, 1973.

Jones, E. *The Life and Work of Sigmund Freud* (edited and abridged by Lionel Trilling & Stephen Marcus). Penguin, 1974.

Psychology

Hildgard, E. R. & Atkinson, R. C. *Introduction to Psychology*, (6th edn) Harcourt, Brace and Jovanich, New York, 1975.

Sociology

Brennan, T. & Parker, N. A. (eds) *The Foundations of Social Casework*. Ian Novak, Sydney, 1966.

Ellard, J. 'The Problems of the Migrant.' *Med. J. Aust.* 1969, 2:1039-43.

Susser, M. W. & Watson, W. *Sociology in Medicine*. Oxford Medical Publications 2nd edn, 1974.

Psychiatric Nursing and its History

Maddison, D. C., Day, P. & Leabeater, B. *Psychiatric Nursing*. E. & S. Livinstone Limited, Edinburgh and London.

Walk, A. 'The History of Mental Nursing.' *J. Ment. Sc.* 1961, 107:2-17.

Hospital and Administrative Psychiatry

Clark, D. *Administrative Therapy*. Tavistock Publications, London, 1964.

Jones, Maxwell. *Beyond the Therapeutic Community*. Yale University Press, New Haven and London, 1968.

Martin, Denis, V. *Adventure in Psychiatry*. Bruno Cassirer, Oxford, 1962.

Sainsbury, M. J. 'Changes in admission centre psychiatry.' *Med. J. Aust.* 1966, 2:172.

Sainsbury, M. J. 'Psychiatric Admissions from Nine Sydney Municipalities or Shires.' *Med. J. Aust.* 1966, 2:215.

General Medicine and Electroencephalography

Davidson, Sir Stanley. *The Priniciples and Practice of Medicine*. E. & S. Livingstone Limited, Edinburgh and London.

Kiloh, L. & Osselton, J. W. *Clinical Electroencephalography*. Butterworth, Washington, 1966.

Lance, J. W. *The Mechanisms and Management of Headache*. Sandoz, Basle; Butterworth, London, 1969.

Penry, J. Kiffin (ed.). *Epilepsy, the Eighth International Symposium*. Raven Press, New York.

Sutherland, J. M. & Tait, H. The Epilepsies—Modern Diagnosis and Treatment. E. & S. Livingstone Limited, Edinburgh and London.

Thanatology

Kubler-Ross, E. *On Death and Dying*. McMillan, New York, 1969.

Milton, G. W. 'The Care of the Dying.' *Med. J. Aust.* 1972, 2:177.

Raphael, B. 'The Presentation and Management of Bereavement.' *Med. J. Aust.*, 1975, 2:909-911.

Sainsbury, M. J. & Milton, G. W. 'The Nurse in a Cancer Ward.' *Med. J. Aust.*, 1975, 2:911-913.

Sandford, N. & Deloughery, G. L. 'Teaching Nurses to Care for the Dying Patient.' *J. P. N. and Mental Health Services*, January 1973.

MADDISON, D., VIOLA, A. & WALKER, W. L. 'Further Studies in Conjugal Bereavement.' *Aust. N.Z. J. Psychiatry*, 1969, 3:63.

INDEX

NOTES

NOTES